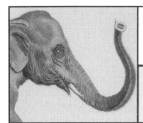

APPLETON &

PRACTICE TESTS

MW01273201

USMLE STEP 3 PRACTICE TESTS

Joel S. Goldberg, DO
Assistant Professor of Medicine
Department of Medicine
MCP/Hahnemann University School of Medicine
Philadelphia, Pennsylvania

Appleton & Lange/McGraw-Hill
Medical Publishing Division

New York   Chicago   San Francisco   Lisbon   London   Madrid   Mexico City   Milan
New Delhi   San Juan   Seoul   Singapore   Sydney   Toronto

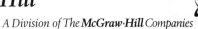

McGraw-Hill

A Division of The McGraw·Hill Companies

Appleton & Lange Practice Tests for the USMLE Step 3

1 2 3 4 5 6 7 8 9 0 CVS/CVS 0 9 8 7 6 5 4 3 2 1

ISBN 0-07-137741-7

Notice

Medicine is an ever-changing science. As new research and clinical experience broaden our knowledge, changes in treatment and drug therapy are required. The authors and the publisher of this work have checked with sources believed to be reliable in their efforts to provide information that is complete and generally in accord with the standards accepted at the time of publication. However, in view of the possibility of human error or changes in medical sciences, neither the authors nor the publisher nor any other party who has been involved in the preparation or publication of this work warrants that the information contained herein is in every respect accurate or complete, and they disclaim all responsibility for any errors or omissions or for the results obtained from use of such information contained in this work. Readers are encouraged to confirm the information contained herein with other sources. For example and in particular, readers are advised to check the product information sheet included in the package of each drug they plan to administer to be certain that the information contained in this work is accurate and that changes have not been made in the recommended dose or in the contraindications for administration. This recommendation is of particular importance in connection with new or infrequently used drugs.

This book was set in Palatino by Rainbow Graphics.
The editors were Catherine A. Johnson and John M. Morriss.
Project management was performed by Rainbow Graphics.
The production supervisor was Lisa Mendez.
The interior design is by Elizabeth Sanders.
Von Hoffman Graphics was printer and binder.

This book is printed on acid-free paper.

Library of Congress Cataloging-in-Publication Data
Goldberg, Joel S.
    Appleton & Lange's practice tests for the USMLE Step 3 / Joel S. Goldberg.—1st ed.
        p. cm.
    Includes bibliographical references.
    ISBN 0-07-137741-7 (alk. paper)
    1. Medicine—Examinations, questions, etc.   I. Title: Appleton and Lange's practice
tests for the USMLE step 3. II. Appleton & Lange. III. Title.
R834.5 .G6472 2003
610'.76—dc21
                                                                                2002028834

For Mickey, Dan, and Kasey

Contents

Preface

This test was designed to be an up-to-date mirror of the USMLE Step 3 examination. The content and question types are designed around the current USMLE guidelines.

The questions are original and brand-new. They have been produced by a faculty of clinicians who are experts in their respective fields and are deeply involved with current teaching programs at their medical institutions. In this manner, you are assured of material that is both appropriate and accurate.

Appleton & Lange Practice Tests for the USMLE Step 3 will help you immensely in your preparation for the USMLE Step 3.

Joel S. Goldberg

Contributors

David Baron, DO
Chairman
Division of Psychiatry
Temple University School of Medicine
Philadelphia, Pennsylvania

Sherri E. Blackstone, MD
Division of Endocrinology, Diabetes, and Metabolic
    Diseases
Jefferson Medical College of Thomas Jefferson
    University
Philadelphia, Pennsylvania

Alexander J. Brucker, MD
Professor of Ophthalmology
Scheie Eye Institute
University of Pennsylvania
Philadelphia, Pennsylvania

Andrew H. Crenshaw, Jr., MD
Assistant Professor
Campbell Clinic of Orthopedic Surgery
University of Tennessee Center for Health Sciences
Memphis, Tennessee

Elise Hardy, MD
Division of Endocrinology, Diabetes, and Metabolic
    Diseases
Jefferson Medical College of Thomas Jefferson
    University
Philadelphia, Pennsylvania

Stephen C. Hauser, MD
Assistant Professor of Medicine
Mayo Medical School
Consultant
Division of Gastroenterology and Hepatology
Department of Internal Medicine
Mayo Medical Center
Rochester, Minnesota

Diane M. Hershock, MD
Assistant Professor of Medicine
Hematology–Oncology Division
Department of Medicine
University of Pennsylvania Cancer Center
University of Pennsylvania Health System
Philadelphia, Pennsylvania

Anne Honebrink, MD
Clinical Assistant Professor
Department of Obstetrics and Gynecology
University of Pennsylvania Health System
Medical Director, Women's Division
Women's and Children's Health Services
Philadelphia, Pennsylvania

Serge A. Jabbour, MD
Clinical Assistant Professor of Medicine
Division of Endocrinology, Diabetes, and Metabolic
    Diseases
Jefferson Medical College of Thomas Jefferson
    University
Philadelphia, Pennsylvania

Samuel L. Jacobs, MD
Associate Professor
Director, Undergraduate Medical Education
Division of Reproductive Endocrinology and
    Infertility
Department of Obstetrics and Gynecology
UMDNJ-Robert Wood Johnson Medical School
Camden, New Jersey

Michael K. Leonard, MD
Instructor of Medicine
Division of Infectious Diseases
Emory University School of Medicine
Atlanta, Georgia

Mary Gail Mercurio, MD
Assistant Professor of Dermatology
Strong Memorial Hospital
University of Rochester Medical Center
Rochester, New York

Richard Malamut, MD
Clinical Assistant Professor of Medicine
Division of Neurology
MCP-Hahnemann University School of Medicine
Philadelphia, Pennsylvania

James E. Nicholson III, MD
Assistant Clinical Professor
Division of Emergency Medicine
Department of Surgery
Duke University Medical Center
Durham, North Carolina

Otis B. Rickman, DO
Instructor in Medicine
Mayo Medical School
Fellow
Division of Pulmonary and Critical Care Medicine
Mayo Graduate School of Medicine
Rochester, Minnesota

Daniel B. Rukstalis, MD
Associate Professor of Surgery
Chief, Division of Urology
Drexel University College of Medicine
Philadelphia, Pennsylvania

Michael G. Stewart, MD, MPH, FACS
Associate Dean of Clinical Affairs
Baylor College of Medicine
Chief
Division of Otolaryngology, Head and Neck
    Surgery
Ben Taub General Hospital
Houston, Texas

Mehmooda Syeed, MD
Division of Endocrinology, Diabetes, and Metabolic
    Diseases
Jefferson Medical College of Thomas Jefferson
    University
Philadelphia, Pennsylvania

Cynthia M. Tracy, MD
Professor of Medicine
Division of Cardiology
Georgetown University Medical Center
Washington, District of Columbia

Acknowledgments

I would like to thank my editor at McGraw-Hill, Catherine Johnson, for her assistance in the editing and production of this text. I would also like to thank Trish Casey for her assistance in the development of this project, along with the many staff members at McGraw-Hill who participated in the preparation of this book.

Finally, I also wish to thank the physicians who participated in this project. They were able to find the time in their busy schedules to help in the creation of this work, which will benefit medical students across the United States.

Practice Test 1
Questions

1. A 50-year-old woman has a history of rheumatoid arthritis. She has a symmetric arthritis on exam. Her spleen is palpable. Her hemoglobin is 8.4 g/dL, mean corpuscular volume (MCV) 99, and reticulocyte count 10%. Her total bilirubin is 3.4, with 0.3 direct and a lactic dehydrogenase (LDH) of 676, which is elevated. The next test that should be ordered to evaluate her anemia is

   (A) iron and total iron-binding capacity (TIBC)
   (B) ferritin
   (C) Coombs' test direct and indirect
   (D) B_{12} and folate
   (E) bone marrow test

2. A 47-year-old man presents with right-sided flank pain. No fever, chills, weight loss, or hematuria are reported. A palpable mass is noted on exam with no costovertebral tenderness. A hemoglobin is 8.2 with an alanine transaminase (ALT) of 180 U/L and an LDH of 300 U/L. Diagnostic studies show a right-sided mass in the kidney with possible extension into the perineal fat. No adenopathy and no evidence of direct invasions is noted. No focal lesions are noted in the liver. The management of this patient should include

   (A) intravenous pyelography
   (B) alpha interferon

   (C) interleukin-2 therapy
   (D) resection of the renal mass
   (E) bone scan

Items 3–6

A 24-year-old woman presents to your office with a chief complaint of right ptosis, diplopia on vertical gaze, and proximal muscle weakness. All symptoms may worsen later in the day. Her past medical history is significant for thyroid disease. A diagnosis of myasthenia gravis is suspected.

3. Confirmation of myasthenia gravis may be assured by all of the following EXCEPT

   (A) injection of edrophonium
   (B) repetitive stimulation during nerve conduction testing
   (C) anti–voltage-gated calcium channel antibodies
   (D) antiacetylcholine receptor antibodies
   (E) all of the above

4. The primary tumor most likely to be associated with myasthenia gravis is

   (A) oat-cell lung cancer
   (B) thyroid carcinoma
   (C) breast cancer
   (D) pituitary adenoma
   (E) thymoma

5. Pharmacologic therapy for myasthenia gravis may involve all of the following EXCEPT

   (A) pyridostigmine
   (B) oral prednisone
   (C) azathioprine
   (D) cyclosporine
   (E) quinidine

6. The patient described above calls you from home at 11:00 P.M. with complaints of shortness of breath, hoarseness, and inability to swallow. Your next suggestion to the patient should be

   (A) urgent admission to the intensive care unit for plasma exchange
   (B) admission to the hospital for intravenous methylprednisolone
   (C) to take one additional pyridostigmine tablet and call back in 1 hour
   (D) to be evaluated in your office early the following morning
   (E) to take an anxiolytic and call you in the morning

END OF SET

7. All of the following have been shown to improve survival in patients with heart failure EXCEPT

   (A) hydralazine plus isosorbide dinitrate
   (B) enalapril
   (C) metoprolol
   (D) digoxin

8. A 55-year-old white woman presents with a displaced distal radius fracture after a same-level fall. The patient undergoes an uneventful reduction, and a splint is applied. The patient's neurologic examination is normal postreduction. During the next 2 hours, the patient begins to complain of numbness in her fingers. Her 2-point discrimination in the median nerve distribution is 5 mm. Her splint is spread open, ice is applied, and the hand is elevated. Thirty minutes later, 2-point discrimination is 10 mm in the median nerve distribution. The next appropriate course of action is

   (A) observation because nerve function will return
   (B) an emergent carpal tunnel release
   (C) electromyography/nerve conduction velocity (EMG/NCV) to document median nerve compression at the wrist
   (D) none of the above

9. A previously healthy 62-year-old woman develops over a few hours the worst headache of her life. She also notes decreased vision in both eyes. She is brought to the emergency room 2 days later. Magnetic resonance imaging (MRI) of the head shows extensive bleeding into a previously undiagnosed large pituitary tumor, consistent with pituitary apoplexy. Which of the following abnormalities is likely on hormone testing, assuming normal pituitary function prior to acute onset of headache?

   (A) low thyroid-stimulating hormone (TSH), low free thyroxine (T_4)
   (B) low follicle-stimulating hormone (FSH) and luteinizing hormone (LH), low estradiol
   (C) abnormal cortisol response to corticotropin stimulation test
   (D) normal cortisol response to hypoglycemia
   (E) A and C

10. Which of the following adverse events occur frequently during treatment of adult growth hormone (GH) deficiency?

    (A) edema
    (B) arthralgias
    (C) myalgias
    (D) paresthesias or carpal tunnel syndrome
    (E) all of the above

Items 11–15

A 53-year-old woman, G2P2, last menstrual period (LMP) 6 months ago, presents to your office for her annual gynecologic exam. She is complaining of hot flashes, vaginal dryness, and insomnia.

11. The most helpful test to make a diagnosis is

   (A) endometrial biopsy
   (B) serum beta human chorionic gon-adotropin (hCG)
   (C) Pap smear
   (D) antiphospholipid antibody studies
   (E) serum FSH

12. All of the following steps would be appropriate in managing her case EXCEPT

   (A) discussing the need for hormone replacement therapy
   (B) determining her risks for osteoporosis
   (C) placing her on anticoagulation therapy
   (D) discussing the risks of future cardiovascular disease
   (E) counseling her about adequate calcium intake

13. Risk factors for osteoporosis include all of the following EXCEPT

   (A) cigarette smoking
   (B) high alcohol intake
   (C) sedentary lifestyle
   (D) obesity
   (E) high animal protein intake

14. The best way to determine if this patient has osteoporosis is to obtain

   (A) serum calcium levels
   (B) DEXA bone density study
   (C) dual-photon absorptiometry
   (D) urinary hydroxyproline ratios
   (E) hip and spine x-rays

15. Estrogen replacement therapy would be contraindicated in women with a history of all of the following EXCEPT

   (A) hypertension
   (B) breast cancer
   (C) active liver disease
   (D) undiagnosed vaginal bleeding
   (E) previous stroke

END OF SET

16. A 36-year-old woman with no past history notices a scaly eruption near her left nipple. She thinks it is from a sports bra she recently started to wear. During her examination, she is found to have a hard, erythematous, crusted lesion approximately 1.5 cm on the left nipple. There is no discharge and no masses within the breast. She is started on antibiotics and given topical emollients and a Medrol dose pack. She returns for follow-up 2 weeks later with minimal improvement. The most appropriate next step in the management of this patient is to

   (A) continue antibiotics and local treatment
   (B) order a mammogram and, if negative, continue with current therapy
   (C) continue local treatment and recommend not wearing the sports bra
   (D) order a mammogram and refer her to a surgeon for possible biopsy
   (E) add an antifungal agent

<u>Items 17–19</u>

A 75-year-old white man with a history of cirrhosis presents to the emergency department via ambulance after his wife found him to be extremely confused today. He had been running a low-grade fever and has a cough productive of yellow sputum. On examination, his temperature is 40.5° C (104.9° F), pulse 130, blood pressure 100/64 mm Hg, respiratory rate 30, and SaO_2 of 89%. Testing reveals a WBC of 16,000, normal electrolyte; chest radiograph reveals a right lower lung zone consolidative infiltrate.

17. What other diagnostic testing is indicated?

   (A) arterial blood gases
   (B) sputum Gram stain and culture
   (C) blood cultures
   (D) none of the above
   (E) all of the above

18. In which setting should this patient be treated?

    (A) outpatient
    (B) nursing home
    (C) general medical ward
    (D) intensive care unit (ICU)
    (E) none of the above

19. What antibiotics are indicated in treating this patient?

    (A) fluoroquinolone
    (B) vancomycin
    (C) third-generation cephalosporin
    (D) A and C
    (E) none of the above

END OF SET

20. A patient being treated with isoniazid (INH), ethambutol, rifampin, and pyrazinamide (PZA) for pulmonary tuberculosis presents to the health department complaining of decreased vision and difficulty in distinguishing colors. The patient is showing toxicity to

    (A) rifampin
    (B) INH
    (C) ethambutol
    (D) PZA

Items 21–24

A 24-year-old obese G3P0020 woman presents to the delivery room after 10 hours of regular contractions. On admission to the delivery room she is found to be completely dilated with the fetal vertex at 0 station. Estimated fetal weight is 3,900 grams both clinically and on ultrasound done in the delivery room. After 2 hours of pushing, she complains of rectal pressure and is found to be crowning. The fetal head delivers from the left occipitoanterior (LOA) position, but gentle downward traction on the newborn's head does not release the anterior shoulder.

21. Immediate management could include all of the following EXCEPT

    (A) application of fundal pressure by an assistant

    (B) performing an episiotomy
    (C) suctioning infant's nose and mouth
    (D) application of suprapubic pressure by an assistant
    (E) removal of maternal legs from stirrups and sharply flexing the legs from the hips onto the abdomen

22. A macrosomic, 4,500-gram infant is eventually delivered. The baby appears initially vigorous and has a 1-minute Apgar of 8, but a 5-minute Apgar is 6, with points off for color, muscle tone, and reflex irritability. The most likely cause for this baby's condition is

    (A) hyperglycemia
    (B) hypoglycemia
    (C) sepsis
    (D) congenital cardiac abnormality
    (E) Down syndrome

23. All of the following are risk factors for shoulder dystocia EXCEPT

    (A) fetal macrosomia
    (B) prolonged second stage of labor
    (C) maternal obesity
    (D) lack of prenatal care

24. The Zavenelli maneuver used with shoulder dystocia describes

    (A) delivery of the posterior shoulder first
    (B) replacement of the fetal head into the pelvis with subsequent performance of cesarean delivery
    (C) deliberate fracture of the fetal clavicle
    (D) rotation of the posterior shoulder 180 degrees to release the impacted anterior shoulder

END OF SET

25. A 22-year-old woman, whom you have been treating for allergy-induced asthma with good control for the last several years, advises you that she wishes to become pregnant. She asks your advice about how to best deal with her asthma in pregnancy. You tell her

(A) that pregnancy and asthma are a risky combination and that she should reconsider her decision to become pregnant

(B) that medications for asthma are contraindicated in pregnancy and that she should immediately stop all of her medications once she becomes pregnant

(C) that most medications used to control asthma are safe to use in pregnancy and that she and her developing fetus are better off continuing to use medications prescribed to control her asthma than having repeated acute asthma attacks

(D) that the use of beta-adrenergic medications such as terbutaline should be avoided in pregnancy since they can bring on preterm labor

26. A patient who suffered head trauma 9 days ago presents with headache, diplopia, unilateral proptosis, and conjunctival vessel engorgement. The most likely diagnosis is

(A) orbital roof blow-in fracture

(B) malar complex fracture

(C) orbital floor blow-out fracture

(D) cavernous sinus thrombosis

(E) carotid cavernous fistula

27. An elderly woman living alone slipped on a wet floor at home, sustaining a hip fracture, and was unable to get up or phone for help. She was found on the floor by her daughter approximately 18 hours later and was transported to the emergency department by EMS. She is awake but mildly confused with a nonfocal neurological exam and appears very dehydrated. X-ray confirms an intertrochanteric fracture of the right hip. An electrocardiogram (ECG) is unchanged from prior tracings showing an old right bundle branch block. Her serum creatinine is 2.2, with a blood urea nitrogen (BUN) of 80. Her creatine kinase (CK) is 15,000 with MB fraction < 5% of the total. The patient normally takes no medications and has no true allergies, but her daughter cautions that even small doses of narcotics given in the course of dental work

several years ago induced a transient delirium. All of the following statements are correct EXCEPT

(A) this patient requires cardiac monitoring

(B) aggressive rehydration is an important part of initial therapy; placement of a Foley catheter with careful monitoring of fluid intake and output is essential and early hemodynamic monitoring may be appropriate in elderly patients

(C) screening studies for disseminated intravascular coagulation (DIC) are appropriate

(D) ketorolac may be given for pain

(E) alkalinization of the patient's urine is needed

28. What condition would be most appropriately treated with a topical steroid?

(A) atopic dermatitis

(B) urticaria

(C) vasculitis

(D) acne

(E) tinea

29. Features of the anticholinergic toxidrome include each of the following EXCEPT

(A) dry mucous membranes

(B) agitation

(C) fever

(D) miosis

(E) vasodilatation

30. What condition would be most appropriately treated with a topical antibiotic?

(A) Lyme disease

(B) urticaria

(C) vasculitis

(D) acne

(E) tinea

31. A patient comes to your office with a chief complaint of burning, retrosternal discomfort that occurs after large meals, especially those that include greasy food, chocolate, or mint. Further data are obtained. All of the following would indicate the need for an upper gastrointestinal tract endoscopy EXCEPT

    (A) the patient is male, 51, and has had these symptoms once or twice a month for "about 10 years"

    (B) the patient is found to have mild microcytic hypochromic anemia

    (C) recently, the patient has noted sticking of food in her chest such as dry chicken and rice

    (D) the patient is female, 32, and these symptoms do not occur except after dietary indiscretions

    (E) the patient is male, 49, and has had these symptoms for "about 1 year" and tried a proton pump inhibitor for 2 months without relief

32. When evaluating and managing a patient with altered mental status, each of the following is an appropriate routine initial intervention EXCEPT

    (A) administration of naloxone

    (B) bedside glucose measurement

    (C) administration of flumazenil

    (D) administration of thiamine

    (E) cardiac monitoring

33. A 62-year-old woman previously in good health is seen for new epigastric discomfort and "difficulty eating." At endoscopy, a 1.5-cm nodular mass/lesion in her antrum is biopsied. A breath test for *Helicobacter pylori* is positive. The pathology is consistent with a malignancy. Which of the following would most likely benefit from chemotherapy?

    (A) mucosa-associated lymphoid tumor (MALToma), low grade, restricted to mucosa by endoscopic ultrasound

    (B) adenocarcinoma of the stomach

    (C) carcinoid tumor of the stomach

    (D) non-Hodgkin's lymphoma, with intra-abdominal lymphadenopathy positive for lymphoma on fine-needle biopsy with endoscopic ultrasound

34. A 60-year-old woman presents with fever and persistent bleeding from a dental extraction done several weeks ago. Her only complaint is fatigue, which she attributes to stress. She does have a history of aplastic anemia and was treated with antithymocyte globulin, cyclosporine, and prednisone 10 years ago with a complete response and no evidence of relapse. On exam, she appeared ill and pale with no lymphadenopathy or hepatosplenomegaly.

    DATA
    Hemoglobin 8.0 g/dL
    MCV 117 fL
    WBC 3,100/μL
    Neutrophils 21%
    Lymphocytes 69%
    Platelets 36,000/μL

    The smear showed hypogranular and hyposegmented neutrophils. Teardrops were also evident. The most likely diagnosis is

    (A) recurrent aplastic anemia

    (B) vitamin B_{12} deficiency

    (C) tuberculosis

    (D) chronic lymphocytic leukemia

    (E) myelodysplasia

35. Which of the following is true about obsessive–compulsive disorder (OCD)?

    (A) Lifetime prevalence is about 2 to 3%, making it the fourth most common psychiatric diagnosis.

    (B) Obsessions are ego syntonic; compulsions are ego dystonic.

    (C) People with OCD do not realize the irrationality of their obsession.

    (D) Carrying out a compulsion increases anxiety.

    (E) The main neurotransmitter pathology involved in OCD is dysregulation of gamma-aminobutyric acid (GABA).

36. Which of the following characteristics are NOT true about post-traumatic stress disorder (PTSD)?

    (A) The emotional stress is of a magnitude that would be traumatic for almost anyone.
    (B) Patients reexperience trauma through dreams and waking thoughts.
    (C) The lifetime prevalence is 1 to 3%.
    (D) The cognitive model of PTSD states that the affected person is unable to process or rationalize the trauma that precipitated the disorder.
    (E) PTSD usually develops within the first month of the trauma.

37. The most important x-ray in determining if a shoulder is dislocated is

    (A) anterior–posterior
    (B) bicipital groove view
    (C) internal rotation view
    (D) external rotation view
    (E) axillary lateral

38. In treating meningitis, which of the following antibiotics would achieve the LEAST dependable levels in the cerebrospinal fluid (CSF)?

    (A) ceftriaxone
    (B) cefuroxime
    (C) ceftazidime
    (D) cefotaxime

39. An adult presents with symptoms of acute frontal sinusitis, as well as headache, fever, nausea, vomiting, and lethargy. In addition to acute frontal sinusitis, which is the most likely diagnosis?

    (A) toxic shock syndrome
    (B) intracerebral abscess
    (C) frontal bone osteomyelitis
    (D) coexisting viral gastroenteritis
    (E) viral syndrome

40. What is the most common site for metastatic disease from prostate cancer?

    (A) liver
    (B) lung
    (C) bone
    (D) lymphatic

41. What is the best initial therapy for advanced prostate cancer metastatic to the bone?

    (A) taxane-based chemotherapy
    (B) external beam radiation therapy to sites of pain
    (C) observation
    (D) medical or surgical castration
    (E) palliative care

42. A patient presenting with fever, hypotension, and severe right upper quadrant pain should be empirically treated with which of the following antibiotic regimens?

    (A) ceftazidime
    (B) levofloxacin
    (C) ampicillin–sulbactam and gentamicin
    (D) ceftriaxone and gentamicin

43. The most common etiology of diarrhea in someone visiting a foreign country is

    (A) *Cryptosporidium*
    (B) *Giardia lamblia*
    (C) *Escherichia coli*
    (D) *Salmonella typhi*

Items 44–45

A 19-year-old white woman presents to the emergency department with a complaint of pain in the right eye. Examination reveals a perilimbal flush and a white lesion of the cornea. The patient has the history of contact lens wear.

44. The most likely diagnosis is

    (A) corneal foreign body
    (B) contact lens overwear syndrome
    (C) corneal abrasion
    (D) corneal ulcer
    (E) none of the above

45. The most appropriate treatment in the emergency department would be

    (A) antibiotics
    (B) reevaluate in 24 hours
    (C) antibiotic with steroid
    (D) antibiotics with steroids and referral to ophthalmologist
    (E) immediate ophthalmology consult

                                    END OF SET

46. A 30-year-old woman who runs 30 miles a week presents for evaluation after 6 months of amenorrhea. A pregnancy test is negative. TSH is normal. Which set of hormones will the patient likely have?

	FSH	LH	Prolactin	Estradiol
I	Low	Low	High	Low
II	Normal	Normal	High	Low
III	Low	Low	Normal	Low
IV	High	High	Normal	Low

    (A) I
    (B) II
    (C) III
    (D) IV

47. Which of the following statements regarding theories of phobias is true?

    (A) In classical conditioning, anxiety is aroused by pairing one frightening stimulus with another frightening stimulus.
    (B) In operant theory, anxiety is a drive that motivates the organism to do what it can to obviate the painful affect.
    (C) Learning theory provides complex explanations and understanding of underlying psychic processes involved with phobias.
    (D) According to psychoanalytic theory, the phobic patient's primary defense is projection of childhood unresolved oedipal situations.
    (E) Freud's theories of phobia are based on Little Albert.

48. A 25-year-old man falls on his outstretched hand and develops immediate pain and swelling over the radial aspect of his wrist. X-rays are normal. The most appropriate treatment is

    (A) tell the patient he has only a ligament sprain
    (B) ice, elevate, avoid heavy lifting, analgesics, and return if pain increases
    (C) treat the patient for a navicular (scaphoid) fracture and repeat x-rays in 10 days
    (D) none of the above

49. A 74-year-old former smoker with chronic obstructive pulmonary disease (COPD) presents to the emergency department with shortness of breath, wheezing, cough, and fever of 24 hours' duration. His vital signs are stable; examination reveals diffuse wheezing, and chest radiograph shows air trapping but clear lung fields. Which of the following treatments is indicated?

    (A) intravenous (IV) steroids
    (B) inhaled beta agonist
    (C) antibiotics
    (D) oxygen
    (E) all of the above

50. A 58-year-old man with long-standing hypertension is seen with complaints of chest pain and dyspnea on exertion. His ECG is as follows. The most helpful test to evaluate his symptoms is

    (A) stress electrocardiogram
    (B) coronary arteriography
    (C) echocardiogram
    (D) stress echocardiogram

Practice Test 1
Answers and Explanations

1. **(C)** The patient has a hemolytic anemia by virtue of her lab tests. The elevated MCV is a reflection of her brisk reticulocytosis, which renders larger erythrocytes. Serum B_{12} and folate are not needed since the reticulocyte count is elevated. The Coombs' test would be indicated because a positive test would confirm immune hemolysis as the cause of this hemolytic anemia.

2. **(D)** This is a patient with Stauffer syndrome, which is a paraneoplastic syndrome associated with renal cell cancer. There is no evidence of a focal abnormality in the liver despite elevated transaminases. The computed tomography (CT) also shows no evidence of direct extension outside the renal capsule. Thus, this patient should undergo surgery.

3–6. **(3-C, 4-E, 5-E, 6-A)** Antiacetylcholine receptor antibodies will be elevated in 85 to 90% of patients with generalized disease but in only 60% of patients with pure ocular myasthenia. Repetitive stimulation will demonstrate the characteristic electrodecremental response of > 10 to 15% between the first and fourth stimuli but will be abnormal in only 70 to 75% of patients. Injection of 10 mg of edrophonium will correct a visible abnormality (such as ptosis) within several minutes of injection. Due to potential cholinergic side effects such as bradycardia, the patient should be monitored and atropine should be readily available. Elevated voltage-gated calcium channel antibodies that attack the presynaptic membrane within the neuromuscular junction may be found in the Lambert–Eaton syndrome.

Malignant thymoma is found in 10% of patients with myasthenia gravis, with the majority demonstrating hyperplasia of the thymus gland. All patients with myasthenia should undergo CT scan of the chest.

Thymectomy should be strongly considered in all patients under the age of 70 due to a 20% chance of complete and permanent remission and a 70% chance of partial remission within 6 months to 2 years after surgery. Quinidine may worsen symptoms of myasthenia and is contraindicated. Other medicines that may worsen the disease include procainamide, all aminoglycosides, all reversible neuromuscular blockers, and high-dose prednisone (when not already on prednisone).

The patient in question 6 is in myasthenic crisis and needs urgent admission to the intensive care unit for plasma exchange. Vital capacity should be obtained and repeated frequently with readings under 1 liter necessitating elective intubation.

7. **(D)** Digoxin reduces the frequency of rehospitalization, but does not improve survival. Several studies have now shown survival benefit with angiotensin-converting enzyme inhibitors and beta blockers in patients with heart failure. An early study (the Vasodilator-Heart Failure Trials) showed benefit over digoxin and diuretics with hydralazine plus isosorbide dinitrate. This regimen remains an option in patients with contraindications to other vasodilators.

8. **(B)** Compression of the median nerve secondary to swelling following a fracture of the

distal radius is a known cause of carpal tunnel syndrome. Peripheral nerve injuries occurring at the time of injury can usually be monitored for return of function in 6 to 12 weeks. EMG/NCV studies are indicated if return of function has not occurred. Nerve injuries secondary to a laceration or associated with an open fracture should be explored. A developing nerve compression syndrome occurring during the course of treatment should be explored emergently.

9. **(B)** Given that the event happened acutely and the patient was seen only 2 days after, hormonal abnormalities will depend on the half-life of each hormone tested and on end-organ responsiveness. TSH will be low, but free T_4 will be normal, because thyroxine has a half-life of 7 days. In the absence of adrenocorticotropic hormone (ACTH), adrenal atrophy will occur in a few weeks (at least 6 weeks); if tested with corticotropin before atrophy, the response will be normal; however, hypoglycemia that stimulates ACTH secretion will lead to abnormal cortisol response (since ACTH is damaged). FSH, LH, and estradiol will be low.

10. **(E)** All of the side effects listed are more commonly seen at GH doses > 4 μg/kg/day.

11. **(E)** This is a classic case presentation of menopause, with amenorrhea, hot flashes, vaginal dryness, and insomnia all being associated with waning estrogen levels. The serum FSH is an indicator of ovarian function and is elevated above 30 mIU/mL after menopause. This is the most helpful test in determining her menopausal status. Pregnancy is highly improbable in this case scenario. Although a Pap smear should be obtained at the time of routine annual gynecologic exam, it is not helpful in making the diagnosis of menopause, other than possibly indicating atrophic processes. An endometrial biopsy would be most helpful in the case of postmenopausal bleeding, and not in the diagnosis of menopause itself. Antiphospholipid antibodies are a part of the

workup of recurrent pregnancy loss. (*Beckmann, 449–453*)

12. **(C)** There is no need to put this patient on anticoagulation therapy. In fact, if she did have a history of prior venous thromboembolic events, she would not be a candidate for estrogen replacement therapy at all. All of the other choices are appropriate. (*Beckmann, 455–458*)

13. **(D)** Obesity is not a risk factor for osteoporosis and may actually be somewhat protective in light of higher circulating estrogen levels in obese women. All of the other choices are indeed risk factors for osteoporosis. (*Beckmann, 453*)

14. **(B)** Dual energy x-ray absorptiometry, or DEXA bone densitometry, is the best way to evaluate a person's bone density. Dual-photon absorptiometry was used in the past but is not as precise as DEXA scans. Serum calcium levels, urinary hydroxyproline levels, and hip and spine x-rays are not accurate reflections of bone density. (*DeCherney, 1036–1038*)

15. **(A)** Estrogen replacement therapy is not contraindicated in women with hypertension and may actually improve their status. All of the other choices are contraindications to estrogen replacement therapy. (*Beckmann, 457–458*)

16. **(D)** This represents Paget's disease of the nipple, which is often a misdiagnosed form of breast cancer presentation. An eczematoid eruption on the nipple is a classic presentation. A negative mammogram does not exclude the diagnosis and thus a biopsy is warranted. Although antibiotics and creams were given, the patient should have been referred for mammography and biopsy almost immediately. The external lesion is a manifestation of intraductal malignancy involving the ducts near the nipple.

17. **(E)** All of the above are indicated. ABGs can help further risk stratify the patient and give

important insight into his acid–base status. It is also important to identify an organism so that pathogen-specific treatment can be given. However, a specific pathogen is identified only 50% of the time.

18. **(D)** He has severe community-acquired pneumonia by both American Thoracic Society and Infectious Disease Society of America criteria and should be managed in an ICU.

19. **(D)** Current guidelines recommend a combination of two drugs for severe community-acquired pneumonia.

20. **(C)** Patients receiving ethambutol should be monitored for signs of ocular toxicity as it can cause optic neuritis. In addition to decreasing visual acuity, it may also cause loss of green and red color discrimination. Isoniazid can cause a peripheral neuropathy, and vitamin B_6 (pyridoxine) needs to be coadministered to prevent this. INH and rifampin both are responsible for drug-induced hepatitis. Elevated uric acid levels may be seen with pyrazinamide therapy.

21. **(A)** The management of shoulder dystocia requires immediate, appropriate management to decrease the chance of injury or death to the baby. Fundal pressure can serve to more firmly impact the anterior shoulder behind the maternal symphysis. All of the other maneuvers described have been used alone or in combination to successfully release an impacted anterior shoulder.

22. **(B)** Maternal obesity and infant macrosomia make the diagnosis of maternal gestational diabetes likely. Once the infant is removed from the elevated glucose in maternal circulation, he or she is likely to become hypoglycemic. While sepsis and congenital heart defects could cause these symptoms and signs, infant hypoglycemia is the most likely cause in this setting.

23. **(D)** While lack of prenatal care puts both mother and fetus at increased risk for poor outcome, it has not been associated independently with shoulder dystocia. All of the other factors listed above each have been independently associated with shoulder dystocia.

24. **(B)** This maneuver has been reported to have been used with success when other maneuvers have failed in the management of shoulder dystocia.

25. **(C)** Pregnancy has unpredictable effects on asthma activity but is one of the most common chronic medical conditions to accompany pregnancy. Most drugs used to treat asthma can be used in pregnancy. Terbutaline is in fact used to try to stop preterm labor.

26. **(E)** This is a classic presentation of carotid cavernous fistula, which typically presents a few days after head trauma.

27. **(D)** The patient has rhabdomyolysis. A substantial number of these patients develop acute renal failure. Aggressive IV hydration and alkalinization of the urine is beneficial in protection of the kidneys. ECG monitoring is important due to the associated metabolic derangements that may result in cardiac dysrhythmias. DIC is a known complication of rhabdomyolysis. Nonsteroidal anti-inflammatory drugs (NSAIDs) like ketorolac are definitely contraindicated in rhabdomyolysis because of their potential to impair renal function.

28. **(A)** Topical steroids are the most common treatment for atopic dermatitis. The other conditions are not helped by topical steroids.

29. **(D)** The typical findings associated with anticholinergic intoxication are often recalled by the saying: "Red as a lobster, blind as a bat, mad as a hatter, dry as a bone, and hot as Hades." This helps us to recall the typical appearance of the patient who is flushed; has difficulty seeing due to paralysis of accommodation and mydriasis; is agitated, tachycardic, and confused; and has dry mucosa and fever. Additionally, they may have a distended bladder and delayed gastric empty-

ing. Miosis is not associated with the anticholinergic toxidrome but is found with intoxication due to opiates, organophosphates, and clonidine.

30. **(D)** Topical antibiotics may be used for acne treatment. The other conditions are not helped by topical antibiotics.

31. **(D)** Patients such as this with a history of typical heartburn (gastroesophageal reflux disease [GERD]), if the history is prolonged and they are over 50, usually men, are at greatest risk of Barrett's esophagus and should undergo a screening endoscopy. Patients with GERD symptomatology and unexplained anemia, especially microcytic hypochromic, gastrointestinal bleeding, dysphagia, or weight loss require investigation including endoscopy. Patients with GERD symptoms not responding to a reasonable course of anti-GERD therapy also require further evaluation, including endoscopy (i.e., to exclude severe ulcerating esophagitis, stricture, other diagnosis). Many persons with heartburn, especially infrequent heartburn that is managed by dietary prudence and/or minimal use of medications, do not require endoscopy.

32. **(C)** Flumazenil, a parenteral benzodiazepine antagonist has been called by some "a drug looking for an indication." This agent may be useful to reverse the effects of excessive benzodiazepine given in the course of conscious sedation. It is not, however, an appropriate agent for routine use in patients presenting with altered mental status (AMS). This agent has the potential to precipitate withdrawal seizures in individuals who have been chronically taking benzodiazepines. It may also cause seizures if administered to a patient who has taken an overdose of a cyclic antidepressant. Bedside glucose determination, cardiac monitoring, and administration of thiamine are each appropriate in the management of patients presenting with AMS. Routine administration of naloxone is also indicated as part of the initial approach to AMS,

although patients who have combined opiates and stimulants such as cocaine or amphetamines may sometimes rapidly emerge from their stupor in a state of violent agitation and require resedation.

33. **(D)** A small adenocarcinoma of the stomach most likely would require surgery, while a small carcinoid tumor of the stomach might be excised endoscopically. Chemotherapy is unlikely to be helpful in the management of these two tumors. MALTomas of the stomach, if low grade and not advanced in stage by endoscopic ultrasound, often respond to the eradication of *H. pylori* alone. Non-Hodgkin's lymphoma of the stomach, a common gastrointestinal primary lymphoma, often is successfully treated with chemotherapy.

34. **(E)** B_{12} deficiency will give hypersegmented polys and have no effect on the platelets. CLL could give an elevated WBC although the differential is suggestive; the anemia is macrocytic with an autoimmune process.

35. **(A)** Obsessions and compulsions are ego dystonic. People with OCD realize that their obsessions are irrational. Carrying out compulsions decreases anxiety. The main neurotransmitter in OCD is serotonin.

36. **(E)** PTSD develops after the first month of trauma.

37. **(E)** A posterior dislocation of the shoulder can appear reduced on any of the above views except the axillary lateral view. If an axillary lateral view is impossible to obtain, a true lateral of the scapula is the next best view.

38. **(B)** Ceftriaxone and cefotaxime both achieve acceptable CSF levels to be used to treat bacterial meningitis. Ceftazidime also achieves adequate levels in the CSF and may be used to treat gram-negative bacterial meningitis. Cefuroxime, a second-generation cephalosporin, does not achieve adequate CSF levels.

39. (B) This is a classic presentation of brain abscess, which is often missed in the presence of other infectious symptoms, such as sinusitis. This patient needs an urgent CT scan with IV contrast to identify the diagnosis.

40. (D) Prostatic cancer appears to spread initially to the regional lymphatics prior to dissemination to the bone. Bone metastases would then be the second most common site of metastatic spread, although more often symptomatic than lymphatic disease.

41. (D) Androgen ablation with either surgical orchiectomy or medical therapies represents the best initial therapy for newly diagnosed bone metastases from prostate cancer. This therapy is expected to prolong survival for 18 to 36 months, depending on the response to treatment.

42. (C) The vignette describes a toxic patent acute cholecystitis or possibly even cholangitis. The patient needs to be covered broadly for organisms that are present in the hepatobiliary tract. This involves anaerobes and gram-negative organisms *(E. coli, Enterobacter)* for the most part. The only regimen listed with anaerobic activity is ampicillin–sulbactam. The gentamicin is for added gram-negative coverage.

43. (C) Travelers to foreign countries must be warned about eating properly cooked food and drinking only safe water as diarrhea may be very common during travel. Actually, diarrhea is the most common illness to develop in a traveler. The most common organism responsible is *E. coli* (enterotoxigenic). Treatment is supportive and an oral quinolone such as ciprofloxacin for 3 days will shorten the course of traveler's diarrhea.

44. (D) Patients who wear contact lenses are known to be at a higher risk than the general population for the development of corneal ulcers. The presence of pain, perilimbal flush, and a white lesion of the cornea constitutes a corneal ulcer until proven otherwise.

45. (E) Corneal ulcers, whether associated with contact lens wear or not, can cause permanent visual impairment. While antibiotic therapy is indicated, the immediate referral to and evaluation by an ophthalmologist is mandatory. Under normal circumstances the ophthalmologist would determine if culturing the ulcer were necessary before initiating antibiotic therapy. Treatment with antibiotics would then be initiated. If an ophthalmologist is not available, patients should be treated with antibiotic therapy and then seen within 24 hours by an ophthalmologist. In that scenario, culturing of the ulcer would be complicated by the fact that the patient had already received antibiotic therapy.

46. (C) Rigorous exercise such as marathon running, ballet, or swimming can result in amenorrhea. The cause is complex, but the typical laboratory tests are low or low-normal levels of FSH, LH, and estradiol. Prolactin is normal.

47. (B) Classical conditioning is anxiety with pairing of a frightening stimulus with a neutral stimulus. Learning theory provides simple and intelligible explanations for aspects of phobia. In psychoanalytical theory, the defense is displacement (sexual conflict is displaced from the person who evokes the conflict to an unimportant object or situation).

48. (C) Nondisplaced fractures of the carpal navicular are common. Initial x-rays are often normal. As the fracture begins to heal, the fracture line usually becomes visible. With persistent pain in the anatomic snuffbox, a bone scan is indicated.

49. (E) All of the options have been shown to be beneficial in treating acute exacerbations of COPD.

50. (D) With left ventricular hypertrophy, resting abnormalities are common and will interfere with the ability to diagnose changes on the ECG during exercise. Coronary arteriography should be undertaken only after ischemia has been demonstrated. A resting echocardiogram will give functional information, but a stress echocardiogram will give dynamic functional information about heart muscle function. Development of wall motion abnormalities during exercise strongly suggests ischemia and coronary artery disease.

Practice Test 2
Questions

DIRECTIONS (Questions 1 through 50): Each of the numbered items or incomplete statements in this section is followed by answers or by completions of the statement. Select the ONE lettered answer or completion that is BEST in each case. ·

1. The following associations are correct EXCEPT

   (A) transudate: pleural/serum protein ratio < 0.5
   (B) exudate: pleural/serum LDH ratio > 0.6
   (C) transudate: pleural LDH < ⅔ upper limits laboratory normal
   (D) exudate: pleural cholesterol > 60 mg/dL
   (E) all of the above are correct

2. A 78-year-old man with a history of resected lung cancer 3 years ago, who quit smoking, now presents with worsening dyspnea. His exam is unremarkable but he is tachycardic at 100. His respirations are normal. His chest x-ray (CXR) is significant for a previous lobectomy. An arterial blood gas (ABG) was normal. An electrocardiogram (ECG) shows sinus tachycardia. The QRS voltage is decreased compared to an old ECG. The next step is

   (A) echocardiography
   (B) cardiac catheterization
   (C) exercise tolerance test
   (D) pulmonary function tests
   (E) apical lordotic views of the chest

3. A 25-year-old right-handed woman in her fifth month of pregnancy complains to you of paresthesias in the fingers of both hands, which wake her at night. She also describes shoulder aching. Examination reveals a negative Tinel's sign at both wrists with ⅘ power of the right abductor pollicis brevis muscle. Your clinical diagnosis is

   (A) cervical myelopathy
   (B) cervical radiculopathy
   (C) brachial plexopathy
   (D) median neuropathy
   (E) musculoskeletal disease

4. The patient described above does not have resolution of her symptoms after cessation of the pregnancy. An electromyogram (EMG) is performed and confirms the presence of bilateral median neuropathy localized to the wrist but demonstrates "severe amounts of acute and chronic denervation in the abductor pollicis brevis muscle." Your therapeutic recommendation should be

   (A) wrist splints
   (B) decompressive surgery at the wrist
   (C) anti-inflammatory medications
   (D) vitamin B_6 (pyridoxine) therapy
   (E) A and C
   (F) A, B, and C
   (G) A, B, C, and D

5. A 35-year-old man with a past history of depression presents to the emergency department complaining of a 3-day history of paresthesias in his hands and feet. He denies pain but has felt clumsy when attempting to button his shirt. He appears quite anxious to you, and his exam is notable only for a resting tachycardia of 112 and an absence of deep tendon reflexes in his arms and legs. Your chief diagnostic consideration at this point should be

   (A) bilateral carpal tunnel syndrome
   (B) panic attack
   (C) Guillain–Barré syndrome
   (D) multiple sclerosis
   (E) vasovagal near syncope

6. A lumbar puncture is performed and reveals highly elevated protein of 345 (normal < 45) with no white or red blood cells and normal glucose. His blood gas is normal, but his vital capacity is 0.9 liters. Your next course of action is

   (A) transfer to intensive care unit (ICU) for observation with repeat ABG
   (B) emergency mechanical ventilation and begin treatment for his condition
   (C) emergency magnetic resonance imaging (MRI) of the vertebral spine and urgent neurosurgical consultation
   (D) oxygen therapy, serial blood gas and vital capacity, and schedule EMG
   (E) immediate transfer to a university medical center for urgent therapy

7. A diagnosis of Guillain–Barré syndrome is made. Immediate therapy may include

   (A) plasma exchange
   (B) intravenous immunoglobulin
   (C) observation for autonomic signs such as gastroparesis or cardiac dysrhythmia
   (D) serial measurement of sodium to watch for syndrome of inappropriate diuretic hormone (SIADH)
   (E) all of the above

8. All of the following are responsible for community-acquired sinusitis in adults EXCEPT

   (A) *Aspergillus fumigatas*
   (B) *Streptococcus pneumoniae*
   (C) *Haemophilus influenzae*
   (D) *Moraxella catarrhalis*
   (E) *Pseudomonas aeruginosa*

9. A 52-year-old man with uncontrolled hypertension for 10 years comes to see you. His blood pressure is 150/90 mm Hg on spironolactone 200 mg/day. His serum potassium is 2.5 mEq/L on potassium supplement 80 mEq/day. The most appropriate test is

   (A) random aldosterone (A) and renin (R)
   (B) stop spironolactone, start doxazosin, then measure A and R 2 weeks later
   (C) stop spironolactone, start doxazosin, then measure A and R 4 weeks later
   (D) stop spironolactone, start doxazosin, then measure A and R 6 weeks later
   (E) computed tomography (CT) scan of the adrenals

10. All of the following are true EXCEPT

    (A) use of warfarin is contraindicated in the first trimester of pregnancy
    (B) patients with protein S deficiency have a higher incidence of arterial thrombosis than venous thrombosis
    (C) patients who have resistance to activated protein C are usually treated with warfarin even though this lowers their protein C levels
    (D) heparin resistance may be seen with antithrombin III deficiency
    (E) patients with hereditary deficiency of protein C may have a paradoxical hypercoagulable state after starting warfarin

11. Lifelong male erectile disorder occurs in what percent of men under age 35?

    (A) 1%
    (B) 10%
    (C) 15%
    (D) 25%

12. The nonsteroidal anti-inflammatory agent Celebrex® (celecoxib) displays cross-allergic sensitivity to which of the following drugs?

(A) cephalosporin antibiotics

(B) aminoglycoside antibiotics

(C) macrolide antibiotics

(D) sulfa-based antibiotics

(E) none of the above

13. A 24-year-old woman is admitted to the hospital after having had a seizure. Her blood pressure is 90/50 mm Hg, serum sodium is 119 mEq/L, serum potassium is 5.5 mEq/L, and there is a mild metabolic acidosis. Acute adrenal insufficiency is suspected. Which statement is NOT true?

(A) The presence of hyperkalemia and metabolic acidosis excludes secondary adrenal insufficiency.

(B) The presence of hyponatremia excludes secondary adrenal insufficiency.

(C) Hyperpigmentation does not occur in secondary adrenal insufficiency.

(D) 60 minutes after 250 µg of corticotropin, a cortisol level of at least 20 µg/dL indicates normal adrenal function

(E) In patients with primary adrenal insufficiency, adrenocorticotropic hormone (ACTH) levels invariably exceed 100 pg/mL.

14. The diffusion capacity of carbon monoxide is impaired in all of these disorders EXCEPT

(A) emphysema

(B) pulmonary fibrosis

(C) pulmonary hypertension

(D) pulmonary edema

(E) neuromuscular diaphragmatic weakness

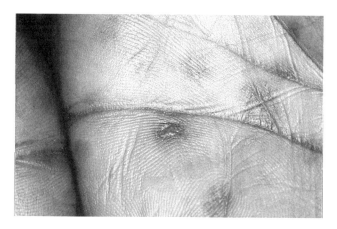

Figure 2.1

Items 15–16

A patient comes to your office complaining of a rash and low-grade fevers over the past few days. The patient is seen in Figures 2.1 and 2.2. On exam you also find epitrochlear lymphadenopathy.

15. Which organism is responsible for his illness?

(A) *Neisseria gonorrhea*

(B) adenovirus

(C) syphilis *(Treponema pallidum)*

(D) *Chlamydia trachomatis*

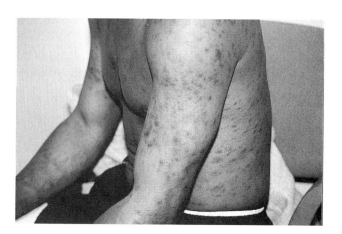

Figure 2.2

16. The best treatment for this patient is

   (A) doxycycline 100 mg once a day for 7 days
   (B) ceftriaxone 250 mg intramuscularly (IM) once
   (C) benzathine penicillin 2.4 million U IM once
   (D) benzathine penicillin 2.4 million U IM once a week for 3 weeks

END OF SET

17. Of the options listed below, the most common congenital infection is

   (A) cytomegalovirus (CMV)
   (B) parvovirus
   (C) varicella zoster
   (D) toxoplasmosis

18. In the United States, pregnant women with positive human immunodeficiency virus (HIV) status should be advised

   (A) to breast feed their babies as long as they are on appropriate medication
   (B) not to breast feed
   (C) to terminate their pregnancy since there is such a high chance of neonatal transmission
   (D) to undergo permanent sterilization to eliminate the risk of pregnancy

19. Dry eyes, xerostomia, and parotid hypertrophy, without evidence of systemic collagen vascular disease, is best classified as

   (A) Sjögren syndrome
   (B) Sjögren's disease
   (C) Miculicz's disease
   (D) sicca syndrome
   (E) Sjögren's disease, secondary type

20. All of the following are risk factors for bacterial cystitis in young men EXCEPT

   (A) intact foreskin
   (B) HIV infection
   (C) intravenous drug use
   (D) anal intercourse

Items 21–22

A 31-year-old woman presents to the emergency room with a complaint of pain in the left eye. The patient indicates that she has been wearing contact lenses for many years. She slept in her contact lenses the night before and experienced pain upon awakening. There is a hazy light reflex on the cornea. There is perilimbal flush.

21. The differential diagnosis includes

   (A) corneal abrasion
   (B) contact lens overwear syndrome
   (C) corneal ulcer
   (D) corneal foreign body
   (E) all of the above

22. Evaluation requires which of the following?

   (A) slit lamp examination
   (B) staining of the cornea with fluorescein
   (C) visual acuity testing
   (D) all of the above
   (E) none of the above

END OF SET

23. Which of the following statements best describes the current role of intravenous (IV) steroids in the management of spinal cord injuries?

   (A) Steroids should be administered as soon as possible for blunt spinal cord injuries seen within the first 8 hours of injury.
   (B) Steroids are indicated for both blunt and penetrating injuries of the spinal cord.
   (C) Steroids are of no proven value in spinal cord injuries.
   (D) Steroids have been shown to worsen the outcome in spinal cord injuries.
   (E) Steroids are indicated in penetrating injuries to the spinal cord seen within 1 hour of injury.

24. Which of the following types of alopecia results in permanent scarring?

    (A) alopecia areata
    (B) androgenetic alopecia
    (C) discoid lupus erythematosus
    (D) telogen effluvium

25. The incidence of which form of skin cancer increases most dramatically among immunosuppressed patients who have undergone organ transplantation?

    (A) basal cell carcinoma
    (B) squamous cell carcinoma
    (C) malignant melanoma
    (D) Kaposi's sarcoma
    (E) dermatofibrosarcoma protuberans

26. A 67-year-old woman is seen in the emergency department with a history of several hours of constant left lower quadrant pain, anorexia, nausea, and fever. On physical exam, she is febrile, but her other vital signs are stable. There is moderate direct tenderness upon palpation of the left lower quadrant of her abdomen with brown, guaiac-positive stool on rectal exam. Which of the following tests is most appropriate in order to make a diagnosis?

    (A) flexible sigmoidoscopy
    (B) colonoscopy
    (C) barium enema
    (D) abdominal–pelvic CT scan
    (E) mesenteric arteriogram

27. A 55-year-old woman without any significant medical history is admitted to the hospital with hematemesis and mild orthostatic hypotension. After stabilization with intravenous fluids, an endoscopy is performed. In the fundus of the stomach, a circular, protruding mass/lesion is noted, with a maximal diameter of 2.5 cm. The surface mucosa overlying this mass is normal (gastric) in appearance, except for a small nipple-like central depressed area, without adherent clot or visible vessel. No other lesions are noted. Which of the following is most appropriate to make a diagnosis under these circumstances?

    (A) endoscopic ultrasound of the mass/lesion with fine-needle aspiration/biopsy
    (B) abdominal ultrasound
    (C) abdominal–pelvic CT scan
    (D) surgical resection
    (E) endoscopic biopsy

28. The Jarisch–Herxheimer reaction is most frequently seen in the setting of treatment of

    (A) malignant melanoma
    (B) secondary syphilis
    (C) erythema multiforme
    (D) psoriasis
    (E) Rocky Mountain spotted fever

29. The indication for antibiotic therapy for asymptomatic bacteriuria in pregnant women is related to

    (A) increased risk of symptomatic bladder infections
    (B) increased incidence of acute pyelonephritis
    (C) risk of fetal infection
    (D) increased incidence of preeclampsia

30. An office cystoscopy is indicated in the evaluation of men with benign prostatic hypertrophy (BPH) in the following situations EXCEPT

    (A) all men with BPH prior to surgery
    (B) in the setting of severe obstructive or irritative voiding symptoms
    (C) the finding of microscopic or gross hematuria
    (D) to rule out the presence of a urethral stricture
    (E) recurrent urinary tract infections

31. An obese 55-year-old woman presents with a 4-hour history of dyspnea and anterior chest pain that is worse when she takes a deep breath. The patient and her husband have just returned from a vacation trip to Australia. She is postmenopausal and taking estrogen replacement. Room air pulse oximetry shows 90% saturation and her temperature is 38° C (100.4° F). Exam reveals a few crackles at both bases, and the patient appears anxious and tachypneic. Chest x-ray shows poor inspiratory effort with platelike atelectasis present bilaterally. The patient's 12-lead ECG is shown in Figure 2.3. Based on the available data, which of the following statements is true?

    (A) The patient needs supplemental oxygen and IV antibiotics and she requires admission.

    (B) The patient has pericarditis and should be further evaluated with an echocardiogram and treated with a nonsteroidal anti-inflammatory drug (NSAID) such as indomethacin.

    (C) The patient has a high clinical probability of pulmonary embolus and should be started on IV heparin while awaiting further evaluation with a pulmonary ventilation–perfusion scan or a helical CT scan of the chest.

    (D) The patient should be given nebulized albuterol and IV methylprednisolone along with supplemental oxygen.

    (E) The data presented are most consistent with viral pleuritis.

32. Each of the following is a potential cause of pulseless electrical activity (PEA) EXCEPT

    (A) cardiac tamponade
    (B) hyperkalemia
    (C) toxic ingestion
    (D) pulmonary embolus
    (E) hyperthermia

33. Miosis and altered mental status may be commonly associated with each of the following EXCEPT

    (A) clonidine overdose
    (B) use of opiates
    (C) pontine hemorrhage
    (D) organophosphate intoxication
    (E) status epilepticus

34. Which of the following diseases will result in a positive serum antineutrophil cytoplasmic antibody (ANCA) test?

    (A) sarcoidosis
    (B) DiGeorge syndrome
    (C) polymorphic reticulosis

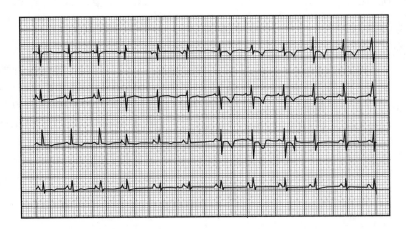

Figure 2.3

(D) relapsing polychrondritis

(E) Churg–Strauss syndrome

35. A 55-year-old man with a 5-year history of hypertension, facial fullness, and truncal obesity presents with several days of midthoracic back pain. Physical examination shows a cushingoid-appearing man with a blood pressure of 160/100 mm Hg. His serum potassium is 3 mEq/L and his fasting glucose is 160 mg/dL. A 24-hour urine free cortisol is 424 μg/day (N: 20–90 μg/day). An x-ray of his spine shows a compression fracture at T8. What would you do now?

(A) overnight dexamethasone suppression test

(B) MRI of the pituitary gland

(C) CT of the adrenals

(D) serum ACTH levels

(E) high-dose dexamethasone suppression test

36. A 50-year-old woman presents with low energy, depressed mood, and loss of interest in activities with a past history of depression. Also, she is finding it difficult to organize her bills. She mentions that she was a very active person; she is rebellious and went to jail several times. Also, she has been at several different companies as the CEO and her last working day was a year ago. What is the LEAST likely diagnosis?

(A) major depressive disorder (MDD)

(B) bipolar disorder

(C) cyclothymia

(D) dysthymia

37. Which of the following is NOT usually associated with a transudate?

(A) congestive heart failure

(B) nephrosis

(C) cirrhosis

(D) hypoalbuminemia

(E) rheumatoid arthritis

38. The abnormality demonstrated by the pulmonary function test shown in Figure 2.4 is

(A) obstruction

(B) restriction

(C) variable extrathoracic obstruction

(D) fixed intrathoracic obstruction

(E) none of the above

	Predicted		Control	
	Normal	Range	Found	%Pred.
Lung Volumes				
TLC (Pleth)	6.34	>4.97	5.76	91%
VC	3.85	>3.01	3.21	83%
RV	2.49	<3.24	2.55	102%
RV/TLC	39.3	<51.5	44.3	113%
FRC			4.2	
Spirometry				
FVC	3.85	>3.01	2.60*	68%
FEV$_1$	2.92	>2.24	1.32*	45%
FEV$_1$/FVC	75.9	>66.7	50.9*	
FEF$_{25-75}$	2.5	>1.4	0.5*	19%
FEF$_{max}$	7.4	>3.9	4.1	56%
MVV	111	>78	43*	39%
Diffusing Capacity				
DLCO(SB)	23.0	>15.0		
VA	6.34	>4.97		
Oximetry			Rest	
O$_2$ Sat	95	≥93	93	
Pulse			95	

*Outside normal range + weight exceeds 95th percentile

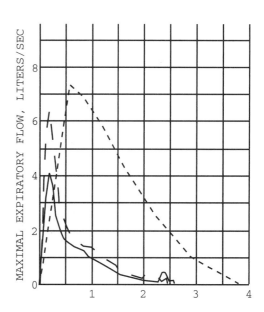

Figure 2.4

39. An appropriate use of intravenous vancomycin would be

    (A) routine surgical prophylaxis for hip replacement
    (B) a hospitalized patient on hemodialysis with gram-positive cocci in two sets of blood cultures
    (C) a patient with *Clostridium difficile* colitis
    (D) home antibiotic therapy every 12 hours for methicillin-sensitive *Staphylococcus aureus* bacteremia

40. The biophysical profile is a test currently used in antepartum fetal surveillance. Its components include all of the following EXCEPT

    (A) nonstress test
    (B) fetal breathing movements
    (C) estimated fetal weight
    (D) gross fetal body movement
    (E) amniotic fluid volume

41. All of the following are risk factors for endometrial cancer EXCEPT

    (A) chronic anovulation
    (B) obesity
    (C) early menopause
    (D) diabetes mellitus
    (E) nulliparity

42. A 70-year-old man is referred for progressive bone pain. He has known prostate cancer with metastatic disease to the skeleton and has been treated in the past with multiple hormonal therapies including a gonadotropin-releasing hormone (GnRH) analogue, androgen blockade, and an adrenal steroid enzyme inhibitor after being refractory to hormonal blockade. The pain is in the chest wall area and is exacerbated by coughing. His ribs bilaterally and hips appear involved as well. Plain films of the spine show diffuse osteoblastic disease in the skeleton with no fractures or spinal collapse. The next diagnostic test you should order is

    (A) a prostate-specific antigen (PSA)
    (B) a bone scan and a CT

    (C) an MRI
    (D) a CT scan
    (E) a bone scan

43. This patient continues to have chest pain and now is incontinent of both bowel and bladder. Which would be the most appropriate therapy at this time?

    (A) orchiectomy
    (B) steroids followed by radiation therapy
    (C) steroids followed by surgical resection of the vertebral body
    (D) mitoxantrone
    (E) strontium 89 and mitoxantrone

Items 44–46

A 30-year-old woman with steroid-dependent asthma presents with a 2-month history of right groin pain with ambulation. Physical examination and x-rays of the hip are normal.

44. The most likely diagnosis is

    (A) avascular necrosis
    (B) osteoarthritis
    (C) ruptured L2 disk
    (D) femoral hernia

45. The most appropriate early treatment for the above patient is

    (A) an NSAID
    (B) crutches
    (C) physical therapy
    (D) narcotic analgesics

46. The most appropriate test for confirming this diagnosis is

    (A) bone scan
    (B) gallium scan
    (C) MRI scan
    (D) CT scan
    (E) ultrasound

END OF SET

47. A 53-year-old man with a history of hypertension is admitted with nausea, vomiting, and epigastric pain. His vital signs on admission are: heart rate 90, BP 90/60, temperature 37.2° C (99° F), and respiratory rate 18. He is cold, clammy, and anxious. An echocardiogram is performed and shows an ejection fraction of 40%. His ECG is shown in Figure 2.5. Correct treatment includes all of the following EXCEPT

(A) heparin
(B) aspirin
(C) nitroglycerin
(D) IV normal saline
(E) thrombolytic

48. Regarding the above patient, his diagnosis most likely is

(A) acute anterior myocardial infarction
(B) acute closure of the left anterior descending coronary artery
(C) acute lateral wall myocardial infarction secondary to closure of the right coronary artery
(D) acute inferior myocardial infarction with right ventricular involvement

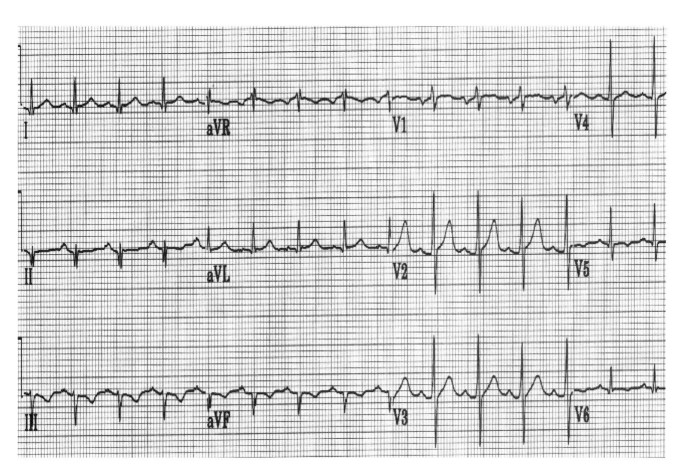

Figure 2.5

49. After intervention, the patient described above does well and has an uncomplicated remainder to his hospital course. He is seen as an outpatient 6 days after discharge from the hospital. He is receiving a beta blocker, a statin, an angiotensin-converting enzyme (ACE) inhibitor, and Plavix. He is pain free and has begun an exercise program and diet. His only complaint is of daily palpitations. Appropriate tests/procedures to consider include

(A) repeat cardiac catheterization

(B) coronary artery bypass grafting (CABG)

(C) 24-hour ambulatory monitor

(D) electrophysiology (EP) study

50. The leading cause of congenital hearing loss is

(A) congenital cytomegalovirus (CMV)

(B) congenital rubella infection

(C) congenital syphilis

(D) congenital varicella syndrome

Practice Test 2
Answers and Explanations

1. **(E)** Light's criteria for exclusion of a transudate include pleural to serum protein ratio > 0.5, pleural to serum LDH > 0.6, and pleural LDH > ⅔ upper limits of laboratory normal. Another criterion frequently used is a pleural cholesterol of > 60 mg/dL. It has high sensitivity and specificity for an exudate.

2. **(A)** This patient probably has a pericardial effusion with tamponade. The best way to demonstrate this is via an echocardiogram. Cardiac catheterization would be revealing but is invasive and time consuming. Lordotic views of the chest are not necessary. Pulmonary function tests would not be needed with no change in CXR or blood gases.

3. **(D)** Carpal tunnel syndrome is common during pregnancy and is generally a self-limited condition that resolves postpartum. The Tinel's sign will be positive only 50% of the time in patients with carpal tunnel syndrome. Shoulder aching is a common associated symptom and should not be mistaken for proximal disease.

4. **(F)** Both wrist splints and anti-inflammatory medications may be useful in alleviating symptoms, but the ongoing denervation suggests a more severe axonal injury requiring more immediate surgical treatment to prevent permanent loss of nerve and muscle function. There have been no controlled studies to demonstrate efficacy of pyridoxine in this clinical setting. Higher-dose pyridoxine is irreversibly toxic to the dorsal root ganglion.

5–7. **(5-C, 6-B, 7-E)** All patients with acute onset of symmetric sensory and/or motor symptoms should at least be considered for a diagnosis of Guillain–Barré syndrome. Absent or reduced deep tendon reflexes will make the diagnosis more likely. Other diagnostic considerations (and especially psychiatric illnesses) can be considered on a more leisurely basis as an outpatient.

The characteristic spinal fluid analysis of very high protein with an absence of cells can help to confirm the diagnosis a few days after onset of symptoms with nerve conductions demonstrating a motor demyelinating polyradiculoneuropathy providing definitive proof of the diagnosis.

In neuromuscular causes of respiratory collapse such as Guillain–Barré and myasthenia gravis, the vital capacity will fall long before there are changes in the ABG. A vital capacity < 1 liter requires emergency ventilatory support. A vital capacity > 1 liter at time of presentation should be repeated frequently, every 1 to 4 hours.

Both immunoglobulin therapy and plasma exchange will decrease the risk of requiring mechanical ventilator and speed time of recovery when initiated within the first 10 to 14 days after onset of symptoms. Intravenous immunoglobulin at a dose of 2 mg/kg over 5 days is easier to administer and has much fewer potential side effects than plasma exchange (hypotension, reduced platelet count, complications of central line placement) and so may be the preferred therapy. SIADH and autonomic neuropathy symptoms are quite common in this condition.

8. **(A)** *S. pneumoniae, H. influenzae,* and *M. catarrhalis* all are responsible for acute sinusitis. *Aspergillus* spp. may cause sinusitis in an immunocompromised host such as a neutropenic patient or a bone marrow transplant recipient. Hospitalized patients, especially those with nasogastric tubes and endotracheal tubes, are at risk for development of nosocomially acquired sinusitis, often due to gram-negative organisms such as *Pseudomonas.*

9. **(D)** In patients suspected of having hyperaldosteronism, the best screening test is random A and R; off all interfering medications, mainly diuretics and ACE inhibitors, for 2 weeks; and spironolactone for 6 weeks. Interference from beta blockers and calcium channel blockers is minimal. Alpha-1 blockers (doxazosin) do not interfere with the testing. If the A/R ratio is < 20, primary hyperaldosteronism is excluded. If the ratio is > 20, then confirmatory tests need to be performed, because there are false positives. A high 24-hour urine aldosterone on high-salt diet confirms the diagnosis. CT scan should not be done before the diagnosis is confirmed.

10. **(B)** Patients with either protein S or C deficiency often have venous thrombosis. Arterial thrombosis may occur infrequently, especially if an anatomical conduit is suspected such as a patent ductus. Similar observations have been made in patients with antithrombin III deficiency or resistance to activated protein C.

11. **(A)** It occurs in about 1% of men under age 35.

12. **(C)** Celebrex® has a cross-allergic potential with sulfa-based antibiotics. Reactions of a severe urticarial and bronchoconstrictive nature have been reported. These often take weeks to develop.

13. **(B)** In secondary adrenal insufficiency, the potassium and acid–base balance are normal, because aldosterone secretion is not affected. However, hyponatremia also occurs in secondary adrenal insufficiency because of cortisol deficiency, increased vasopressin secretion, and water retention. Normal plasma ACTH rules out primary but not secondary adrenal insufficiency. In primary adrenal insufficiency, ACTH levels invariably exceed 100 pg/mL.

14. **(E)** Diffusing capacity is impaired in any disorder that increases the distance between alveolus and capillary or that decreases the surface area available for gas exchange. In neuromuscular weakness, there is no pulmonary parenchymal or vascular abnormality.

15. **(C)** Syphilis presents with three distinct clinical syndromes. In primary syphilis, a chancre (a painless papule) is present at the site of inoculation. About 2 to 8 weeks after the chancre appears, the patient develops secondary syphilis, the period in which the spirochetes disseminate. The patient may experience fever; a rash with protean characteristics, often involving the palms and soles; condylomata lata (highly infectious lesions found in intertriginous areas); and central nervous system (CNS), renal, and hepatic involvement. Almost any system may be affected. Epitrochlear lymphadenopathy is classically associated with syphilis during the secondary phase. Tertiary or late syphilis is the slowly progressive stage that can affect almost all organ systems if syphilis goes untreated and may occur years after the initial infection.

16. **(C)** For primary and secondary syphilis, benzathine penicillin is the recommended treatment. For latent syphilis infection, three doses of benzathine penicillin are needed. Penicillin is the recommended treatment for all stages. One must consider penicillin desensitization therapy in the penicillin-allergic patient, especially in cases of pregnancy or CNS manifestations. Doxycycline may be an alternative therapy.

17. **(A)** 0.2 to 2.2% of all neonates are infected with CMV. Parvovirus, zoster, and toxoplasmosis are less common.

18. **(B)** While current medication regimens coupled with early detection have dramatically reduced the incidence of neonatal transmission of HIV, breast milk can carry HIV and pass it on to the feeding infant. HIV-positive mothers should therefore be advised to avoid breast feeding.

19. **(D)** Sjögren's disease or syndrome involves some aspect of systemic inflammation or a defined collagen vascular disease. The combination of dry eyes, dry mouth, and parotid hypertrophy is appropriately called "sicca syndrome."

20. **(C)** Intravenous drug use may predispose young men to HIV infection but is not, in and of itself, a risk factor for bacterial cystitis.

21. **(E)** A patient who presents with pain in the eye and the history of contact lens wear should be considered for all of the options listed in that all can occur with contact lens wear and can be associated with pain.

22. **(D)** All ocular examinations should include a slit lamp examination. Although this patient was seen in the emergency department, most emergency departments do have slit lamps to examine the front of the eye. Visual acuity testing is done on all patients with ocular complaints. The staining of the cornea is absolutely essential in evaluating corneal abnormalities. If the patient has a corneal abrasion, corneal ulcer, or foreign body, the cornea will stain in a focal, well-defined area. Contact lens overwear syndrome can be associated with a diffuse epithelial stain, which helps to differentiate it from focal staining seen in corneal abrasions, ulcers, and foreign bodies. These are best seen with a slit lamp.

23. **(A)** High-dose methylprednisolone has been demonstrated to be of value in the treatment of blunt injuries to the spinal cord if initiated within 8 hours of injury. Steroids are not indicated in the treatment of penetrating injuries of the spinal cord.

24. **(C)** Lupus erythematosus is an autoimmune disorder that often affects the scalp and causes alopecia. It is characterized by oval, scarring areas of alopecia that are white and atrophic centrally with an active erythematous margin.

25. **(B)** Transplant patients receiving antirejection drugs demonstrate a 65-fold increased risk of squamous cell carcinoma.

26. **(D)** The patient history and physical exam are most consistent with acute diverticulitis. Flexible sigmoidoscopy and colonoscopy are unsafe and should *not* be performed as insufflation of air can convert a small perforation (an inflamed diverticulum) into a large perforation. Once the patient recovers and is well, colonoscopy should be performed to rule out a mucosal lesion (i.e., colon cancer). A barium enema without air insufflation can be performed safely in the hands of an experienced radiologist but does not give as much diagnostic information as a CT scan. About one in four persons with acute diverticulitis can have a guaiac-positive stool. This does not require immediate evaluation. Although left lower quadrant pain can be a feature of ischemic colitis, often with blood in the stool and/or diarrhea, the fever in this case makes this diagnosis less likely, and angiography is not helpful or diagnostic anyway in suspected left-sided ischemic colitis.

27. **(D)** This patient, previously healthy, has bled from a lesion in her upper stomach that is submucosal, based on its appearance. It is highly unlikely that an endoscopic biopsy, which is superficial and usually mucosal, will be diagnostic. Abdominal ultrasound may not even identify the lesion, nor be diagnostic. A CT scan is more likely to locate the lesion and give a more accurate estimate of its diameter than that determined by endoscopy, which often is an underestimate. If the lesion contains significant fat (i.e., possibly a lipoma), the CT scan may recognize this. Endoscopic ultrasound is useful in sizing the lesion and determining what layers of

the stomach wall are involved, and may be able to give a reasonable determination of whether the lesion is benign or malignant. Fine-needle aspiration/biopsy may also help define the histologic nature of the lesion but will not always be diagnostic of benign versus malignant, as these submucosal tumors often are gastrointestinal stomal tumors (GISTs), and they often require complete surgical removal to best make that distinction. Finally, if these are large (i.e., > 4 cm) *or* if they exhibit any "bad behaviors," such as bleeding or progressive growth over time, they should be removed. In this case, with bleeding, surgery is indicated and is most likely to be diagnostic.

28. **(B)** The Jarisch–Herxheimer reaction is an acute febrile reaction associated with shaking chills, myalgias, and malaise that follows penicillin treatment of secondary syphilis. It is thought to be due to release of treponemal lipopolysaccharides that act like an endotoxin.

29. **(B)** Pregnant women with symptomatic bacteriuria have an increased incidence of acute pyelonephritis that, in turn, is associated with increased fetal mortality.

30. **(A)** Hematuria (in the absence of infection), severe voiding symptoms, a possible urethral stricture, and recurrent urinary tract infections are all indications for an office cystoscopy. A cystoscopy is not necessary performed simply as a preop screening test.

31. **(C)** The clinical information provided is strongly suggestive of pulmonary embolus. The ECG shown exhibits the S1Q3T3 pattern and anterior ischemia. The S1Q3T3 pattern includes: prominent S-wave in lead I, Q-wave in lead III, and T-wave inversion in lead III. The ECG can provide valuable clues to the diagnosis of pulmonary embolism but taken by itself is nondiagnostic. The most frequent ECG changes associated with pulmonary embolism are nonspecific ST and T-wave changes and PVCs. New onset of a right bundle branch block is suggestive of

pulmonary embolism as is the S1Q3T3 pattern. The S1Q3T3 pattern is present in 12 to 20% of cases of pulmonary embolism. A completely normal ECG is very uncommon in cases of pulmonary embolism.

32. **(E)** When we encounter PEA, we should consider carefully the possible causes and their treatment. Likely etiologies include: acidosis, hypoxemia, hyperkalemia, hypovolemia, hypothermia, toxic ingestions (tricyclics, calcium channel blockers, beta blockers), tension pneumothorax, cardiac tamponade, myocardial infarction, and pulmonary embolus. Hyperthermia does not cause PEA.

33. **(E)** Miosis is commonly associated with use of opiates and with intoxication due to clonidine and organophosphates. Miosis is also observed with pontine hemorrhage. Mydriasis is commonly seen with generalized seizures.

34. **(E)** The ANCA test is used to diagnose Wegener's granulomatosis, but Churg–Strauss syndrome can also cause the ANCA test to be positive.

35. **(D)** Since the 24-hour urine free cortisol is diagnostic of Cushing's (more than three times the upper limit of normal), there is no need to do an overnight dexamethasone suppression test. The next step would be to measure ACTH levels to classify Cushing's as ACTH dependent or ACTH independent; then high-dose dexamethasone suppression test (pituitary Cushing's will suppress, but not ectopic) and imaging can be done to locate the etiology of Cushing's.

36. **(D)** Dysthymia is a chronic depressed mood with euphoria or no euthymia between depressed states.

37. **(E)** Inflammatory and connective tissue diseases are usually exudates. Rheumatoid arthritis also characteristically has a very low glucose.

38. **(A)** The high TLC, low FEV_1 and low FEV_1/FVC ratios are consistent with obstruction. The loop typically has a scooped appearance in the middle flow ranges.

39. **(B)** As the problems of antimicrobial resistance and nosocomial infections increase, more strict attention must be made regarding the use of antibiotics. Vancomycin is the last defense against methicillin-resistant *S. aureus*, which is a serious, usually nosocomial infection. Vancomycin-resistant strains of *Enterococcus* already exist and are a menace to treat. Vancomycin should never be used to treat an infection that could be treated with another antibiotic just for the sake of convenience. Vancomycin should be used empirically only for a serious infection in which the risk of methicillin-resistant *S. aureus* is high, as in hemodialysis patients or in meningitis when there is concern for penicillin-resistant pneumococcus.

40. **(C)** All of the other parameters listed, plus observation of fetal tone, are used in the biophysical profile.

41. **(C)** Early menopause is not a risk factor for the development of endometrial cancer, but rather late menopause and early menarche are risk factors for the development of endometrial cancer. This is because an early menarche and late menopause result in a longer reproductive life span, and thus prolong the total exposure time to estrogen. Chronic anovulation and nulliparity are also associated with a longer reproductive life span and thus lead to increased risk of endometrial cancer. Obesity is associated with higher endogenous estrogen levels throughout a woman's lifetime because of peripheral conversion of androstenedione to estrone in the fat tissue. Diabetes mellitus is also considered a risk factor for endometrial cancer. *(Beckmann, 542)*

42. **(C)** The patient has symptoms suggestive of thoracic cord compression that needs to be evaluated. This is most effectively done with an MRI. The degree of pain is not predictive, nor is the absence of an identifiable level on sensory examination or motor loss. There is no overt neurologic dysfunction, but cough-related pain may be suggestive of epidural disease and needs to be worked up. A bone scan can show the extent of disease but not rule out epidural involvement. CT also does not have the precision of an MRI. A PSA would add little at this point.

43. **(B)** This is evolving cord compression and needs to be emergently treated with steroids and radiation. Mitoxantrone has shown little antitumor benefit but can be used for palliation, as can strontium. Neither will relieve cord compression. A laminectomy can be considered in some isolated cases but due to its diffuse nature, it is unclear whether the spine could be stabilized.

44. **(A)** Avascular necrosis of the femoral head is a common complication of prolonged cortisone therapy, and patients should be informed of this potential side effect. Steroid therapy should be used with caution but not withheld when absolutely necessary. Other causes are sickle cell disease, alcohol use, deep-sea diving with inadequate decompression, trauma, and Gaucher's disease. Often, a causative disease or agent is not evident.

45. **(B)** Protected weight bearing of the hip to prevent segmental collapse of the weight-bearing surface of the femoral head is most important while workup is in progress. Dead bone is invaded by blood vessels and is absorbed. Before the tissue can be replaced with new bone, this weakened area below the cartilage surface can collapse.

46. **(C)** An MRI scan will show avascular bone in the weight-bearing area of the femoral head on both T1 and T2 weighted images. The opposite hip should also be examined, as the first stage of the disease is an asymptomatic hip with positive MRI findings. A bone scan will be positive but is not specific. A gallium scan will be positive with frank severe arthritis. A CT scan will be normal, unless plain x-rays are abnormal.

47–48. (47-C, 48-D) This patient has had an acute inferior myocardial infarction with right ventricular involvement. Hypotension is common with right ventricular involvement because of the inability for the damaged RV to pump blood to the left side of the heart. Treatment with nitroglycerin reduces preload and would result in even more severe hypotension. Volume support is needed. The right coronary artery supplies the right ventricle and inferior myocardial wall in most people.

49. (C) The patient has had an extensive myocardial infarction and has depressed left ventricular function. He is at risk for postinfarct ventricular arrhythmias. Since he has not had alarming arrhythmias noted and his symptoms occur daily, a 24-hour ambulatory monitor is indicated. If an abnormality is seen on the monitor or if he had shown severe depression in his ejection fraction, an EP study might be indicated as a next step. He does not have symptoms to suggest ischemia, so catheterization and CABG are not indicated.

50. (A) Widespread vaccination has made congenital rubella infection very rare. Congenital varicella and syphilis are fortunately rare and are not associated with deafness.

Practice Test 3
Questions

DIRECTIONS (Questions 1 through 50): Each of the numbered items or incomplete statements in this section is followed by answers or by completions of the statement. Select the ONE lettered answer or completion that is BEST in each case.

Items 1–3

After a fall while horseback riding, a 37-year-old woman is evaluated at your hospital with a computed tomography (CT) scan of the abdomen. The scan shows no evidence of a ruptured spleen but a 2.5-cm right adrenal mass. The patient's medical history, review of systems, and physical examination are unremarkable.

1. All of the following are true EXCEPT

   (A) send plasma aldosterone and renin activity to exclude hyperaldosteronism
   (B) perform overnight dexamethasone suppression test to exclude Cushing's
   (C) collect 24-hour urine for catecholamines and metanephrines to exclude pheochromocytoma
   (D) repeat CT scan in 3 to 6 months to assess change in tumor size
   (E) 1 to 5% of normal people have similar CT scan finding

2. The 24-hour urine collection mentioned above showed high levels of catecholamines and metanephrines, consistent with a pheochromocytoma. Which statement is NOT true regarding pheochromocytomas?

   (A) Ten percent are malignant.
   (B) The best diagnostic test is plasma catecholamines.
   (C) Levels are affected by tricyclic antidepressants.
   (D) Hypertension can persist for as many as 4 to 8 weeks postoperatively.
   (E) Ten percent recur after surgical removal.

3. The patient is scheduled to have surgery. Pre- and perioperative management of pheochromocytoma might include all of the following EXCEPT

   (A) phenoxybenzamine
   (B) propranolol
   (C) nitroprusside
   (D) phentolamine
   (E) amiloride

END OF SET

4. A 30-year-old man from South America has a sudden onset over 10 days of easy bruising, gum bleeding, and hematuria. He was seen in the emergency department and found to have significant bruising over his torso and extremities, as well as mucosal pallor. His initial lab work showed a white blood count (WBC) of 33,000/µL, many immature myeloid forms, hemoglobin of 7.8 gm/dL, platelet count of 26,000/µL, prothrombin time/partial thromboplastin time (PT/PTT) of 18 and 41, fibrinogen of 110 mg/dL, and elevated D dimers. A bone marrow was performed, which was markedly hypercellular with cells being heavily granulated with myeloperoxidase-positive granules. Flow cytometry and cytogenetics were sent. Which of the following is correct?

   (A) The patient has acute promyelocytic leukemia (APML) and disseminated intravascular coagulation (DIC).
   (B) The low platelet count is the only reason for bleeding.
   (C) The most likely cytogenetic abnormality is t8,21 mutation.
   (D) The only therapy that will induce remission is high-dose cytarabine.
   (E) The patient has a < 10% chance of cure.

5. A number of sexual problems may be associated with depression. Which of the following is seldom a problem associated with depression?

   (A) decreased libido
   (B) erectile dysfunction
   (C) delayed orgasm
   (D) premature ejaculation

6. All of the following comorbid disorders have been reported among patients with bipolar disorder II EXCEPT

   (A) substance abuse or dependence
   (B) anxiety disorders
   (C) schizophrenia, paranoid type
   (D) personality disorders

7. A 24-year-old Hispanic man with acquired immune deficiency syndrome (AIDS) presents to

the emergency department with fever, chills, dyspnea, and cough. He has been noncompliant with antiretroviral therapy; however, he does take trimethoprim–sulfamethoxazole three times a week. Physical exam reveals tachypnea, tachycardia, an SaO_2 of 87% on room air, and bilateral crackles. Laboratory testing reveals WBC of 1.8×10^9/L, with a left shift. Chest radiograph reveals diffuse bilateral alveolar infiltrates. Sputum methenamine silver stain shows oval-shaped structures with a "crushed Ping-Pong ball" appearance. The next most appropriate step would be to

   (A) perform a bronchoscopy to get better samples
   (B) begin patient on amphotericin B
   (C) start cefipime 2 g every 12 hours
   (D) begin IV trimethoprim–sulfamethoxazole and corticosteroids
   (E) begin inhaled pentamidine

Items 8–11

A 72-year-old man (Figure 3.1) presents to your office complaining of tremor. Your examination demonstrates a slow tremor of the right hand much worse at rest than on sustention. You are concerned about a diagnosis of Parkinson's disease.

8. All of the following clinical signs may be compatible with a diagnosis of Parkinson's disease EXCEPT

   (A) generalized dyskinesia
   (B) bradykinesia
   (C) lead-pipe rigidity
   (D) postural instability
   (E) subcortical dementia

9. You decide to initiate medical therapy for this patient's presumed Parkinson's disease with levodopa/carbidopa. The patient's wife calls you 1 week later convinced that your patient has developed side effects from the medicine. These include all of the following EXCEPT

   (A) hallucinations
   (B) gastric distress
   (C) difficulty swallowing

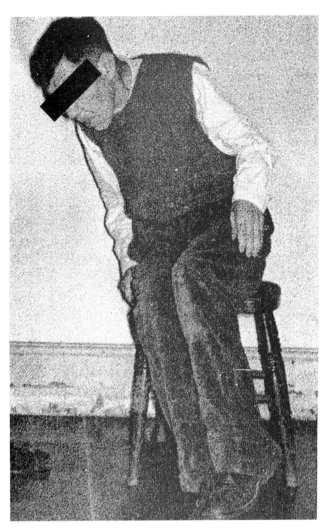

Figure 3.1

(A) dehydration

(B) central dysautonomia

(C) residual medication effect

(D) neurally mediated syncope

(E) sick sinus syndrome

11. All of the following therapies may be useful in treating this patient EXCEPT

(A) increased fluid intake

(B) increased salt intake

(C) propranolol

(D) fludrocortisone

(E) midodrine

END OF SET

12. In discussing the health risks of her morbid obesity with a patient, which of the following statements would be correct?

(A) Obesity directly contributes to heart disease by increasing the risk of Type 1 diabetes.

(B) Obesity raises the level of high-density lipoprotein (HDL).

(C) It can result in left ventricular hypertrophy.

(D) It can be reversed by weight loss.

(E) It results in high blood pressure as a result of changes in the pulmonary vasculature.

(D) orthostatic hypotension

(E) dyskinesia

10. Pergolide, a dopamine agonist, is added to the patient's medical regimen. The patient's wife now calls you complaining that the patient has significant light-headedness when attempting to get out of bed in the morning hours. You evaluate the patient and find a supine blood pressure of 190/100 with a drop to 110/70 immediately upon standing. The patient is asymptomatic during this tilt and his heart rate does not change from 72 beats per minute. You discontinue the pergolide without change in the patient's drop in blood pressure or light-headedness. The most likely diagnosis is

13. A 46-year-old man is admitted to the intensive care unit (ICU) with new-onset seizures. After he is stabilized, a magnetic resonance imaging (MRI) scan is obtained, which reveals multiple ring-enhancing lesions as depicted in Figure 3.2. The human immunodeficiency virus (HIV) serology comes back positive and his CD4 count is 9/mm^3. What is the most likely diagnosis, based on the presentation, that he should be treated for?

(A) metastatic lesions

(B) primary central nervous system (CNS) lymphoma

(C) *Toxoplasma gondii*

(D) *Cryptococcus neoformans*

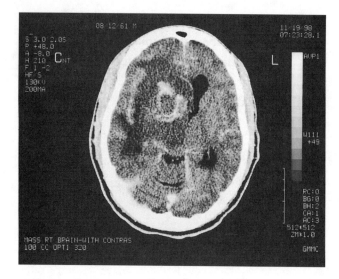

Figure 3.2

14. A 28-year-old G2P1001 woman presents to the emergency department with heavy vaginal bleeding at 32 weeks' gestation. Which of the following is NOT indicated in this patient's initial evaluation?

    (A) fetal monitoring
    (B) maternal vital signs
    (C) vaginal exam
    (D) transabdominal ultrasound

15. All of the following are used to calculate an Apgar score on a newborn EXCEPT

    (A) heart rate
    (B) respiratory effort
    (C) muscle tone
    (D) temperature
    (E) skin color

Items 16–17

You are asked to consult on a 45-year-old man with cyanosis in the postanesthesia recovery area after esophagogastroduodenoscopy (EGD). His SaO_2 is 97% on an FIO_2 50%. An arterial blood gas (ABG) reveals a PO_2 of 94 mm Hg, PCO_2 35 mm Hg, pH 7.41, and calculated SaO_2 82%.

16. What is the most likely diagnosis?

    (A) pulmonary embolus
    (B) hypoventilation
    (C) esophageal rupture
    (D) methemoglobinemia
    (E) myocardial infarction

17. What is the most appropriate treatment for the above condition?

    (A) heparin
    (B) positive pressure ventilation
    (C) thoracotomy
    (D) methylene blue
    (E) thrombolytics

END OF SET

18. Which of the following statements is NOT true regarding *Streptococcus agalactiae* (Group B streptococcus)?

    (A) It is an etiology of neonatal sepsis.
    (B) It may cause bacteremia in diabetics.
    (C) Pregnant women should be screened for the presence of Group B streptococcus in the female reproductive tract.
    (D) It is increasingly resistant to penicillin.

19. What is the finding in the right ear on the audiogram in Figure 3.3?

    (A) conductive hearing loss
    (B) mixed hearing loss
    (C) sensorineural hearing loss
    (D) normal hearing
    (E) factitious hearing loss

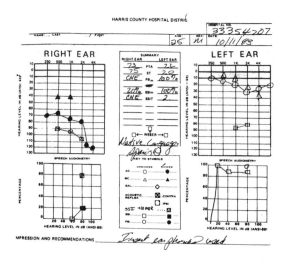

Figure 3.3

20. What is the finding in the left ear on the audiogram in Figure 3.4?

   (A) conductive hearing loss
   (B) mixed hearing loss
   (C) sensorineural hearing loss
   (D) normal hearing
   (E) factitious hearing loss

21. What is the recurrence rate of renal stones?

   (A) 10% in 10 years
   (B) 50% in 5 years
   (C) 0% in 5 years
   (D) stones are rarely completely eradicated

<u>Items 22–23</u>

A 78-year-old patient presents with a complaint of loss of vision in the left eye. The patient's retinal examination is shown in Figure 3.5.

22. The differential diagnosis includes

   (A) central retinal vein occlusion
   (B) central retinal artery occlusion
   (C) papilledema

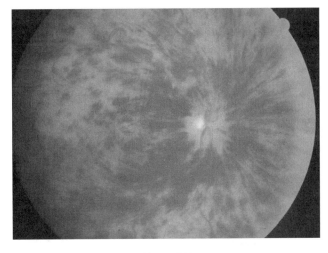

Figure 3.5

   (D) commotio retinae
   (E) HIV retinopathy

23. The workup in this patient includes

   (A) lumbar puncture
   (B) sedimentation rate
   (C) complete blood count
   (D) all of the above
   (E) none of the above

END OF SET

24. A 5-year-old child weighing 20 kg is brought in with vomiting and diarrhea and is noted to be pale, tachycardic, and lethargic. Several attempts to place a peripheral IV are unsuccessful. Which of the following choices represents the preferred intervention at this point?

   (A) subclavian vein access with administration of a 300-cc bolus of normal saline (NS)
   (B) femoral vein access with administration of a 400-cc bolus of normal saline with 5% dextrose (D_5NS)
   (C) intraosseous access with administration of a 400-cc bolus of NS
   (D) saphenous vein cutdown with administration of a 200-cc bolus of NS
   (E) intraosseous access with administration of a 200-cc bolus of NS

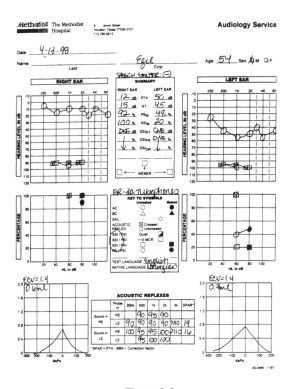

Figure 3.4

25. Among patients > 70 years of age presenting to the emergency department with abdominal pain, about 40% will require surgery. Which of the following choices represents the most common cause of abdominal pain in this group of patients?

    (A) viral gastroenteritis
    (B) appendicitis
    (C) constipation
    (D) biliary tract disease
    (E) urinary tract infection

26. In treating epistaxis, which is the most common location of bleeding, and what is the anatomic area usually bleeding?

    (A) anterior bleeding, nasal septum
    (B) anterior bleeding, inferior turbinate
    (C) anterior bleeding, nasal floor
    (D) posterior bleeding, sphenopalatine artery
    (E) posterior bleeding, nasopharynx

27. The most important late effect of exposure to ionizing radiation is

    (A) increased incidence of cancer
    (B) increased GI disorders
    (C) neurovascular syndrome
    (D) peripheral blood lymphopenia

28. What is the most common head and neck manifestation of sarcoidosis?

    (A) lacrimal gland hypertrophy
    (B) parotid gland hypertrophy
    (C) intranasal mass
    (D) cervical adenopathy
    (E) subglottic stenosis

Items 29–30

A 76-year-old man with a long history of benign prostatic hypertrophy (BPH) and voiding symptoms presents to the office with a complaint of 1 week of a dribbling urinary stream and a sense of lower abdominal fullness.

29. What is the most appropriate diagnostic test to make the diagnosis of urinary retention?

    (A) physical examination with digital rectal examination
    (B) bladder ultrasound
    (C) intravenous pyelogram (IVP)
    (D) placement of urethral catheter
    (E) pelvic CT scan

30. Once the diagnosis of a distended bladder is confirmed by bladder ultrasound, all of the following treatments would be reasonable EXCEPT

    (A) placement of a urethral catheter for bladder drainage for 3 to 5 days
    (B) administration of alpha blockers such as tamulosin without a urethral catheter
    (C) institution of self-clean intermittent catheterization
    (D) immediate transurethral prostatectomy
    (E) administration of finasteride

END OF SET

31. When reviewing the history of a patient who presents to the emergency department for evaluation of chest pain, the single most important risk factor for myocardial infarction is

    (A) age
    (B) obesity
    (C) smoking
    (D) hyperlipidemia
    (E) diabetes mellitus

32. Which cell is responsible for collagen production?

    (A) endothelial cell
    (B) fibroblast
    (C) keratinocyte
    (D) Langerhans' cell
    (E) mast cell

33. A patient is found to have malabsorption by a 72-hour fecal fat analysis. An endoscopic (upper GI) small bowel biopsy is performed. Which of the following disorders, if present, is most likely to be found *and* diagnosed by this test?

    (A) small bowel bacterial overgrowth
    (B) celiac disease
    (C) small bowel lymphoma
    (D) Zollinger–Ellison syndrome
    (E) Whipple's disease
    (F) eosinophilic gastroenteritis

34. A 22-year-old woman with acute myelogenous leukemia 11 days postinduction chemotherapy develops fever, anorexia, right-sided abdominal pain, and infrequent loose stools. An abdominal x-ray reveals a dilated right colon. Which is the most likely diagnosis?

    (A) appendicitis
    (B) ectopic pregnancy
    (C) cytomegalovirus (CMV) infection
    (D) typhlitis
    (E) hepatic flexure obstruction

35. All of the following patients should undergo colonoscopic examination EXCEPT

    (A) 22-year-old woman with left-sided ulcerative colitis since age 6
    (B) 12-year-old male foster child with extra teeth and benign jaw tumors
    (C) 49-year-old woman on ibuprofen with one guaiac-positive stool
    (D) 42-year-old woman, history of ovarian cancer age 25, mother with colon cancer age 49, sister with colon cancer age 56
    (E) 37-year-old man with extensive Crohn's colitis since age 26

36. Which of the following drugs has the greatest potential for increasing a patient's risk of developing a sunburn?

    (A) tetracycline
    (B) erythromycin
    (C) doxycycline

    (D) penicillin
    (E) cephalexin

37. In a normal early pregnancy (up to 70 days postconception), the serum level of human chorionic gonadotropin (hCG) should double every

    (A) 12 to 24 hours
    (B) 4 days
    (C) 2 days
    (D) 7 days

38. A 34-year-old man has just returned from a mission trip to Kenya. He is complaining of 3 days of fever/chills, headache, and myalgias. He had been prescribed chloroquine before his trip. He was living in a small village and ate all the local food. On exam he has a temperature of 40.3° C (104.5° F), heart rate of 126 bpm, and respiratory rate of 16/min. The physical exam is unremarkable otherwise. What would be the most appropriate laboratory test to make his diagnosis?

    (A) erythrocyte sedimentation rate
    (B) complete blood count with a manual differential
    (C) thick and thin smears for malaria
    (D) two sets of blood cultures
    (E) serology for *Brucella*

39. A patient with known hypertrophic cardiomyopathy has symptoms of chest pain and dizziness on exertion. He comes to discuss therapeutic options. The following may be said regarding his condition:

    (A) Hypertrophic cardiomyopathy can be treated or reduced by aggressive antihypertensive therapy.
    (B) The patient may require aortic valve replacement because of obstruction at the valve level.
    (C) The patient may suffer kidney damage related to excess growth hormone.
    (D) The patient can be cured by myectomy.
    (E) The patient can be treated by beta blockers or calcium channel blockers.

40. A 57-year-old woman with breast cancer is seen in the emergency department due to anorexia, nausea, and vomiting. She has been more lethargic and confused over the last few days as well. Her exam was unrevealing and no focal neurological changes were noted. Her hemoglobin was 10.5, blood urea nitrogen (BUN) 12, creatinine (Cr) 1.1, albumin 2.6, and calcium (Ca) 16. The next step would be

(A) calcitonin
(B) furosemide to promote renal excretion of calcium
(C) mithramycin
(D) pamidronate
(E) hydration and pamidronate

41. A patient suffering from metastatic disease to the skeleton is most likely to be

(A) a 65 year old with a 3-month history of pain in the midthoracic region and a lytic lesion on x-ray involving a pedicle
(B) a 21 year old with a 2-year history of pain in the shoulder and a lesion in the greater tuberosity of the humerus
(C) a 72 year old with generalized osteopenia, multiple vertebral compression deformities, and a highly elevated serum parathyroid hormone (PTH)
(D) a 12 year old with an incidentally discovered eccentric lytic lesion with sclerotic margins in the distal tibial metaphysis

42. The best explanation of premenstrual syndrome is

(A) luteal phase progesterone deficiency
(B) decreased luteal phase endorphin levels
(C) abnormal prostaglandin metabolism
(D) unknown
(E) salt retention causing activation of the renin–angiotensin system

43. A patient presents with a 2-day-old ankle sprain. On examination there is moderate lateral ankle swelling and ecchymosis. When the foot is pulled forward on the ankle, there is a 1-cm shift of the talus anteriorly (anterior drawer sign). What is the most appropriate treatment?

(A) cortisone injection
(B) ankle strapping
(C) early active exercise
(D) elevation and ice packs
(E) short leg walking cast

44. A 34-year-old businessman presents to your office with fever, cough, night sweats, arthralgias, malaise, and dyspnea. He recently returned from a prolonged business trip in Arizona. Which of the pathogens is causing his symptoms?

(A) histoplasmosis
(B) blastomycosis
(C) aspergillosis
(D) coccidioidomycosis
(E) cryptococcosis

45. A surgeon has been called to evaluate a 22-year-old man with severe pain in his right leg. There may have been minor trauma yesterday while playing softball. On exam he is toxic appearing with a temperature of 40.2° C (104.4° F) and a blood pressure of 86/36 mm Hg. The right leg is erythematous, warm, and painful to touch. A small abrasion is draining clear fluid. His WBC is 24,000/mm^3, Cr 1.8 mg/dL, and aspartate transaminase (AST) 98 mg/dL. Besides immediate surgical debridement, what antibiotic(s) should be administered?

(A) vancomycin
(B) nafcillin and clindamycin
(C) nafcillin
(D) clindamycin
(E) piperacillin/tazobactem

46. A very obese 65-year-old man with a history of poorly controlled hypertension and a "leaky heart valve" presents at midnight with sudden onset of unilateral flank pain and he is found to have microscopic hematuria (25 RBCs/HPF). He is afebrile, with blood pressure 180/105 and pulse 90. Serum Cr is normal. He reports a prior history of renal stones at age 48. Which of the following statements is true?

(A) Nephrolithiasis is the most likely cause of these findings. After the patient's pain is relieved with IV narcotics, it is reasonable to send him home for the night with an outpatient imaging procedure (helical CT or IVP) sometime within the next few days.

(B) Abdominal aortic aneurysm (AAA) must be excluded by a definitive imaging technique prior to disposition of this patient from the emergency department.

(C) Bacterial endocarditis may be excluded from the differential diagnosis since the patient is currently afebrile.

(D) Microscopic hematuria rarely occurs with AAA.

47. Which of the following injectable drugs has been associated with localized lipodystrophy?

(A) B_{12}
(B) epinephrine
(C) triamcinolone
(D) haldol
(E) dopamine

48. The most common type of skin cancer is

(A) melanoma
(B) squamous cell carcinoma
(C) basal cell carcinoma
(D) sebaceous carcinoma

49. The most important histological prognostic marker for melanoma is

(A) brisk lymphocytic infiltrate
(B) disruption of the normal dermal architecture
(C) tumor thickness/level of invasion
(D) pigment density

50. Figure 3.6 represents which congenital uterine anomaly?

(A) bicornuate uterus
(B) uterine septum
(C) uterine didelphus
(D) Rokitansky–Hauser syndrome

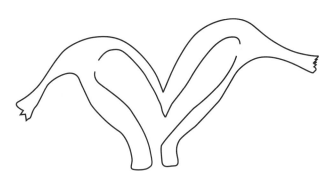

Figure 3.6

Practice Test 3
Answers and Explanations

1. **(A)** Adrenal incidentalomas have a prevalence of 1 to 5% on abdominal CT scans. Two major issues need to be addressed: size of the tumor and hormonal secretion.
   - *Size:* Tumors more than 4 cm (especially more than 6 cm) carry a higher risk of malignancy (adrenal carcinoma); therefore, most adrenal tumors larger than 4 cm should be removed. Other experts take a cutoff of 5 or 6 cm as indication for surgery. Certainly, before surgery, pheochromocytoma needs to be ruled out.
   - *Hormonal secretion:* In all adrenal incidentalomas, 24-hour urine collection for catecholamines and metanephrines should be done, even if the patient is completely asymptomatic, because pheochromocytomas can be lethal if undiagnosed. In normotensive people, there is no need to screen for hyperaldosteronism. Because autonomous glucocorticoid production without specific signs and symptoms of Cushing's (subclinical or preclinical Cushing's) is found in 5 to 20% of adrenal incidentalomas, overnight dexamethasone suppression test should be done in all these patients. Twenty-four-hour urine free cortisol is less sensitive in the specific case of subclinical Cushing's, where cortisol secretion is not high enough yet to give abnormal urine free cortisol. Patients who are found to have pheochromocytoma or hyperaldosteronism need to have surgery. Most experts agree now that subclinical Cushing's may worsen underlying conditions, such as osteoporosis, hypertension, obesity, and diabetes. In the presence of any of those conditions, surgery is also indicated. The natural history of subclinical Cushing's is unclear; probably, most of these patients would not progress to clinical Cushing's.
   - If surgery is not done (size < 4 cm, non-functioning adenoma), imaging at periodic intervals is indicated: Repeat CT scan at 3 to 6 months, then every year for a few years. Hormonal reevaluation is also repeated every year for a few years.

2. **(B)** A "rule of 10" has been quoted for pheochromocytomas: 10% are bilateral, 10% are malignant, 10% are familial, 10% occur in children, 10% are extra-adrenal, and 10% recur after surgical removal. The best diagnostic test is 24-hour urine collection for catecholamines and metanephrines; testing for plasma catecholamines results in many false positives. Persistent hypertension after surgery may be related to resetting of baroreceptors, hemodynamic changes, structural changes in blood vessels, or coincident essential hypertension.

3. **(E)** Initial therapy includes alpha-1 blocker, like phenoxybenzamine. After adequate alpha blockade, beta blockers are added to control heart rate and tachyarrhythmias. These should be continued for almost 2 weeks preoperatively. Perioperative hypertension is best managed with a short-acting intravenous agent, such as nitroprusside or phentolamine. Since patients with pheochromocytomas are volume depleted, diuretics such as amiloride are contraindicated.

4. **(A)** This is a typical presentation for APML or acute myelocytic leukemia (AML) M3. The finding of heavily granulated, myeloperoxidase-positive immature myeloid cells is very consistent with APML. DIC is also highly suggestive of this disease. The cytogenetic abnormality associated with M3 is t15,17, and thus remission can be induced with the use of ATRA (all-*trans* retinoic acid) as well as systemic chemotherapy with cytarabine and an anthracycline. The complete response rate is approximately 80%, with cure rates greater than 50%.

5. **(D)** Premature ejaculation is seldom a problem associated with depression.

6. **(C)** Glenda M. MacQueen, M.D., Ph.D, L. Travor Yound, M.D., Ph.D, Bipolar Disorder: symptoms, course and response to treatment.

7. **(D)** *Pneumocystis carinii* is a common respiratory pathogen in HIV. Silver stains on sputum of AIDS patients have a high sensitivity for *P. carinii.* The appearance is as described in this question. Intravenous trimethoprim–sulfamethoxazole and corticosteroids are the treatment of choice. Inhaled pentamidine has many toxic side effects and is used only for patients intolerant of trimethoprim–sulfamethoxazole.

8–11. **(8-A, 9-C, 10-B, 11-C)** Parkinson's disease is defined as a combination of lead-pipe rigidity, bradykinesia (including masked face), postural instability, and rest tremor. Cogwheel rigidity is produced by a tremor superimposed on increased tone and is commonly seen in this disease. A subcortical dementia includes a slowness of thought along with reduced memory and concentration.

   Dyskinesia, while not a part of Parkinson's disease, may be seen as a sign of too much dopamine. It may also be seen in more advanced Parkinson's disease as part of the "on–off" phenomenon. Dyskinesia is also a common manifestation of medication effect such as that caused by the phenothiazines and butyrophenones (tardive dyskinesia).

   A severe reduction in systolic blood pressure from supine to standing with no change in heart rate is characteristic of dysautonomia. This is commonly associated with Parkinson's disease and dopaminergic medications, or as part of generalized autonomic dysfunction including bowel/bladder symptoms, decreased perspiration, and gastric reflux. This latter condition is known as multiple system atrophy (formerly called Shy–Drager syndrome) and has a more rapid progression with poor response to dopamine therapy.

   Increased fluid and salt are very important in relieving the symptoms of orthostatic hypotension, but it must be realized that the drop in blood pressure cannot be corrected and that the therapeutic goal is relief of symptoms. Midodrine is a peripherally active alpha-1 agonist that does not cross the blood–brain barrier (no CNS side effects) and produces relief of symptoms within 1 hour with a half-life of 3 to 4 hours. This allows titration of dose and timing of dose to the patient's symptoms, which are generally worse in the morning hours.

12. **(C)** Obesity increases the risk of heart disease either indirectly by causing changes that increase the risk of heart disease or directly. Indirect causes of heart disease in obesity include elevation in low-density lipoprotein (LDL) and triglycerides, reduction in HDL, elevation in blood pressure, and increasing the risk of Type 2 diabetes. Direct effects include development of compensatory left ventricular hypertrophy, which ultimately can cause congestive heart failure. Direct and indirect effects of obesity on heart disease can be minimized through weight loss but may not be completely reversible.

13. **(C)** Patients with AIDS are at risk for serious CNS manifestations. The three most common structural lesions are *Toxoplasma gondii,* primary CNS lymphoma, and PML (progressive multifocal leukoencephalopathy). PML is associated with JC virus. The most common lesion is caused by infection with *Toxoplasma gondii.* Radiographically, it presents with ring-enhancing lesions—often multiple. The presence of positive *Toxoplasma* serology also

aids in making the diagnosis. The common approach to CNS lesions in AIDS is to treat for toxoplasmosis for 2 weeks (especially if the patient has positive serology for *Toxoplasma*), repeat imaging, and then obtain a brain biopsy if there is no improvement. The only treatment available for PML is to initiate antiretroviral therapy. This lesion can be very rapid in its progression. Occasionally, *Cryptococcus neoformans* or *Mycobacterium tuberculosis* may cause focal lesions, but they are very rare.

14. **(C)** Placenta previa is in the differential diagnosis of third trimester bleeding. If placenta previa is present, a vaginal exam can promote heavier bleeding, which can threaten both maternal and fetal well-being.

15. **(D)** The Apgar score awards 0 to 2 points each for heart rate, respiratory effort, muscle tone, reflex irritability, and color. The newborn's temperature is not used in the calculation of the score.

16. **(D)** Recognize the difference in measured oximetry and calculated oximetry in someone with methemoglobinemia (MHB). Benzocaine spray is frequently used as topical anesthetic prior to EGDs. MHB is produced when drugs such as local anesthetics, sulfa drugs, or dapsone change iron in hemoglobin from ferrous to ferric states making oxygen unable to bind. The pulse oximeter is characteristically normal; however, the calculated oxygen saturation on the blood gas is low. The blood may also be described as chocolate brown.

17. **(D)** Methylene blue donates an electron and reduces iron from ferric to ferrous.

18. **(D)** Group B streptococcal infection has historically been a very serious threat in neonates and expectant mothers. It is responsible for both neonatal sepsis and puerperal sepsis. There are new guidelines for screening and treating expectant mothers who have Group B streptococcus in their vaginal flora. Infection with Group B streptococcus may also be associated with diabetes and breast cancer

(due to lymphatic obstruction). It remains very susceptible to penicillin.

19. **(B)** The combination of sensorineural hearing loss (bone conduction—solid triangles) and conductive hearing loss (air conduction—solid circles) makes this a mixed hearing loss.

20. **(C)** When a bone-conduction line is not shown, it is because it is identical to the air-conduction line. Therefore, the lack of a gap between air and bone conduction makes this a sensorineural hearing loss.

21. **(B)** The majority of renal and ureteral calculi are completely eradicated with therapy. However, there is a 50% rate of recurrent stone formation within 5 years.

22. **(A)** Central retinal vein occlusions have a classic appearance of obscuration of the disc margins, retinal hemorrhages that appear to be radiating from the nerve head, engorged veins, and tortuous vessels. Marked hemorrhages within the macula are common.

23. **(E)** Patients presenting with bilateral vascular occlusive disease must be worked up for hematologic disorders. Young patients with unilateral central vein occlusions should be considered for evaluation. These studies include hyperviscosity syndromes, clotting disorders, elevated homocystine levels, and antiphospholipid antibodies.

   Only rarely is there an association between a hematologic disorder and a unilateral central retinal vein occlusion in an older individual. Unilateral central retinal vein occlusions are a frequent finding in older individuals. Risk factors associated with central retinal vein occlusions are the presence of hypertension and glaucoma.

24. **(C)** This child is in shock and he desperately needs aggressive fluid resuscitation. Intraosseous access is the preferred route of fluid resuscitation if peripheral IV access cannot be obtained immediately. Appropriate fluids for initial resuscitation are either normal saline

or Ringer's lactate with an initial bolus of 20 cc/kg. Dextrose is given by a separate bolus as 2 to 4 cc/kg of 25% dextrose in water ($D_{25}W$) for children in this age group only if they are hypoglycemic by bedside glucose determination.

25. **(D)** Contrary to popular belief, elderly patients presenting to the emergency department (ED) are seldom there as a result of simple constipation. This is a high-risk population both for intra-abdominal pathology and for extra-abdominal causes of pain referred to the abdomen. Morbidity and mortality among elderly patients seen in the ED for abdominal pain is quite similar to the morbidity and mortality associated with chest pain in this same age group.

26. **(A)** Eighty to ninety percent of nosebleeds are anterior, and most of those emanate from Kiesselbach's area, which is a rich plexus of vessels on the anterior nasal septum.

27. **(A)** The most important late effect is an increased risk of many different types of cancer. Acute radiation syndrome includes nausea, vomiting, and diarrhea, followed by several days to weeks of little symptoms. GI symptoms return during weeks 2–5.

28. **(D)** Large studies have shown cervical adenopathy to be the most common head and neck manifestation.

29. **(B)** A bladder ultrasound would be a quick and noninvasive test to determine the amount of urinary residual within the bladder. The diagnosis of a distended bladder could also be made with an IVP, a CT scan, or the placement of a Foley catheter, but these tests are more expensive and invasive.

30. **(E)** Each of the treatments, with the exception of the administration of finasteride, has a chance of resolving the acute urinary retention. Finasteride will not take effect for 6 to 12 months.

31. **(E)** While each of the listed risk factors for ischemic heart disease is important, diabetes mellitus carries the largest relative risk. Diabetics seen in the ED for chest pain, abdominal pain, vomiting, and a wide array of non-specific symptoms such as "weakness and dizziness" deserve an ECG and careful consideration of the possible presence of myocardial ischemia or infarction.

32. **(B)** The fibroblast synthesizes collagen, the principal component of the dermis.

33. **(E)** Whipple's disease is always found on upper GI/endoscopic small bowel biopsy *and* has pathognomonic features. Small bowel bacterial overgrowth and Zollinger–Ellison syndrome have a patchy distribution, and the pathologic findings are nonspecific. Eosinophilic gastroenteritis and small bowel lymphoma have pathognomonic features but are patchy in distribution, and can be missed on small bowel biopsies. Celiac disease, if present, always will be found on biopsy of the upper small bowel, but the pathologic features are not specific/pathognomonic.

34. **(D)** Typhlitis typically affects the cecum and right colon, with dilatation and decreased, loose bowel movements, in acutely neutropenic patients postchemotherapy. Appendicitis would be unlikely to cause this radiologic picture. Cytomegalovirus of the colon would be unusual this soon post-induction chemotherapy. Ectopic pregnancy and obstruction are not likely diagnoses in this patient.

35. **(B)** This child may have familial polyposis coli/Gardner's syndrome, and screening is indicated, but it should be flexible sigmoidoscopy and not colonoscopy (high yield, less traumatic for adolescent). Left-sided ulcerative colitis for over 15 years and ulcerative colitis beyond the splenic flexure or substantial colonic Crohn's disease for over 7 to 10 years require screening colonoscopy. The history in option D suggests hereditary nonpolyposis colorectal cancer syndrome, type II, which mandates colonoscopic screening, as does the history of colon cancer itself in a first-degree relative younger than 50 (her mother, at age 49, hence screening of first-degree relatives by age 39, 10 years earlier).

Genetic and gynecologic screening also would be indicated. Patient C has evidence of occult bleeding, which requires colonoscopy whether or not she is on nonsteroidal anti-inflammatory drugs (NSAIDs).

36. **(C)** Doxycycline is a frequent cause of phototoxic drug reactions.

37. **(C)** When a normal pregnancy is present, the level of serum hCG should double approximately every 2 days.

38. **(C)** A patient with fever who has returned from a malaria-endemic country must be presumed to have malaria while working to exclude other diagnoses. A complete travel history must be obtained. This patient was given chloroquine, but Kenya, as well as other parts of Africa, have chloroquine-resistant malaria, and alternate methods of malaria prophylaxis are needed. The diagnosis of malaria is made by looking for gametocytes and intraerythrocytic ring forms in thick and thin smears of the blood.

39. **(E)** Hypertrophic cardiomyopathy has a genetic component, and there is no known way to prevent it from occurring or to cure it. Beta blockers and calcium channel blockers reduce the heart rate and the force and contraction of the heart muscle.

40. **(E)** Pamidronate should be used with vigorous hydration due to dehydration. Furosemide will promote renal excretion of calcium but will not correct a calcium of 16. Mithramycin is a historically good drug but has been replaced by pamidronate. Calcitonin can rapidly lower calcium if there are life-threatening complications, but tachyphylaxis is a concern.

41. **(A)** The patient in option B probably has a primary bone tumor that is most likely benign or not aggressive due to length of time symptoms have been present. The patient in option C probably has a parathyroid adenoma. The patient in option D most likely has a nonossifying fibroma, which is a benign process.

42. **(D)** The exact cause of PMS is unknown. There are no good studies within evidence-based medicine that have demonstrated a definite etiologic agent in the development of PMS. All of the other items have been postulated as explanations for PMS, but never proven. *(Beckmann, 475–477)*

43. **(E)** A positive anterior talar drawer sign indicates a tear of the anterior talofibular ligament. The opposite ankle should also be examined, as some patients will have congenital joint laxity. The ligament tear will take at least 6 weeks to heal. A cast will control swelling, protect the joint from further injury, and allow weight bearing. At 3 weeks postinjury, a removable walking boot can be applied if the ankle is more stable to examination. Active exercises can be started then. Grade I and II ankle sprains can be treated with ankle strapping or a removable boot and early active exercises.

44. **(D)** Recognize travel to the desert Southwest as a risk factor for coccidioidomycosis.

45. **(B)** The person described is presenting with necrotizing fasciitis likely secondary to group A streptococcus infection. The patient is quite toxic and is already exhibiting multiorgan failure. Urgent debridement is indicated as well as antibiotic therapy to cover for gram-positive organisms (*Streptococcus* and *Staphylococcus*) and an agent to help turn off toxin production. Clindamycin acts to inhibit protein synthesis and thus may shut down toxin production.

46. **(B)** Older men, especially those with hypertension, who present with flank pain have a leaking AAA until proven otherwise and must have appropriate imaging to exclude this diagnosis. If hemodynamically stable, consider helical CT scan. Alternatively, a bedside ultrasound is a reliable way to identify AAA, although it is usually not helpful in identifying leakage. Up to a third of patients with AAA show microscopic hematuria, which limits the use of this finding in separating these patients from those who may

have nephrolithiasis. Less commonly, bacterial endocarditis may produce septic emboli to the kidney with resulting hematuria.

47. **(C)** Injections of insulin, iron, steroids, and diphtheria–pertussis–tetanus may result in localized lipodystrophy.

48. **(C)** Basal cell carcinoma is the most common form of skin cancer.

49. **(C)** Tumor thickness is the most important prognostic factor in melanoma.

50. **(A)** While all of the options represent congenital disorders of fusion of the müllerian ducts, the diagram shown in Figure 3.6 is of a bicornuate uterus.

Practice Test 4
Questions

DIRECTIONS (Questions 1 through 50): Each of the numbered items or incomplete statements in this section is followed by answers or by completions of the statement. Select the ONE lettered answer or completion that is BEST in each case.

1. A 17-year-old boy noted pain in his upper left arm for the past month. On exam, he was found to have a 3- to 4-cm ill-defined fixed mass in the mid-left upper extremity. X-rays of the arm revealed a mass extending from the mid-humerus, confirmed by bone scan and angiography. A chest CT was negative. Biopsy was consistent with an osteosarcoma. What is the next step in the management of this patient?

   (A) radiation therapy followed by chemotherapy
   (B) amputation at the shoulder followed by adjuvant chemotherapy
   (C) amputation at the shoulder with observation afterward
   (D) limb-sparing surgery followed by postoperative radiation
   (E) preoperative chemotherapy followed by limb-sparing surgery, then adjuvant chemotherapy

2. All of the following drugs can worsen hyponatremia due to the syndrome of inappropriate antidiuretic hormone (SIADH) EXCEPT

   (A) carbamazepine
   (B) demeclocycline
   (C) clofibrate
   (D) phenothiazines
   (E) vincristine

Items 3–5

A 27-year-old woman with a history of irregular periods presents for annual exam. She is currently sexually active and has never used anything for birth control. She has never been pregnant, nor does she desire to get pregnant currently, and her last menstrual period (LMP) was 6 weeks ago. Physical exam reveals an obese, mildly hirsute white female in no acute distress. Her pelvic exam reveals a normal-sized uterus with top-normal-size adnexa bilaterally.

3. Which of the following is the LEAST likely diagnosis?

   (A) polycystic ovarian disease
   (B) pregnancy
   (C) exercise-induced amenorrhea
   (D) hyperthecosis
   (E) congenital adrenal hyperplasia

4. Which lab test results would be most helpful to establish the most likely diagnosis in this case?

   (A) low luteinizing hormone:follicle-stimulating hormone (LH:FSH) ratio
   (B) normal thyroid-stimulating hormone (TSH)
   (C) elevated testosterone
   (D) low progesterone
   (E) elevated fasting insulin

5. Assuming she is not pregnant, what would be the best management in light of the fact that she does not desire fertility at this time?

   (A) observation and routine follow-up in 1 year
   (B) regular ovulation induction with clomiphene citrate
   (C) regulating her menses with oral contraceptives
   (D) periodic administration of tamoxifen to induce menses
   (E) endometrial biopsy

                                    END OF SET

6. A 56-year-old man presents with a 2-cm subareolar lump on his breast. He has a mammogram, which is negative. What would be the next course of action?

   (A) observation
   (B) diagnostic mammography
   (C) thermography
   (D) ultrasound
   (E) biopsy

7. A 55-year-old man has a 2-week history of confusion. He has a history of three packs of cigarettes a day for 30 years and was diagnosed with limited-stage small cell lung cancer 5 years ago. On exam he was confused, but otherwise his exam was unremarkable. His serum calcium was 12 mg/dL. A chest x-ray revealed a 4-cm mass in the region of his prior tumor. CT showed a right hilar mass. After hydration and bisphosphonate therapy, the serum calcium declined to 9.1 mg/dL. His liver tests were normal. All of the following tests are inappropriate EXCEPT

   (A) pulmonary function tests
   (B) bone marrow
   (C) fine-needle aspirate
   (D) computed tomography (CT) of the abdomen
   (E) bronchoscopy

8. Causes of nephrogenic diabetes insipidus include all of the following EXCEPT

   (A) hypercalcemia
   (B) hypokalemia
   (C) lithium
   (D) chlorpropamide
   (E) sickle cell disease

Items 9–10

A 16-year-old boy with a lifelong history of asthma presents to your office for a routine checkup. He tells you his asthma is in good control. His medication regimen consists of albuterol as needed and salmeterol twice daily. He uses his albuterol at night two to three times per week and uses it four times per day for wheezing. He denies feeling short of breath or having increased wheezing but has noticed increased cough.

9. What class of asthma does he fit into?

   (A) mild intermittent
   (B) mild persistent
   (C) moderate persistent
   (D) severe persistent
   (E) none of the above

10. Which medicine must be added to his regimen?

   (A) inhaled steroid
   (B) nebulized albuterol
   (C) montelukast
   (D) theophylline
   (E) no additions necessary

                                    END OF SET

Items 11–12

A 77-year-old woman presents to your office with recurrent episodes of vertigo worsened when she turns her head to the left. She has severe nausea and vomiting during these attacks, which occur several times a day. There had been similar symptoms, lasting for several weeks at a time, multiple times in the past 10 years.

11. The most likely diagnosis is

   (A) brain stem transient ischemic attack (TIA)

(B) cerebellar TIA

(C) benign positional vertigo

(D) acoustic neuroma

(E) Ménière's disease

12. You initiate meclizine 25 mg tid without therapeutic effect. In reviewing the following choices, you exclude which as likely to be ineffective?

(A) prednisone

(B) prochlorperazine

(C) diazepam

(D) metoclopramide

(E) vestibular exercises

END OF SET

13. A patient comes to the hospital on meperidine for chronic back pain and Zantac for gastroesophageal reflux disease (GERD). He is depressed. All of the following would be an appropriate antidepressant EXCEPT

(A) selective serotonin reuptake inhibitor (SSRI)

(B) tricyclic antidepressant

(C) monoamine oxidase inhibitor (MAOI)

(D) selective norepinephrine reuptake inhibitor (SNRI)

(E) bupropion (Welbutrin)

14. The side effects of testosterone administration include all of the following EXCEPT

(A) sleep apnea

(B) gynecomastia

(C) lower extremity edema

(D) peliosis hepatis

(E) increased triglycerides

15. Regarding heart failure, which of the following statements is true?

(A) The 5-year mortality rate for men and women is equivalent.

(B) Approximately 4.8 million individuals have heart failure.

(C) Digoxin and diuretics reduce mortality in patients with heart failure.

(D) Coronary heart disease alone causes most cases of heart failure.

16. The pathogenesis of some bacterial diseases is due to toxins produced by the bacteria and not the result of direct tissue invasion or destruction. The following bacteria produce toxins that are pathogenic EXCEPT

(A) *Streptococcus pneumoniae*

(B) *Streptococcus pyogenes*

(C) *Staphylococcus aureus*

(D) *Clostridium difficile*

17. In a restaurant, someone calls for assistance from a physician, and you respond. The patient is choking; has a weak, ineffective cough; and can make only a high-pitched noise on inhalation. What is the most appropriate first course of action?

(A) do not intervene; wait for the patient to expel the foreign body

(B) finger sweep of the pharynx

(C) three firm back blows

(D) the Heimlich maneuver

(E) cricothyroidotomy with a sharp knife

18. What is the definition of a complicated urinary tract infection (UTI)?

(A) recurrent bacterial cystitis in women

(B) infection in the presence of structural or functional abnormalities of the urinary tract

(C) urinary tract infection associated with a high fever

(D) urinary tract infection in men

Items 19–20

A 65-year-old man presents with symptoms of malaise. His medical history and review of systems are negative. His ocular history is positive for ocular toxoplasmosis. The patient is presently being treated for an acute inflammatory process of the retina and is on pyrimethamine, sulfa, and steroids.

19. Which study should be performed immediately in this patient?

(A) toxoplasmosis titer
(B) blood sugar
(C) sedimentation rate
(D) antinuclear antibodies
(E) complete blood count (CBC)

20. Which of the following should be added to the patient's regimen?

(A) vitamin B$_{12}$
(B) iron
(C) vitamin C
(D) folinic acid
(E) riboflavin

END OF SET

21. Among patients who have a known seizure disorder not primarily related to alcohol, the single most common cause of recurrent seizure activity leading to treatment in the emergency department (ED) is

(A) occult central nervous system (CNS) trauma
(B) missed doses of anticonvulsant medication
(C) CNS infections
(D) fluid and electrolyte disturbances
(E) cocaine abuse

Items 22–23

A 43-year-old man had been hospitalized a week earlier for an elective operation. He now comes to the ED complaining of fever, rigors, headache, cough, and diarrhea. His symptoms came on suddenly about 24 hours ago. He is toxic appearing, with a temperature of 39° C (102.2° F), heart rate 118 bpm, respirations 24/min, and oxygen saturation 92% on room air. His oropharynx is injected and the neck is supple. He has diffuse crackles in his lungs. Laboratory studies reveal a white blood count (WBC) of 18,000/mm^3 (23% band forms, 70% neutrophils), hematocrit 34%, and platelets 105,000. Chemistries are significant for sodium of 124 mg/dL and creatinine 1.8 mg/dL. The chest radiograph is seen in Figure 4.1. He is initially placed on ceftriaxone but worsens over the next 24 hours.

22. Which of the following tests is most likely to make a diagnosis of the etiology of his pneumonia?

(A) blood cultures
(B) bronchoscopy with bronchoalveolar lavage to send for Gram stain
(C) urine for detection of *Legionella pneumophila* antigen
(D) blood specimen for *Mycoplasma* serology

23. The most appropriate antibiotic to add to this man's regimen is

(A) amikacin
(B) amphotericin
(C) azithromycin
(D) vancomycin

END OF SET

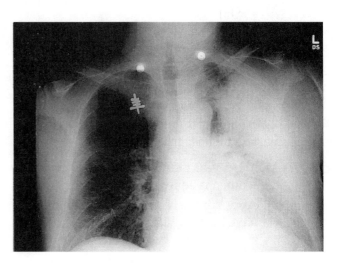

Figure 4.1

24. A 70-year-old man is brought to the ED by his son for evaluation of an episode of generalized weakness with near syncope. He denies chest pain, emesis, diarrhea, or fever. Current medicines include a nonsteroidal anti-inflammatory drug (NSAID) for osteoarthritis and hydrochlorothiazide and a beta blocker for hypertension. He denies prior hospitalizations or surgery. Exam shows a temperature of 37° C (98.6° F), pulse 80, blood pressure 114/88, and respirations 24/min. Room air pulse oximetry shows 93% oxygen saturation. The patient appears pale, and his oral mucosa is slightly dry. Neuro exam is nonfocal. Chest is clear. Heart sounds are normal with no murmur present. Abdomen is nontender. Rectal shows brown heme-positive stool. Lab: hemoglobin (Hgb) 12.8 g, WBC 12,100, blood urea nitrogen (BUN) 55, and creatinine 1.5. Electrocardiogram (ECG) shows nonspecific T-wave changes. Which of the following represents the most appropriate initial management?

    (A) Administer 1 to 2 liters of normal saline (NS) IV, stop hydrochlorothiazide, and then discharge for follow-up by his primary care doctor in 2 to 3 days.

    (B) Admit to a monitored bed for serial ECGs and cardiac enzymes.

    (C) Establish adequate IV access and place a nasogastric (NG) tube.

    (D) Order a head CT.

    (E) Obtain a chest x-ray and blood cultures.

25. Which of the following is the most common location of melanoma in African-American patients?

    (A) face
    (B) genitalia
    (C) nailbed
    (D) trunk
    (E) oral mucosa

26. What internal cancer in women most frequently metastasizes to the skin?

    (A) breast
    (B) lung
    (C) ovary
    (D) colon
    (E) kidney

27. The best marker for procainamide-induced lupus is

    (A) antinuclear antibody (ANA)
    (B) anti-Ro Ab
    (C) anti-Sm Ab
    (D) anti-nRMP Ab
    (E) antihistone Ab

28. A previously healthy 27-year-old man develops bloody diarrhea. In interviewing this patient, all of the following questions are important and relevant EXCEPT

    (A) "Have you recently had contact with a young puppy?"

    (B) "Have you taken any antibiotics in the past 4 to 6 weeks?"

    (C) "Have you gone camping lately and ingested stream water?"

    (D) "Have you drunk apple cider from a roadside stand lately?"

    (E) "Do you use recreational drugs, such as cocaine?"

29. All of the following statements regarding carbon monoxide toxicity are true EXCEPT

    (A) significant carbon monoxide toxicity is frequently associated with metabolic acidosis

    (B) all patients with suspected carbon monoxide toxicity should be initially treated with 100% oxygen via nonrebreather mask

    (C) this entity should be included in the differential diagnosis when multiple patients who all reside in the same home present at the same time with flulike symptoms

    (D) pregnant women and small children are particularly susceptible to the adverse effects of carbon monoxide intoxication

    (E) intravenous methylene blue will rapidly reduce the carboxyhemoglobin level and should be routinely administered

30. A 65-year-old woman suddenly develops severe, persistent, periumbilical abdominal pain. On physical examination, while she is in pain, there is little abdominal tenderness upon palpation of her abdomen. Which of the following best fits with her clinical presentation?

    (A) history of atrial fibrillation, hypertension, and mild congestive heart failure

    (B) previous appendectomy, cholecystectomy, and laparotomy for lysis of adhesions

    (C) insulin-dependent diabetes mellitus complicated by retinopathy, nephropathy, and lower-extremity peripheral neuropathy

    (D) history of cholelithiasis and pneumobilia

31. A 32-year-old woman with systemic scleroderma comes to your office complaining of dysphagia. All of the following questions you ask her are likely to result in a "yes" answer EXCEPT

    (A) "Have you experienced extreme cold sensitivity of your hands, with red, white, or bluish discoloration?"

    (B) "When you try to swallow liquids, do they come out your nose?"

    (C) "Do you often experience a painful, burning sensation in the center of your chest?"

    (D) "Do you experience periodic hoarseness?"

32. A 38 year old with chronic pancreatitis could have all of the following on questioning EXCEPT

    (A) a history of cholelithiasis on previous abdominal sonograms

    (B) a history of prolonged, heavy alcohol use

    (C) a family history of several close relatives with chronic pancreatitis

    (D) a personal history of hypothyroidism and Sjögren syndrome

33. What is the cutaneous marker of insulin resistance?

    (A) erythema nodosum

    (B) acanthosis nigricans

    (C) pyogenic granuloma

    (D) pyoderma gangrenosum

    (E) pretibial myxedema

34. An overweight teenage boy presents with a 2-week history of knee pain after trying out for the football team. Physical exam and x-rays of his knee are normal. The next step in workup of this patient would be

    (A) magnetic resonance imaging (MRI) scan of the knee

    (B) diagnostic arthroscopy of the knee

    (C) temporary immobilization of the knee

    (D) physical examination of the hip

35. All of the following are causes of the abnormality seen in Figure 4.2 EXCEPT

    (A) hypertrophic pulmonary osteoarthropathy

    (B) chronic bronchitis

    (C) cyanotic congenital heart disease

    (D) cystic fibrosis

    (E) idiopathic pulmonary fibrosis

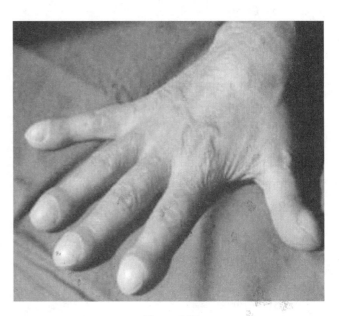

Figure 4.2

36. A 30-year-old man with known acquired immune deficiency syndrome (AIDS) is seen because of chest pains and shortness of breath. All of the following have been associated with AIDS EXCEPT

   (A) pericarditis
   (B) cor pulmonale
   (C) cardiomyopathy
   (D) myocarditis
   (E) ruptured chordae tendineae

37. In the treatment of a 38-year-old woman recently diagnosed with hypertension prior to pregnancy who is now 12 weeks pregnant, all of the following antihypertensive agents may be appropriate to use EXCEPT

   (A) propranolol
   (B) hydralazine
   (C) lisinopril
   (D) methyldopa

38. A cystic mass is present on the dorsum of a 28-year-old woman's wrist. The most likely diagnosis is

   (A) ganglion cyst
   (B) giant cell tumor
   (C) leiomyosarcoma
   (D) metastatic tumor
   (E) none of the above

39. A 34-year-old man with AIDS presents to the ED complaining of hematuria and right-sided flank pain for the past 6 hours. His HIV regimen consists of zidovudine (AZT), lamivudine (3TC), indinavir, and ritonavir. His presentation is most likely a side effect secondary to which of his antiretrovirals?

   (A) AZT
   (B) 3TC
   (C) indinavir
   (D) ritonavir

40. When using ultrasound to date a pregnancy, the most accurate measurement is

   (A) fetal crown–rump length measured between 7 and 14 weeks

   (B) fetal femur length measured between 12 and 22 weeks
   (C) fetal biparietal diameter measured between 17 and 26 weeks
   (D) fetal abdominal circumference measured between 20 and 30 weeks

Items 41–42

Four months after left superficial parotidectomy for a benign tumor, a patient notes "sweating" from the left cheek when eating spicy food. It is fairly profuse and is not decreasing in volume or frequency.

41. What is the most likely diagnosis?

   (A) salivary fistula
   (B) occlusion of parotid duct
   (C) crocodile tears syndrome
   (D) Frey syndrome
   (E) recurrent tumor

42. The patient is extremely bothered by the symptoms and requests definitive treatment. Which of the following is the best treatment for the condition?

   (A) intra-oral ligation of parotid duct
   (B) surgical wound exploration
   (C) vidian neurectomy
   (D) tympanic neurectomy
   (E) complete parotidectomy

END OF SET

43. Cardiac catheterization is NOT indicated in a patient with

   (A) aortic stenosis and syncope
   (B) tetralogy of Fallot
   (C) chest pain after an equivocal exercise stress test
   (D) a cardiomyopathy
   (E) atypical chest pain as a first-line study

44. A 35-year-old woman presents with numbness and pain in the little and ring fingers that awakens her from sleep. There is no history of trauma. She has decreased sensation in the little and the medial (ulnar) half of the ring finger. The most likely diagnosis is

    (A) ruptured cervical disk
    (B) carpal tunnel syndrome
    (C) cubital tunnel syndrome
    (D) radial tunnel syndrome

45. A 67-year-old previously healthy smoker with hemoptysis presents to your office for a second opinion regarding a mass seen on his chest radiograph. It is located in the right upper lung zone and is 3×3 cm. A CT scan reveals no adenopathy and no other lesions. He has no comorbidities. What do you recommend?

    (A) repeat chest radiograph in 1 month
    (B) repeat CT scan in 3 months
    (C) transthoracic needle aspiration (TTNA)
    (D) chemotherapy
    (E) consultation with a thoracic surgeon

Items 46–47

A 27-year-old man with no known past history presents to your office with a 3-day history of right jaw pain, loss of taste, and progressive weakness of the entire right side of his face. You consider a diagnosis of idiopathic Bell's palsy but wish to exclude other possible causes of a facial nerve palsy.

46. Other possible causes would include all of the following EXCEPT

    (A) Lyme disease
    (B) multiple sclerosis
    (C) herpes zoster
    (D) diabetes
    (E) sarcoidosis

47. The expected therapeutic benefit of oral prednisone in the treatment of idiopathic Bell's palsy would include

    (A) speeding recovery time
    (B) lessening degree of residual weakness

    (C) relieving pain
    (D) A and C
    (E) A, B, and C

END OF SET

48. Based on clinical research, which of the following have been shown to be improved by cognitive behavioral therapy?

    (A) depression
    (B) anxiety
    (C) post-traumatic stress disorder (PTSD)
    (D) schizophrenia
    (E) A, B, and C only
    (F) all of the above

49. A 34-year-old African-American man develops hemolysis after taking trimethoprim–sulfamethoxazole to treat pneumonia. What would the peripheral smear from this patient show?

    (A) sickle cells
    (B) target cells
    (C) bite cells
    (D) microspherocytes
    (E) macro-ovalocytes

50. In primary empty sella syndrome, the most frequent finding on hormonal evaluation is

	Prolactin	Growth Hormone	Gonadotropins	ACTH
I	High	Low	Low	Low
II	Normal	Low	Low	Low
III	Normal	Normal	Normal	Low
IV	High	Normal	Normal	Normal
V	Normal	Normal	Normal	Normal

    (A) I
    (B) II
    (C) III
    (D) IV
    (E) V

Practice Test 4
Answers and Explanations

1. **(E)** The patient has an osteosarcoma of the humerus with no evidence of distant metastases. The issue with this disease is local control as well as systemic eradication of micrometastatic disease. Preoperative chemotherapy provides the advantage of more effectively treating distant micrometastatic disease and may make limb-sparing surgery easier due to downsizing of the tumor if there is a response to chemotherapy. Disease-free survival at 2 years has been shown to be increased from 20% with surgery alone to 60% with adjuvant chemotherapy. The patient is therefore a good candidate for limb-sparing surgery as well as chemotherapy.

2. **(B)** All the drugs mentioned enhance arginine vasopressin (AVP) release except demeclocycline, which is used in the treatment of SIADH and works by inhibiting the action of vasopressin at the kidney level.

3. **(C)** This is a classic presentation of Stein–Leventhal syndrome, or polycystic ovarian disease (PCOD). This is a state of hyperandrogenic chronic anovulation associated with oligo/amenorrhea, hirsutism, and obesity. Hyperthecosis is a severe variant of this condition and usually presents with more severe hirsutism, acne, and even skin hyperpigmentation in the intertriginous folds, known as acanthosis nigricans. Another possibility here is congenital adrenal hyperplasia (CAH), which also may have this clinical presentation. CAH is caused by an adrenal enzymatic defect, resulting in higher androgen levels, hirsutism, and oligo/amenorrhea. Furthermore, in light of the fact that she is having unprotected sex and her LMP was 6 weeks ago, pregnancy must be ruled out, although it is not highly probable. The least likely diagnosis here is exercise-induced amenorrhea, which is not associated with obesity or hirsutism. Moreover, it is not likely that an obese person exercises to the point of shutting off the hypothalamic–pituitary–ovarian axis. *(Beckmann, 441–442)*

4. **(C)** An elevated testosterone is often seen in women with PCOD. In addition, there is often an LH:FSH ratio of > 2:1. Although women with PCOD often have fasting hyperinsulinemia, it is a nonspecific finding and not pathognomonic for PCOD. A low progesterone is very nonspecific and merely indicates that the person had not ovulated at the time the level was drawn. It does not diagnose a state of chronic anovulation. The TSH level is usually normal in women with PCOD and is used as a diagnostic tool in thyroid evaluation. *(Beckmann, 441–442)*

5. **(C)** It is very important to regulate this woman's menses, so that she is not at risk for prolonged exposure of the endometrium to unopposed estrogen. This could theoretically lead to higher risk of endometrial hyperplasia and eventually carcinoma later in life. Because she is young and sexually active, regulating her menses with the oral contraceptive is the most logical choice, in order to protect her from unwanted pregnancy as well. Since she is not interested in fertility currently, ovulation induction with clomiphene citrate would not be indicated at this time. Endome-

trial biopsy would be indicated only if this patient were over 35 years of age, in order to rule out endometrial hyperplasia. Tamoxifen is not used to induce menses at all. It has a role in the treatment of breast cancer, and may actually put a patient at risk for endometrial carcinoma as well. *(Beckmann, 441–442)*

6. **(E)** Men are also at risk for breast cancer, and mammograms can be associated with a false-negative result. Observation would clearly be wrong in this 56-year-old man. Neither thermography nor ultrasound can exclude malignancy, and thus a biopsy is warranted.

7. **(E)** The patient had a history of small cell lung cancer and now has a recurrence in the prior tumor bed. It would be quite unusual for a patient to develop a recurrence of the same tumor after definitive treatment 5 years prior, and it is also unusual to have hypercalcemia associated with small cell lung cancer. It is possible that this represents non–small cell lung cancer, in which hypercalcemia is common and is a frequent cause of death in those patients who survive small cell lung cancer. It may be treated by surgical resection if this indeed is a lesion. Thus, the patient should have a bronchoscopy for tissue biopsy. The other choices are not appropriate as the first and critical diagnostic test. A fine-needle aspirate would not be the test of choice for a central lesion since it would be difficult to reach and adequately biopsy unless a bronchoscopy is done.

8. **(D)** Chlorpropamide enhances the action of AVP on renal tubules, as opposed to the other causes listed.

9. **(D)** He has continual symptoms with frequent exacerbations as well as frequent nighttime symptoms, which places him in the severe persistent category.

10. **(A)** Inhaled steroids are the cornerstone of asthma management and must be used. The other therapies may also be appropriate, but the steroid is imperative.

11–12. **(11-C, 12-A)** The lack of associated tinnitus and hearing loss with the recurrent attacks excludes Ménière's disease and the episodic nature of the symptoms excludes neoplasm. The onset of symptoms with position change is highly suggestive of a peripheral localization in the vestibular nerve or labyrinth. There is no evidence to suggest a benefit for prednisone in the treatment of acute attacks of benign positional vertigo. Low-dose benzodiazepines may be the most effective therapy in this condition.

13. **(C)** Meperidine (Demerol) when mixed with MAOIs can lead to fatal seizures.

14. **(E)** Administration of testosterone can cause:
    - Sleep apnea, through increased collapse of the upper airways or as a consequence of increased hematocrit
    - Gynecomastia, from increased aromatization to estrogens
    - Edema, from sodium retention
    - Peliosis hepatis and hepatoma
    - Low high-density lipoprotein (HDL), occasionally high low-density lipoprotein (LDL); no effect on triglycerides

15. **(B)** Approximately 4.8 million individuals have heart failure, and 400,000 to 700,000 new cases are diagnosed annually. Digoxin and diuretics improve symptoms but do not improve survival. The 5-year mortality rate for men with heart failure is 50% and for women 35%. While coronary heart disease is an important cause of heart failure, the risk is much greater in patients with concomitant risk factors like hypertensive heart disease and diabetes.

16. **(A)** Pneumococcal infections are caused by direct bacterial invasion (e.g., pneumonia, meningitis, and bacteremia). *S. pyogenes* and *S. aureus* can both elicit toxins responsible for toxic shock syndrome. *Clostridium difficile, C. tetanus,* and *C. botulinum* all release toxins that are responsible for their pathogenic effects.

17. **(D)** While it is sometimes appropriate to not intervene—if the patient can talk and breathe but is coughing—in this case the patient is moving little air, and the Heimlich maneuver is appropriate. Back blows and finger sweep of the pharynx are no longer recommended under these circumstances.

18. **(B)** Although urinary tract infections are uncommon in men in the absence of structural abnormalities, the definition of a complicated UTI requires the identification of such structural or functional abnormalities. These include hydronephrosis, urinary tract calculi, and urinary retention.

19. **(E)** Pyrimethamine (Daraprim) is used for the treatment of toxoplasmosis. Daraprim is a known cause of aplastic anemia, malaise, nausea, and many other side effects. Its mechanism of action is the selective inhibition of plasmodial dehydrofolate reductase (folate antagonist). CBC must be done regularly while patients are using Daraprim. All patients using Daraprim should take supplemental folinic acid to decrease the risk of anemia.

20. **(D)** Folinic acid must be used in patients using Daraprim. The addition of folic acid is used to decrease the risk of anemia that is secondary to Daraprim.

21. **(B)** The most common reason for recurrent seizures in patients with a known seizure disorder who are seen in the ED is a subtherapeutic anticonvulsant level. This is usually the result of noncompliance but may be due to other factors such as vomiting, intercurrent illness, or drug interactions. Provided the patient does not show new neurological abnormalities, significant fever, prolonged or atypical seizure activity, prolonged postictal state with ongoing altered mental status, or significant new trauma, the value of a CT scan or lab studies beyond an anticonvulsant level is doubtful.

22. **(C)** The patient described is presenting with *Legionella* pneumonia. *Legionella* has been shown to be acquired nosocomially. Infection with *Legionella pneumophila* accounts for most cases. About half of all cases present with gastrointestinal manifestations, especially diarrhea. Headache is also a common symptom. Hyponatremia is seen more frequently in Legionnaires' disease than other types of pneumonia. The organism is very difficult to see on Gram stain and requires special culture media to grow in the lab.

23. **(C)** There is no standardized in vitro susceptibility testing for *Legionella* spp. Traditionally erythromycin has been the drug of choice. However, the newer macrolide agents (i.e., azithromycin) and the quinolones (i.e., levofloxacin) have good activity against *Legionella* clinically and have much fewer side effects than high-dose erythromycin.

24. **(C)** This man experienced gastrointestinal (GI) bleeding due to a gastric ulcer. When the NG tube is placed, 500 cc of coffee-ground material is returned. The paucity of upper GI symptoms is, unfortunately, not uncommon among elderly patients. This man's volume depletion is partially masked by his relatively slow pulse rate resulting from the beta blocker he takes for his hypertension. The NSAID he takes for his osteoarthritis significantly increases his risk for GI bleeding. A rectal exam is very helpful in this case and is a necessary part of the evaluation of every elderly patient with a nonspecific "weak and dizzy" presentation. The normal initial Hgb value can also be a nasty distraction. A falling hemoglobin due to hemorrhage may require some time to equilibrate. One potential cause of disproportionate elevation of the BUN relative to the creatinine is blood in the GI tract due to hemorrhage.

25. **(C)** Acral lentiginous melanoma is the most common form of melanoma in African-American patients. It usually appears as a brown or black macule arising on palm, sole, or nailbed.

26. **(A)** Cutaneous metastases of internal malignancies are relatively uncommon. Of those that occur, the most frequent primary site among women is the breast.

27. **(E)** Drug-induced lupus is generally milder than idiopathic systemic lupus erythematosus (SLE). Common culprits include procainamide, hydralazine, and isoniazid. The antinuclear antibody seen in SLE is anti-histone. Drug-induced lupus usually resolves with discontinuation of the drug.

28. **(C)** Stream water often is infected with *Giardia lamblia,* which is a common cause of acute diarrhea, but not bloody diarrhea, as *Giardia* is not invasive or cytotoxic. Puppies, especially if purchased at a mall or from puppy mills, can be infected with *Campylobacter jejuni,* which can cause acute bloody diarrhea. Recent antibiotics are a risk factor for *Clostridium difficile* colitis, with bloody diarrhea. Apple cider from roadside stands often is not pasteurized, and can be contaminated with *Escherichia coli* O157H7, which can cause bloody diarrhea. Finally, cocaine abuse can be complicated by acute ischemic colitis, with bloody diarrhea.

29. **(E)** IV methylene blue is indicated for treatment of methemoglobinemia but not for carbon monoxide toxicity.

30. **(A)** An elderly person with sudden, acute onset of severe, persistent abdominal pain should be considered to have acute mesenteric ischemia until proven otherwise. Severe pain out of proportion to the degree of tenderness on physical examination of the abdomen is a key finding. Cardiac arrhythmias, such as atrial fibrillation and congestive heart failure with poor pump function, predispose to embolization. Previous abdominal surgeries are a risk for adhesions which, by history, cause obstructive symptomatology (intermittent waves of crampy abdominal pain). Insulin-dependent diabetes mellitus can be complicated by diabetic radiculopathy, but the abdominal pain would not present in such an acute manner and would unlikely be periumbilical. Cholelithiasis, particularly in elderly women, can be complicated by gall-stone ileus, due to fistulous passage of a *large* stone from the gallbladder or biliary tree into the intestine (hence, pneumobilia), where it may cause an obstruction (especially in the terminal ileum). The pain, in this case, due to obstruction, usually is intermittent and crampy.

31. **(B)** Systemic scleroderma often is complicated by diminished motor function of the smooth muscle portion of the esophagus, including the lower esophageal sphincter. Raynaud's phenomenon is almost always present in scleroderma patients with esophageal involvement. Heartburn due to gastroesophageal reflux is common in patients with scleroderma, and may be accompanied by esophageal dysphagia, with or without a stricture. Periodic hoarseness secondary to gastroesophageal reflux also may occur in these patients. Oropharyngeal dysphagia is not typical of scleroderma, as the striated muscle of the pharynx, upper esophageal sphincter, and upper body of the esophagus are not affected.

32. **(A)** Gallstones are a common reason for acute pancreatitis but do not cause chronic pancreatitis. Alcohol, familial pancreatitis, and autoimmune pancreatitis all can cause chronic pancreatitis, manifest as pancreatic exocrine insufficiency with or without gross structural changes of the pancreas (i.e., atrophy, ductal dilatation).

33. **(B)** Insulin resistance is associated with acanthosis nigricans, which is clinically characterized by velvety, hyperpigmented plaques most commonly occurring in neck creases and axillae.

34. **(D)** Knee pain is often referred from a problem with the hip. The most likely diagnosis in the above patient would be an avulsion fracture of either the anterior superior iliac spine or greater trochanteric apophysis, a stress fracture of the femoral neck, or a slipped capitofemoral epiphysis.

35. (B) Chronic bronchitis is not a cause of clubbing.

36. (E) Ruptured chordae tendineae are seen in severe mitral valve prolapse. Pericarditis or inflammation of the pericardium (the thin sac surrounding the heart) has been associated with AIDS. Pleural effusion is a fluid buildup in the space between the lungs and chest wall. Pulmonary hypertension leading to cor pulmonale has been seen with AIDS. Dilated cardiomyopathy in some AIDS patients is associated with a lack of selenium. Congestive heart failure has been associated with AIDS. Myocarditis, an inflammation of the heart muscle, has been seen with AIDS. Many people who develop myocarditis recover in a few weeks with few to no side effects and no long-term complications, although some will develop cardiomyopathy.

37. (C) Angiotensin-converting enzyme (ACE) inhibitors such as lisinopril have been shown to cause severe fetal complications, including death, oligohydramnios, fetal growth restriction, neonatal anuria, and hypotension. All other medications can be used in pregnancy if appropriate for the control of chronic hypertension.

38. (A) Ganglion cyst is the most common tumorous condition of the wrist. The cyst will be filled with a clear, gelatinous fluid. The etiology is uncertain; however, some of these cysts will communicate with the wrist joint, leading to the assumption of a joint capsular herniation. Approximately 50% of these can be eliminated with a cortisone injection followed by subcutaneous rupture of the mass.

39. (C) Indinavir, a protease inhibitor, may cause crystal-induced nephropathy. Patients receiving indinavir must drink more than a liter of water a day to prevent crystal formation. If this occurs, it is usually treated with hydration and analgesic agents until the symptoms resolve. The patient should be reeducated to increase his fluid intake. Rarely does the patient have to discontinue the drug.

40. (A) Early crown–rump length measurement has the smallest range of error as well as the smallest range of gestational age of all the measurements listed.

41. (D) Gustatory sweating (Frey syndrome) is commonly seen after parotidectomy and is caused by regrowth of the parasympathetic nerves from the excised gland into sweat glands of the skin. It is often self-limited and minimally symptomatic.

42. (D) If additional treatment is needed, lysis of the parasympathetic nerves will cure the condition; they are found in the tympanic plexus in the middle ear. Vidian neurectomy is used for profuse rhinorrhea unresponsive to medical treatment.

43. (E) There are two basic reasons for performing a cardiac catheterization. The first is to gain information about the heart and major arteries. This information is used to decide whether surgery is needed and feasible and to clearly define the nature and extent of the cardiac problem. The second basic reason to perform a cardiac catheterization is to help establish a diagnosis, for example, when a patient is experiencing chest pain after other tests have been performed.

44. (C) This patient has numbness in the sensory distribution of the ulnar nerve in the hand. The most common compression point in the upper extremity is where the nerve passes behind the medial epicondyle of the distal humerus within the cubital tunnel. Symptoms appear at night with hyperflexion of the elbow during sleep. Holding the elbow hyperflexed generally reproduces the symptoms. Also tapping the nerve at the posteromedial aspect of the elbow produces "electric-like" sensations in the ulnar nerve distribution in the hand. Initial treatment consists of anti-inflammatory medication and an elbow extension night splint.

45. (E) This patient is at high risk for malignancy due to his age, sex, hemoptysis, and smoking status. Serial radiological studies are inappropriate; chemotherapy is not indicated without tissue. Due to the high likelihood of malignancy and good operative status, a surgical approach is most appropriate, and there is a high chance for surgical cure. The TTNA is an unnecessary extra step.

46–47. (46-B, 47-D) Multiple sclerosis is a disease of the central nervous system and would not produce a peripheral nerve lesion. In endemic areas, Lyme disease may be the most common cause found for facial nerve palsies. Herpes zoster involves both cranial nerves VII and VIII in the Ramsay Hunt syndrome. The typical zoster lesions are found in the external ear canal, and prognosis for full recovery is worse.

Prednisone therapy does not change the eventual residual deficit, but 80 to 90% of patients will make a full recovery within 1 year after onset of symptoms.

48. (F) Cognitive behavior therapy has been shown to decrease symptoms of depression, anxiety, PTSD, and schizophrenia in a number of studies.

49. (C) The smear would likely demonstrate chunks of membrane removed and appearing as "bite" cells.

50. (E) Empty sella is a common incidental finding, which can occur as a result of a congenital diaphragmatic defect (primary empty sella) or as a result of damage to the diaphragm by surgery, radiotherapy, or pituitary tumor infarction (secondary empty sella). The most common finding is a normal hormonal profile.

Practice Test 5
Questions

DIRECTIONS (Questions 1 through 43): Each of the numbered items and incomplete statements in this section is followed by answers or by completions of the statement. Select the ONE lettered answer or completion that is BEST in each case.

1. All of the following are appropriate antibiotic regimens for *Enterococcus faecium* bacteremia EXCEPT

   (A) vancomycin and gentamicin
   (B) ampicillin and gentamicin
   (C) ampicillin and streptomycin
   (D) cefazolin and gentamicin

<u>Items 2–4</u>

The labor curve in Figure 5.1 was plotted on a 28-year-old G1P0 woman at term with an uneventful pregnancy. She presented to the delivery room shortly before initiation of recording of her labor curve with regular, painful contractions every 3 minutes and intact membranes.

2. According to the labor curve, the patient is experiencing

   (A) arrest of descent
   (B) arrest of active phase
   (C) latent phase
   (D) normal labor

DILITATION													
10CM													
9CM													
8CM													
7CM													
6CM													
5CM													
4CM												X	
3CM								X		X	X		
2CM				X		X							
1CM	X	X											
TIME	1AM	3AM	5AM	7AM	9AM	11AM	1PM	3PM	5PM	7PM	9PM	11PM	1AM

Figure 5.1

Assume that the patient is experiencing uncomfortable contractions every 3-5 minutes from 1 AM on. She has intact membranes and maternal vital signs and fetal heart monitor tracing are stable and reassuring.

3. Assuming that the fetal monitor strip is reassuring and maternal condition is stable, appropriate immediate management options include all of the following EXCEPT

   (A) maternal sedation
   (B) cesarean section
   (C) pitocin augmentation of labor
   (D) artificial rupture of membranes (AROM)
   (E) continued observation

4. A factor that has been shown to prolong the duration of latent phase labor is

   (A) large fetal size
   (B) maternal blood pressure
   (C) maternal sedation
   (D) maternal pelvic shape

END OF SET

5. Regarding nuclear pharmacologic stress testing, which statement is NOT correct?

   (A) Dipyridamole, adenosine, dobutamine, and dopamine are used clinically to perform pharmacological stress tests.
   (B) Coronary vasodilatation may be suboptimal with dobutamine because of an inadequate heart rate and blood pressure response.
   (C) Dobutamine can cause a hypotensive response.
   (D) Dipyridamole and adenosine are direct coronary vasodilators.

6. A 55-year-old white woman presents with a displaced distal radius fracture after a same-level fall. The patient undergoes an uneventful reduction, and a splint is applied. The patient's neurologic examination is normal postreduction. During the next 2 hours, the patient begins to complain of numbness in her fingers. Her 2-point discrimination in the median nerve distribution is 5 mm. Her splint is spread open, ice is applied, and the hand is elevated. Thirty minutes later, 2-point discrimination is 10 mm in the median nerve distribution. What is the next appropriate course of action?

   (A) observation because nerve function will return
   (B) an emergent carpal tunnel release
   (C) electromyography/nerve conduction velocity (EMG/NCV) to document median nerve compression at the wrist
   (D) none of the above

7. Which of the following medications is NOT indicated to treat panic disorders?

   (A) beta blockers
   (B) selective serotonin reuptake inhibitors (SSRIs)
   (C) monoamine oxidase inhibitors (MAOIs)
   (D) benzodiazepines
   (E) tricyclics

8. A 27-year-old man fell off the roof of his house while repainting it and was somewhat disoriented and dizzy when he was found. His family brought him to the emergency department (ED) for evaluation. His neurologic examination was normal. However, magnetic resonance imaging (MRI) of the head showed a 7-mm pituitary adenoma. He was discharged with instructions to follow up with you. When you see him in your office, his vitals are normal and his physical examination is unremarkable. All of the following tests would be appropriate EXCEPT

   (A) overnight dexamethasone suppression test
   (B) prolactin
   (C) insulin-like growth factor-1 (IGF-1)
   (D) thyroid-stimulating hormone (TSH), free thyroxine (T_4)
   (E) cortisol

9. A 33-year-old woman complains of increasing weakness and fatigue. She had a bone marrow transplant 17 years ago for acute myelogenous leukemia. She had severe gastrointestinal (GI) bleeding at the time, requiring extensive transfusions. She had no evidence of graft versus host disease and her immunosuppressive therapy was subsequently stopped within 1 year. She now pre-

sents with ascites, splenomegaly, and tender hepatomegaly.

DATA

Hemoglobin	9.0 g/dL
WBC	3,200/μL
Platelet count	73,000/μL
Prothrombin time	INR 2.4
Total bilirubin	4.3 mg/dL
Alkaline phosphate	500 U/L
ALT/AST	90/108 U/L

What is the most likely diagnosis?

(A) post-transplant lymphoproliferative disorder (PTLD)

(B) veno-occlusive disease of the liver

(C) human immunodeficiency virus (HIV)

(D) chronic graft versus host disease

(E) hepatocellular carcinoma

10. When dealing with contaminated traumatic wounds, the most important factor for avoiding infection is

(A) tetanus prophylaxis

(B) appropriate antibiotic therapy

(C) adequate debridement

(D) delayed closure of the wound

(E) use of monofilament nonadsorbable sutures for the skin

11. A 35-year-old male RN presents to the ED with 3 days of sore throat, nasal congestion, and cough productive of yellow sputum. Physical exam is remarkable only for mild erythema of the oropharynx. Chest radiograph is negative. What treatment do you recommend?

(A) azithromycin

(B) amoxicillin

(C) levofloxacin

(D) doxycycline

(E) none of the above

12. A 34-year-old white female nonsmoker presents to the ED with 2 days of sore throat, productive cough, nasal congestion, sharp chest pain with inspiration, and dyspnea. Physical exam is normal other than a mildly reddened oropharynx. Which test is critical in establishing a diagnosis?

(A) complete blood count (CBC)

(B) erythrocyte sedimentation rate (ESR)

(C) chest radiograph

(D) electrocardiogram (ECG)

(E) nuclear lung scan

13. A 48-year-old woman with no symptoms of diabetes mellitus is found on routine testing to have a fasting plasma glucose of 132 mg/dL. According to the new diagnostic criteria for diabetes, you should

(A) inform her that she has diabetes and arrange for her to attend diabetes education classes

(B) inform her that she has diabetes and a medication is necessary to normalize her sugars

(C) order an HbA1c (glycohemoglobin)

(D) inform her that she has impaired fasting glucose

(E) none of the above

Items 14–15

A 47-year-old man with a long history of alcohol abuse presents to the ED with the subacute onset of confusion and unsteady gait. Your exam demonstrates limitation of horizontal gaze with upbeat nystagmus and ataxia of gait.

14. The most likely diagnosis is

(A) Wernicke's encephalopathy

(B) Korsakoff syndrome

(C) cerebellar infarction

(D) postictal state

(E) alcohol intoxication

15. The immediate management of this patient should be

   (A) intravenous (IV) heparin
   (B) IV tissue plasminogen activator (tPA)
   (C) IV phenytoin
   (D) intramuscular (IM) thiamine
   (E) observation only

END OF SET

16. A 47-year-old woman is admitted via the ED with atrial fibrillation of unknown duration. Her pulse is 149 beats per minute and her blood pressure is 170/100. She is anxious and agitated. She appears thin and has dry hair and brittle nails. Her family notes that she has been acting strangely for several weeks, often appearing "overenergized" but unable to concentrate or sleep. Her physical exam shows neck fullness. Possible diagnoses include

   (A) Hashimoto's thyroiditis
   (B) Graves' disease
   (C) multinodular goiter
   (D) acute psychosis

17. Acute treatment for the arrhythmia in the patient described above might include

   (A) digoxin
   (B) oral amiodarone
   (C) propranolol (Inderal)
   (D) urgent cardioversion

18. The following antibiotics have activity against *Pseudomonas* EXCEPT

   (A) piperacillin
   (B) imipenem
   (C) ceftriaxone
   (D) amikacin

19. A patient who has just returned from Connecticut is worried about Lyme disease. What would you tell him is the most characteristic symptom?

   (A) headache
   (B) arthralgias

   (C) a macular rash with central clearing
   (D) diffuse myositis

20. What is the most appropriate treatment for allergic fungal sinusitis?

   (A) IV antifungal medication
   (B) oral antifungal medication
   (C) aggressive surgical debridement of all affected tissue, including resection of normal tissue
   (D) surgical aeration of sinuses and limited removal of inflammatory tissue
   (E) oral antihistamine

Items 21–24

A 78-year-old patient presents with the fundus lesion shown in Figure 5.2.

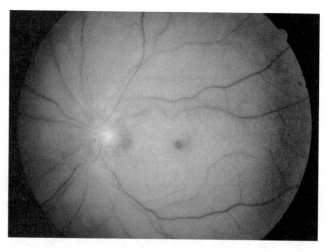

Figure 5.2

21. The diagnosis you suspect is

   (A) central retinal artery occlusion
   (B) toxoplasmosis
   (C) papilledema
   (D) central retinal vein occlusion
   (E) sarcoidosis

22. The workup for this patient should include

    (A) sedimentation rate
    (B) toxoplasmosis titer
    (C) angiotensin-converting enzyme (ACE)
    (D) rapid plasma reagin (RPR)
    (E) prostate-specific antigen

23. If the sedimentation rate is above 100, which of the following diagnoses can be made?

    (A) embolic central retinal artery occlusion
    (B) nonarthritic ischemic optic neuropathy
    (C) arthritic anterior ischemic optic neuropathy
    (D) giant cell arteritis
    (E) sarcoidosis

24. If the patient has an elevated sedimentation rate, which medication should be given immediately?

    (A) penicillin
    (B) prednisone
    (C) aspirin
    (D) coumadin
    (E) clindamycin

END OF SET

25. Which of the following should be consumed with caution in a patient taking multiple medications?

    (A) bananas
    (B) peanuts
    (C) grapefruit juice
    (D) oatmeal
    (E) lemonade

26. Oral contraceptives are used in acne vulgaris primarily to

    (A) normalize follicular hyperkeratinization
    (B) decrease sebaceous gland activity
    (C) provide an anti-inflammatory effect
    (D) reduce *Propionibacterium acnes* proliferation

27. A 4-year-old boy is brought to the pediatrician because he has been having trouble walking for a few days. The mother notices that he has had low-grade fevers. About 2 weeks ago, he was sick but the mother thought he had the flu. On exam, he is sick appearing. His oropharynx appears injected. His knees and ankles are swollen, warm to touch, and very tender. The lungs are clear, and he has a 3/6 diastolic murmur heard best at the apex. The skin is warm, and a macular serpiginous rash is found on the trunks and extremities. Initial laboratory findings include a normal CBC, but the erythrocyte sedimentation rate is 96 mm/hr. What would be the most appropriate diagnostic test?

    (A) two sets of blood cultures
    (B) throat culture for *Streptococcus pyogenes*
    (C) C-reactive protein determination
    (D) technetium bone scan
    (E) skin biopsy of the rash

Items 28–30

A 58-year-old man has been diagnosed with localized prostate cancer on prostate biopsy performed for an elevated serum PSA of 8.5 ng/mL.

28. What additional information is required before discussing treatment options?

    (A) clinical status of inguinal lymph nodes
    (B) Gleason grade of cancer on biopsy
    (C) serum acid phosphatase level
    (D) serum testosterone levels
    (E) cystoscopic appearance of the prostate

29. The patient is now considering options for therapy. Therapeutic alternatives include

    (A) radical nerve-sparing prostatectomy
    (B) external-beam radiation therapy with hormonal ablation
    (C) implantation of radioactive seeds
    (D) prostatic cryoablation
    (E) all of the above

30. The patient is interested in a radical prostatectomy. What would be the expected rate of urinary incontinence following the procedure?

(A) 0%
(B) 5%
(C) 25%
(D) 50%

END OF SET

31. A previously healthy 3-year-old boy who developed nasal congestion yesterday awakened his parents at 3:00 A.M. with difficulty breathing and is now brought to the ED. He is anxious but not toxic in appearance, is sitting upright in his mother's lap, and has resting stridor, a barking cough, tachypnea, and use of accessory muscles of respiration. Temperature is 38° C (100.4° F) and room air pulse oximetry shows 94% saturation. Capillary refill time is 1 second. Auscultation of the lungs reveals transmitted upper airway sounds but no rales or wheezes. His immunizations are up to date. Which of the following actions is appropriate?

(A) Nebulized albuterol should be given.
(B) A portable chest x-ray should be ordered.
(C) Subcutaneous epinephrine should be given.
(D) A third-generation cephalosporin should be given.
(E) A single dose of dexamethasone should be administered.

32. A 57-year-old man presents with enlarged hands and feet, bilateral carpal tunnel syndrome, hypertension, and sleep apnea. Acromegaly is suspected. Which of the following tests is diagnostic of acromegaly?

(A) lack of suppression of growth hormone (GH) measured by immunoradiometric assay (IRMA) to < 5 ng/mL during an oral glucose tolerance test (OGTT)
(B) baseline GH of 6 ng/mL (N: 0–5)
(C) lack of rise of GH in response to thyrotropin-releasing hormone (TRH)

(D) high levels of insulin-like growth factor-2 (IGF-2)
(E) lack of suppression of GH measured by IRMA to < 1 during an OGTT

33. A 54-year-old healthy male nonsmoker is diagnosed with community-acquired pneumonia. Which of the following is the appropriate treatment?

(A) amoxicillin
(B) trimethoprim–sulfamethoxazole
(C) cephalexin
(D) azithromycin
(E) none of the above

34. Resistance to the quinolone class of antibiotics involves alterations of the

(A) cell wall
(B) ribosome
(C) deoxyribonucleic acid (DNA)
(D) microtubules

35. Which of the following findings on physical examination is most suggestive of sinonasal mucormycosis?

(A) nasal septal perforation
(B) boggy nasal mucosal edema
(C) necrotic lesions on turbinate mucosa
(D) purulent nasal discharge
(E) fungal debris in nasal cavity

36. A biopsy is taken of nasal tissue. Which of the following pathological findings is consistent with mucormycosis?

(A) nonseptate hyphae
(B) septate hyphae
(C) branching hyphae
(D) hyphae invading soft tissue
(E) hyphae staining positive for GMS

37. Meperidine (Demerol) is a narcotic analgesic agent that has historically been widely used in the ED setting. In most cases, however, there are more appropriate narcotic agents available for the management of moderate to severe pain. Each of the following undesir-

able pharmacological properties is characteristic of meperidine EXCEPT

(A) release of histamine may aggravate bronchospasm in patients with reactive airway disease

(B) meperidine has been shown to induce spasm of the sphincter of Oddi

(C) normeperidine, a metabolite of meperidine with a relatively long half-life, is a potent central nervous system (CNS) stimulant, which may cause agitation and, occasionally, seizure activity. This metabolite tends to accumulate with repeated dosing of meperidine, especially in patients with renal insufficiency

(D) meperidine can precipitate serotonin syndrome, a potentially lethal condition, if given to patients who are taking monoamine oxidase inhibitors (MAOIs)

38. The most important risk factor for recurrence of an anterior shoulder dislocation is

(A) time of reduction

(B) age of the patient

(C) presence of an axillary nerve injury

(D) fracture of the greater tuberosity

(E) vascular injury

39. A 60-year-old African-American woman presents with microangiopathic hemolytic anemia, intermittent seizures, and a low platelet count. What other findings would be expected?

(A) hypothermia

(B) neutropenia

(C) an elevated partial thromboplastin time (PTT)

(D) hepatic encephalopathy

(E) fever

40. A 24-year-old woman comes to your office complaining of fatigue, loss of appetite, and loss of interest in most things. She has been unable to find a job since she lost hers 3 weeks ago. She and her boyfriend broke up 2 months ago. The most important intervention is to

(A) prescribe an antidepressant

(B) prescribe a benzodiazepine

(C) ask about suicidal thoughts

(D) tell her that this is a normal response to stress

(E) admit her to a hospital

41. Which of the following disorders would NOT typically involve panic attacks?

(A) social phobia

(B) specific phobia

(C) obsessive–compulsive disorder (OCD)

(D) post-traumatic stress disorder (PTSD)

(E) panic disorder

42. A 30-year-old woman presents for a yearly physical. She has no complaints and her history is unremarkable. Her family history is significant for both her mother and maternal aunt with melanoma in their early 30s. The patient had several blistering sunburns as a child and has moderate to extensive freckling on examination. She has numerous flat brown moles, some 1 to 2 cm with irregular borders. The most appropriate management includes

(A) monthly cutaneous self-examinations, with physician exams every 3 to 4 months and photography

(B) minimize exposure to the sun

(C) immediate biopsies of several large moles

(D) prophylactic vitamin A

(E) removal of all moles > 5 mm in diameter

43. You diagnose a 56-year-old man with Type 2 diabetes. Which of the following statements is NOT correct?

(A) His HbA1c (glycohemoglobin) goal should be < 7%.

(B) You should measure his lipid panel.

(C) The patient needs an ophthalmic exam.

(D) You do not need to get a spot urine microalbumin before a year from now.

(E) Fasting glucoses should be < 120 mg/dL.

DIRECTIONS (Questions 44 through 50): The following set of matching questions in this section consists of a list of lettered options followed by several numbered items. For each numbered item, select the appropriate lettered option. Each lettered option may be selected once, more than once, or not at all.

Items 44–50

Match the clinical description and treatment with the appropriate diagnosis below.

   (A) normal vaginal secretion
   (B) bacterial vaginosis
   (C) candidiasis
   (D) trichomoniasis
   (E) mucopurulent cervicitis

44. White, "cottage cheesy" discharge, negative whiff test, vaginal pH < 4.5

45. Thin, homogeneous gray-white discharge, positive whiff test, vaginal pH > 4.5

46. White, clear, flocculent discharge, negative whiff test, vaginal pH 3.8–4.2

47. Greenish-yellow frothy discharge, "strawberry spots," vaginal pH > 4.5

48. Treated with metronidazole 2 g at once

49. Treated with miconazole

50. Treated with metronidazole 500 mg bid × 7 days

END OF SET

Practice Test 5
Answers and Explanations

1. **(D)** Enterococcal infections are becoming increasingly common, especially in the hospitalized setting where enterococcal resistance to vancomycin is of great concern. If the isolate is sensitive to ampicillin, this is the drug of choice. For serious infections (e.g., bacteremias and endocarditis), vancomycin should be combined with an aminoglycoside for synergy. Never should a cephalosporin be used to treat an enterococcal infection.

2. **(C)** Until acceleration of dilatation (at least 1.2 cm/hr) occurs and/or more than 5 cm of dilatation has been achieved, the patient remains in the latent phase of labor. Twenty hours is the upper limit of normal for latent phase in a nulliparous patient.

3. **(B)** Disorders of the latent phase should be managed expectantly as long as mother and baby are stable. They are not associated with an increased incidence of dystocia or active-phase disorders once active labor begins. Once the upper limits of normal latent phase have been reached without onset of more active labor, observation, sedation, or augmentation and/or AROM (as long as the vertex is well applied to the cervix) all are appropriate management options.

4. **(C)** While maternal sedation can help with the treatment of a prolonged latent phase, it can conversely make the latent phase last longer if administered earlier in the latent phase. Preeclampsia is actually associated with shorter labors. While large fetal size and maternal pelvic shape can affect the duration of the active phase, they have not been shown to be associated with a prolonged latent phase.

5. **(A)** Dipyridamole, adenosine, and dobutamine are commonly used during nonpharmacologic stress testing. Dopamine, a vasoconstrictor, would not be an appropriate agent. Dipyridamole and adenosine are direct coronary dilators and give maximal coronary vasodilatory effects.

6. **(B)** Compression of the median nerve secondary to swelling following a fracture of the distal radius is a known cause of carpal tunnel syndrome. Peripheral nerve injuries occurring at the time of injury can usually be monitored for return of function in 6 to 12 weeks. EMG/NCV studies are indicated if return of function has not occurred. Nerve injuries secondary to a laceration or associated with an open fracture should be explored. A developing nerve compression syndrome occurring during the course of treatment should be explored emergently.

7. **(A)** Beta blockers are not indicated for panic disorder; antidepressants and benzodiazepines are.

8. **(E)** Pituitary incidentalomas are common. Their incidence is 10 to 20% of CT/MRI imaging in normal individuals. Screening for hormonal oversecretion should be done in all patients, including prolactin, IGF-1 (acromegaly), overnight dexamethasone suppression test (Cushing's—1 mg of dexamethasone is given at 11:00 P.M., and cortisol is measured at 8:00 A.M. the next day; normal people

should suppress their cortisol to < 3 μg/dL), TSH and free T_4 (TSH-secreting adenoma), and finally luteinizing hormone (LH), follicle-stimulating hormone (FSH), and alpha-subunit (gonadotroph adenomas). The reason for this extensive screening is that many of these tumors can be clinically silent for many years; still, some experts are more conservative, and in the absence of clinical suspicion, they would send only prolactin level, because prolactinomas are the most common of the hormone-secreting tumors.

Patients with macroadenomas should be screened for hypopituitarism: A.M. cortisol and ACTH (corticotropin), TSH and free T_4, and testosterone (if low, add LH and FSH) in men and menses by history in women. Also, patients with macroadenomas should have visual field testing.

In the absence of hormonal oversecretion, hypopituitarism, and visual compromise, no treatment is indicated. Patients are followed by periodic imaging.

9. **(E)** The patient had extensive transfusions to support bleeding during the transplant period. One of the long-term complications of blood transfusions is hepatitis C infection with cirrhosis. In this setting, hepatocellular carcinoma can develop 10 to 20 years after being infected. PTLD has been reported after transplant but usually in the setting of immunosuppression. Patients undergoing either allogeneic or autologous bone marrow transplant can have various abnormalities of the liver at certain times after transplant. Early during transplant, veno-occlusive disease can be an issue, with weight gain, ascites, jaundice, and renal insufficiency. It is not a long-term consequence of transplant. Chronic graft versus host disease can develop as well. HIV testing is indicated in any patient with unexplained symptoms and a history of blood transfusions. HIV can be associated with concomitant hepatitis C infection.

10. **(C)** An adequate mechanical debridement of a traumatic wound is the most important step in management. The simple soaking of a

hand wound in Betadine solution, commonly practiced in emergency departments, is insufficient. Traumatic wounds should be anesthetized, scrubbed, then irrigated thoroughly. If the wound edges still appear contaminated or devitalized, a sharp debridement should be performed. Grossly contaminated wounds and wounds associated with fractures should be closed on a delayed basis.

11. **(E)** This patient has acute bronchitis, and antibiotics are not indicated at this time.

12. **(C)** The most important decision to make in this case is whether she has pneumonia. The chest radiograph is critical for establishing this diagnosis and for distinguishing it from acute bronchitis, which is a common cause of antibiotic abuse.

13. **(E)** A diagnosis of diabetes is made if the fasting plasma glucose is at least 126 mg/dL. This should be confirmed by repeat testing on a different day. A fasting glucose of 110 to 125 mg/dL defines impaired fasting glucose. HbA1c should not be ordered before a diagnosis of diabetes is made.

14–15. **(14-A, 15-D)** This patient presents with the classic signs seen in a patient with Wernicke's encephalopathy. Korsakoff syndrome manifests as a pure amnestic syndrome, and the signs described could not localize to the cerebellum alone and are not seen in a postictal state. Thiamine replacement daily for 3 days may produce an improvement in symptoms.

16. **(B)** Graves' disease causes a diffuse vascular goiter and elevated T_3 and T_4 and a low TSH. Hashimoto's thyroiditis causes hypothyroidism. There is no evidence for a multinodular goiter or acute psychosis.

17. **(C)** Typically, rate control is difficult to achieve in atrial fibrillation secondary to thyrotoxicosis. The best response is achieved with beta blockers, which are used as an adjunct in the management of the thyrotoxic state. Oral amiodarone would not be desirable here. Because of its potential effect on

thyroid metabolism, this could confound management. Digoxin is unlikely to be effective. The patient is hemodynamically stable and does not require urgent cardioversion. Since the patient has been in atrial fibrillation for an unknown period of time, clots may have already formed in the left atrium and extended anticoagulation initiated prior to cardioversion.

18. **(C)** Ceftriaxone is a broad-spectrum, third-generation cephalosporin; however, it does not have activity against *Pseudomonas*. The extended-spectrum penicillins, ceftazidime, fourth-generation cephalosporins, aminoglycosides, carbapenems/monobactem, and selected quinolones all have antipseudomonal activity.

19. **(C)** Lyme disease, caused by *Borrelia burgdorferi*, is a tick-borne illness usually occurring in the summer. It may present as a viral-like illness with fever and arthralgias. More than half of the patients complain of a rash with central clearing (erythema migrans) as the first symptom. Patients may also experience fever, headache, fatigue, and arthralgias. Treatment with oral doxycycline or amoxicillin is effective.

20. **(D)** The pathophysiology of allergic fungal sinusitis is different from fulminant, invasive, or chronic sinusitis: The primary problem is the body's allergic response to fungal allergens, so aggressive surgical resection or antifungal medications are not needed. Aeration and limited debridement of the sinuses, along with systemic steroids, are the appropriate treatments.

21. **(A)** Central retinal artery occlusions are classic for having a cherry red spot. This red central lesion actually represents normal reflex from the pigment epithelium. The surrounding retina, however, is whitened by the infarction secondary to the occlusion of the central retinal artery that supplies blood to the inner layers of the retina.

22. **(A)** A sedimentation rate must be done in all patients with central retinal artery occlusions. Giant cell arteritis may be a readily diagnosed and treatable cause for central retinal artery occlusions, and the sedimentation rate is essential to the workup of patients presenting with this condition. Additional workup may include carotid artery and cardiac valve studies as well as temporal artery biopsy that can be performed in the immediate future.

23. **(D)** An elevated sedimentation rate is indicative of giant cell arteritis but can be elevated in many other conditions. For this reason, patients must be worked up completely for giant cell arteritis and this includes a temporal artery biopsy. Immediate prednisone therapy is indicated for patients with giant cell arteritis. One should not forget, however, that there may be other causes for a patient to develop a central retinal artery occlusion even in the face of an elevated sedimentation rate. The workup includes carotid and aortic valve studies.

24. **(B)** Patients with elevated sedimentation rates and symptoms of lethargy, pain in the temporal region, jaw claudication, or central retinal artery occlusions must be treated immediately with prednisone even if this precedes a full workup. Further workup including temporal artery biopsy and carotid artery and cardiac echo studies should still be done even after the prednisone therapy has been initiated.

25. **(C)** Grapefruit juice elevates serum concentrations of certain drugs metabolized by cytochrome P-450–dependent pathways by diminishing their first-pass metabolism.

26. **(B)** Oral contraceptives are used in acne vulgaris to reduce androgen-stimulated sebum production from the sebaceous gland.

27. **(B)** The child is exhibiting signs of acute rheumatic fever secondary to pharyngitis caused by Group A streptococcus (*S. pyo-*

genes). The major criteria are referred to as the Jones criteria: arthritis, carditis, subcutaneous nodules, erythema marginatum, and Sydenham's chorea, in addition to evidence of an antecedent *S. pyogenes* infection. Often, the patient still has evidence of pharnygitis and can be culture positive for *S. pyogenes*.

28. **(B)** The pathologic Gleason grade of the cancer is necessary in order to determine optimal therapy. Serum acid phosphatase may be interesting but is unlikely to be helpful in a man with a PSA level < 20 ng/mL. Serum testosterone levels and cystoscopy offer no additional information.

29. **(E)** Each of the treatments listed above would be considered reasonable options for this patient with clinically localized prostate cancer. The current published literature is unable to determine the optimal treatment for this disease so men can and must choose between competing options.

30. **(B)** Although published clinical reports have found a highly variable rate of urinary incontinence after radical prostatectomy, the current expectation is that 5% of men will suffer from significant urinary incontinence following this procedure.

31. **(E)** The history and exam are most consistent with viral croup of moderate severity. Epiglottitis is unlikely based on his nontoxic appearance and prior adequate immunizations. Bacterial tracheitis is also unlikely based on the history and nontoxic appearance. Appropriate therapy for viral croup may include supplemental oxygen, cool mist, nebulized racemic epinephrine, and a single dose of dexamethasone. Albuterol, subcutaneous epinephrine, and antibiotics are inappropriate. A chest x-ray is unlikely to influence the management of this case.

32. **(E)** An excellent screening test for acromegaly is IGF-1 (not IGF-2), which is high except in poorly controlled diabetes, starvation, and liver failure, all of which can underestimate IGF-1 levels. The gold standard test re-

mains the OGTT, in which lack of suppression of GH to < 1 if measured by IRMA or < 2 if measured by radioimmunoassay (RIA) is diagnostic of acromegaly. Acromegalic patients, unlike normal subjects, exhibit a paradoxical GH rise to TRH stimulation, but this test has false positives. Random GH levels are useless, because there is a lot of overlap with normal people.

33. **(D)** This patient can be treated as an outpatient. The most likely causative organism is *Streptococcus pneumoniae*, which has a high rate of resistance to all of the medications listed except azithromycin. Current guidelines recommend administration of a macrolide or doxycycline or fluoroquinolone to outpatients with community-acquired pneumonia.

34. **(C)** Quinolone antibiotics inhibit bacterial DNA synthesis by inhibiting DNA gyrase and topoisomerase IV. Both of these enzymes are involved in DNA replication and maintaining the structure of DNA. Quinolones acting on both enzymes is a two-pronged approach. Bacteria acquire resistance to the quinolones by spontaneous mutations that occur in DNA gyrase and topoisomerase and alterations in the cell membrane permeability.

35. **(C)** Black necrotic lesions on the turbinate or nasal mucosa are highly suggestive of mucormycosis in an immunocompromised patient.

36. **(A)** This is the characteristic appearance of mucormycosis; tissue invasion is not needed on the pathological specimen to make the clinopathologic diagnosis.

37. **(B)** Meperidine is seldom the agent of choice for analgesia in the ED. Traditionally, meperidine has been reported to be less likely to cause spasm of the sphincter of Oddi than morphine among patients being treated for pancreatitis and biliary tract disease, although the validity of this observation has been recently questioned.

38. (B) Males between the ages of 17 and 25 are at increased risk for recurrent anterior dislocation. Posterior dislocations are usually associated with seizure disorders.

39. (E) This presentation is consistent with thrombotic thrombocytopenic purpura. Fever and renal failure are most common.

40. (C) It is important to assess the woman's risk of suicide by asking her if she has thought about killing herself, has a plan, has access to the means (pills, gun, rope, bridge, etc.), has rehearsed how she would do it, has had prior attempts, and has family history of suicide.

41. (C) Panic attacks occur in many disorders such as social phobias, specific phobias, PTSD, and panic disorders.

42. (A) The patient has familial atypical mole and melanoma syndrome, with one or more first- or second-degree relatives with a history of melanoma. These patients have a high risk for melanoma. Optimal management includes monthly self-examinations. Random biopsies are not necessary, but removal of atypical or changing moles is. There is no evidence that vitamin supplementation reduces the risk of any cancer.

43. (D) Patients with Type 2 diabetes may already have complications from their diabetes at the time of the diagnosis, including nephropathy, retinopathy, neuropathy, and heart disease. Screening for nephropathy, through urine microalbumin, should be done as soon as the diagnosis is made.

44. (C) This is the classic description of candidiasis. *(Beckmann, 325)*

45. (B) This is the classic description of bacterial vaginosis. *(Beckmann, 325)*

46. (A) This is the description of the normal vagina. *(Beckmann, 325)*

47. (D) This is the classic description of trichomoniasis. *(Beckmann, 325)*

48. (D) This is the treatment of trichomoniasis. *(Beckmann, 329–330)*

49. (C) This is the treatment for candidiasis. *(Beckmann, 331)*

50. (B) This is the treatment for bacterial vaginosis. *(Beckmann, 328–329)*

Practice Test 6
Questions

DIRECTIONS (Questions 1 through 50): Each of the numbered items or incomplete statements in this section is followed by answers or by completions of the statement. Select the ONE lettered answer or completion that is BEST in each case.

1. A 25-year-old woman has amenorrhea and galactorrhea. Her serum prolactin level is 60 ng/mL (N: 0–19). Conditions that might cause these findings include all of the following EXCEPT

   (A) a pituitary microprolactinoma
   (B) a pituitary macroprolactinoma
   (C) primary hypothyroidism
   (D) pregnancy
   (E) chronic renal failure

2. A 10-year-old girl is brought to your office because her teacher at school has noticed that she is sometimes "inattentive." Her parents have noted staring spells and rapid blinking lasting several seconds. The patient is unaware of these lapses. Similar episodes had been diagnosed in her 12-year-old brother. An electroencephalogram (EEG) demonstrates generalized 3-Hz spike-and-wave discharges. The best anticonvulsant in this setting is

   (A) valproic acid
   (B) phenobarbital
   (C) phenytoin
   (D) carbamazepine
   (E) gabapentin

3. In the management of supraventricular tachycardia, drugs with effects on the atrioventricular (AV) node may be clinically useful. All of these medications below slow conduction at the level of the AV node EXCEPT

   (A) digoxin
   (B) diltiazem
   (C) adenosine
   (D) amiodarone
   (E) lidocaine

4. A college-age student is brought to the emergency department (ED) after experiencing a seizure in class. During the day, he had been acting inappropriately according to his friends. There was no history of illicit drug use. On exam he is difficult to arouse. A magnetic resonance imaging (MRI) scan is performed and reveals bilateral temporal lobe enhancement. A lumbar puncture was performed, which showed a white blood count (WBC) of 230 (10% neutrophils, 90% lymphocytes), a red blood count (RBC) of 525, glucose 55 mg/dL, and protein 75 mg/dL. What is the most likely diagnosis?

   (A) mumps encephalitis
   (B) tuberculous meningitis
   (C) herpes simplex virus (HSV) encephalitis
   (D) tertiary syphilis

5. A 4-year-old child presents with unilateral foul-smelling purulent rhinorrhea. The most likely diagnosis is

   (A) chronic sinusitis
   (B) nasal foreign body
   (C) choanal atresia
   (D) nasal encephalocele
   (E) acute rhinitis

6. A previously healthy 30-year-old man presents with sharp intermittent chest pain of 12 hours' duration that is somewhat worse with deep inspiration, as well as low-grade fever and dry cough. Cardiac auscultation reveals a harsh rub heard only in the sitting position. His electrocardiogram (ECG) is shown in Figure 6.1. Based on the information provided, which of the following interventions would be most appropriate?

   (A) Administer intravenous (IV) heparin.
   (B) Administer tissue plasminogen activator (tPA).
   (C) Administer nitroglycerin.
   (D) Order an echocardiogram.
   (E) Order a ventilation–perfusion scan of the lungs.

7. What is the indication for computed tomography (CT) or MRI imaging in the staging of men with clinically localized prostate cancer?

   (A) serum prostate-specific antigen (PSA) > 25 ng/mL
   (B) all men with clinically localized prostate cancer
   (C) presence of chronic back pain
   (D) gross hematuria

8. A woman with a long history of amenorrhea, galactorrhea, and headaches is diagnosed with a macroprolactinoma. Prolactin levels are 1,500 ng/mL, and MRI shows a 3-cm pituitary adenoma abutting the optic chiasm, causing visual field abnormalities. The most appropriate management is

   (A) transsphenoidal surgery
   (B) radiation therapy
   (C) bromocriptine
   (D) pergolide
   (E) bromocriptine for 2 weeks, then transsphenoidal surgery

9. A 17-year-old girl presents with a 2-day history of fever with pain and swelling of the knee. On examination there is a 4+ effusion with increased heat in the knee. The knee is aspirated, and a 60,000 WBC/mm³ is obtained. Differential count reveals that 90% of these are polymorphonuclear leukocytes. No organisms are seen on Gram stain. The most likely cause of this patient's knee swelling is

   (A) *Neisseria gonorrhoeae*
   (B) *Staphylococcus aureus*
   (C) gouty arthritis
   (D) rheumatoid arthritis
   (E) lupus arthritis

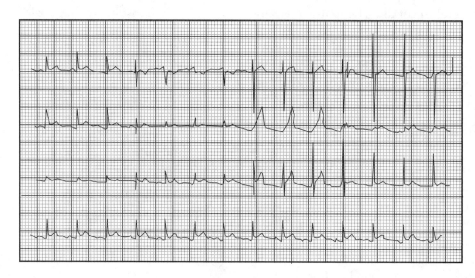

Figure 6.1

10. Characteristics of restrictive cardiomyopathy include all the following EXCEPT

   (A) diastolic dysfunction
   (B) left ventricular chamber enlargement
   (C) biatrial enlargement
   (D) variably reduced systolic function

11. How is the best way to make a diagnosis of osteomyelitis in a patient with a diabetic foot infection?

   (A) Culture material by swabbing the base of the ulcer.
   (B) Obtain a plain-film radiograph of the foot.
   (C) Perform an intraoperative bone culture.
   (D) Measure the erythrocyte sedimentation rate (ESR).

Items 12–16

A 25-year-old G4P2012 woman with a last menstrual period 6 weeks ago, positive home pregnancy test 3 weeks ago, and a positive serum beta human chorionic gonadotropin (hCG) in your office 3 days ago was seen yesterday in the ED with spotting and was advised that "everything looks okay" and to follow up with you the next day. She presents to your office today with a 2-hour history of heavy bleeding and severe cramping, both of which have subsided greatly after passage of a fist-sized "clot" just prior to leaving her house for your office. She and her husband had been actively trying to conceive for the past several months.

Exam in your office shows a tearful woman in no acute physical distress. Vital signs show temperature 36.8° C (98.4° F), blood pressure 110/70, pulse 90, and respirations 18.

Physical exam shows her abdomen to be benign with no tenderness or masses, and on pelvic exam there is minimal bleeding from her cervical os, which is closed. Her uterus is mildly tender, firm, and top normal size, and no adnexal masses or tenderness is present.

When you contact the ED, you find that their exam the day before showed a long, closed cervix with a 6-week-sized uterus. The attending in the ED performed a brief transvaginal ultrasound showing an intrauterine sac and fetal pole with no definite fetal heart motion.

12. What would have been the most correct diagnosis at the time the patient left the ED?

   (A) threatened abortion
   (B) missed abortion
   (C) incomplete abortion
   (D) ectopic pregnancy
   (E) inevitable abortion

13. The chart below outlines serial serum beta hCG levels obtained on this patient. Exam on day 6 showed a top-normal-sized, nontender uterus with a closed cervix and interval bleeding reported by the patient (and confirmed on your exam) to be less than a light day of her usual period. Based on these levels and your exam, appropriate management of this patient includes

Day 1	Day 3	Day 4	Day 6
2,560 IU	4,320	2,100	1,050
Initial office testing	ED	Office visit with recent heavy bleeding and passage of large "clot"	Follow-up visit with decreased bleeding and no cramps

   (A) immediate diagnostic laparoscopy
   (B) immediate dilation and evacuation
   (C) methotrexate injection
   (D) close observation with instructions to the patient to contact you or return to the ED with any heavy vaginal bleeding, cramping, or fever

14. The patient delivered her other babies in another state and has just recently become your patient. Hemoglobin in your office on day 4 is 12.5 g. Assuming that no other laboratory testing was done in the ED and that no old records are available, what other bloodwork should be obtained immediately on this patient?

   (A) hepatitis B surface antigen (HBsAg)
   (B) blood type and Rh
   (C) maternal chromosome testing
   (D) 1-hour 50-g glucose tolerance test (GTT)
   (E) rubella antibody levels

15. At follow-up visit, your patient continues to be tearful and admits to worrying that sexual intercourse the night prior to initiation of bleeding caused her miscarriage. She also notes that prior to having intercourse, she and her husband had a disagreement over whether or not she should continue to work at her job as a nurse throughout the pregnancy, and she wonders what effect this had. Appropriate response to this concern includes

(A) telling your patient that she was not that far into her pregnancy and that she should be grateful that this happened earlier rather than later

(B) telling your patient that while intercourse early in pregnancy is not a common cause of miscarriage, it may have contributed in this case and she will have to be more careful next time

(C) telling your patient to pull herself together and just try again next cycle—this is nature's way of keeping abnormal babies from being born

(D) telling your patient that while searching for a cause and blaming one's self or partner is a normal part of the grief reaction caused by a miscarriage, there is no evidence that sexual intercourse or having a fight with one's spouse affects miscarriage and that having sex or fighting with her husband *did not* cause her miscarriage

16. During the above discussion, your patient and her husband ask you how likely they are to deliver a viable baby with their next pregnancy. Given that she has had two normal pregnancies and one elective abortion, your answer is

(A) 75%
(B) 66%
(C) 85%
(D) 98%

END OF SET

17. When is a prostate biopsy indicated in a male patient?

(A) in the presence of an elevated PSA or an abnormal prostate nodule on digital rectal examination (DRE)
(B) a man with severe voiding symptoms
(C) gross hematuria
(D) recurrent urinary tract infections
(E) an enlarged prostate on DRE

18. The various methods for improving the sensitivity and specificity of a serum PSA test for identifying prostate cancer include all the following EXCEPT

(A) transition-zone PSA density
(B) ratio of free to total serum PSA levels
(C) change in PSA levels over time (PSA velocity)
(D) pre- and post-DRE serum PSA levels

19. A 19-year-old woman is seen for syncope. Since age 12, she has had episodes of syncope with exertion or fright. One such recent episode occurred when the fire alarm went off in her dorm at 3:00 A.M. She has a family history of sudden death. The ECG is shown in Figure 6.2. She is taking no medications and denies illicit drug use. The most likely diagnosis is

(A) Brugada syndrome
(B) Wolff–Parkinson–White (WPW) syndrome
(C) congenital prolonged QT syndrome
(D) idiopathic ventricular fibrillation

20. A 78-year-old woman is brought to your office by her daughter, who is concerned that her mother has not been her usual self since the death of her husband 2 weeks ago. She has lost 6 pounds, becomes tearful when remembering him, is forgetful, and claims that he talks to her. The daughter has seen her mother talking to herself. The mother most likely suffers from

(A) bereavement
(B) major depression

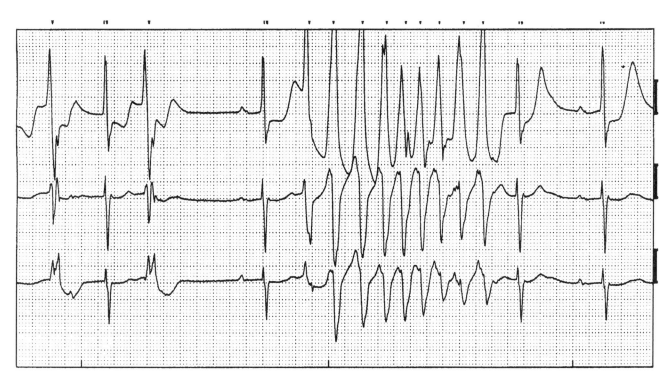

Figure 6.2

(C) dementia

(D) late-onset schizophrenia

(E) alcohol abuse

21. A 25-year-old woman presents with menorrhagia. She has bruised easily all her life. She has no family history of bleeding issues. Her exam is normal and labs are normal except for an activated partial thromboplastin time (aPTT) of 45, a bleeding time of 14 min and von Willebrand's factor (vWF) antigen of 23%, vWFR: Co of 20%, and factor VIII:antihemophilic factor (factor VIII activity) of 25%. She required dilatation and curettage. What is the best initial therapy to prevent perioperative bleeding?

(A) cryoprecipitate

(B) desmopressin (DDAVP)

(C) fresh-frozen plasma (FFP)

(D) factor VIII concentrate

(E) vWF concentrate

22. A 25-year-old man with Type 1 diabetes presents with persistent morning hyperglycemia for the past few months. He is on the following insulin regimen: neutral protamine Hagedorn (NPH) 15 units and Humalog (Lispro) 8 units in the morning; NPH 12 units and Humalog 10 units at dinner time. His last HbA1c is 8%. His prelunch, predinner, and bedtime sugars are in the 90s to low 100s, but his morning sugars are in the 200 range. What is the next step?

(A) Increase morning Humalog to 12 units.

(B) Increase evening NPH to 15 units.

(C) Increase evening NPH to 18 units.

(D) Move NPH to bedtime.

(E) none of the above

Items 23–26

A 59-year-old male smoker presents to your office complaining of dyspnea at two blocks, which has been worsening over a 6-month period. Physical exam shows stable vital signs except for respiratory rate of 26 and SaO_2 of 84% on room air. His jugular venous pressure (JVP) is 7 cm of H_2O, no murmurs or gallops, he is barrel chested with clear and equal bilateral lungs, and there is no peripheral edema.

23. What is the most likely diagnosis?

   (A) congestive heart failure (CHF)
   (B) chronic obstructive pulmonary disease (COPD)
   (C) pulmonary embolus
   (D) pneumothorax
   (E) angina

24. Which treatment will improve his survival?

   (A) angiotensin-converting enzyme (ACE) inhibitor
   (B) heparin
   (C) oxygen
   (D) chest tube
   (E) metoprolol

25. What test will confirm the diagnosis?

   (A) coronary angiogram
   (B) pulmonary function testing
   (C) chest radiograph
   (D) Doppler ultrasound of the legs
   (E) echocardiogram

26. Which of the following treatments is he unlikely to benefit from?

   (A) inhaled ipratropium
   (B) annual influenza vaccination
   (C) Pneumovax vaccination
   (D) inhaled corticosteroids
   (E) pulmonary rehabilitation

END OF SET

27. Which of the following is a classic physical finding in necrotizing otitis externa (sometimes called malignant otitis externa)?

   (A) bulging tympanic membrane
   (B) retracted tympanic membrane
   (C) inflammation of only the cartilaginous portion of the external ear canal
   (D) exposure of bone in the bony portion of the external ear canal
   (E) granulation tissue at the junction of the bony and cartilaginous portions of the external ear canal

28. A previously healthy 40-year-old man experienced a flulike illness of several days' duration 3 weeks ago, which improved without medical attention. He reports, however, feeling "run down" since then. Over the past 3 days, he has developed clumsiness and weakness of his legs with frequent stumbling. He now presents to the ED because he is unable to walk. He is afebrile, with a pulse of 90 and blood pressure of 130/70. His chest is clear. Heart tones are normal. Abdomen is nontender. Exam of the lower extremities reveals absence of the deep tendon reflexes, profound muscular weakness, and sensory impairment bilaterally. Each of the following statements regarding the patient's present condition is true EXCEPT

   (A) potential ventilatory problems associated with this illness are best detected with arterial blood gas (ABG) determination
   (B) lumbar puncture (LP) typically shows a normal opening pressure and cerebrospinal fluid (CSF) cell count with an elevation of the CSF protein
   (C) neurology consultation is needed
   (D) autonomic instability may be associated with this disorder
   (E) because of a significant potential for progression, these patients require admission

29. Which of the following is a precursor lesion of squamous cell carcinoma?

   (A) basal cell carcinoma
   (B) dermatofibroma
   (C) actinic keratosis
   (D) compound nevus
   (E) seborrheic keratosis

30. A 48-year-old man is diagnosed with rheumatoid arthritis. His physician wants to treat him with medications. All of the following are risk factors for this patient's developing gastroduodenal mucosal injury, with or without hemorrhage, EXCEPT

   (A) treatment with aspirin and prednisone
   (B) personal patient history of gastric ulcer, and ibuprofen treatment
   (C) treatment with aspirin and ibuprofen
   (D) treatment with prednisone and methotrexate and history of Mallory–Weiss tear

31. Which of the following laboratory tests is most unlikely to be abnormal in persons with active celiac disease?

   (A) serum immunoglobulin A (IgA)
   (B) serum antigliadin antibody
   (C) serum alanine transaminase (ALT)
   (D) serum antiendomysial antibody
   (E) serum gastrin
   (F) HLA-DR3

32. Which of the following is a feature of Wegener's granulomatosis?

   (A) uveitis
   (B) oral ulcers
   (C) erythema nodosum
   (D) scarring alopecia
   (E) ichthyosis

33. A 3-year-old girl complains of pain in the right elbow area immediately after an older sibling pulled her to an upright position by the arm as she was falling from a couch. The child appears relatively comfortable in her mother's lap now but holds the affected ex-

tremity in a rigid posture close to the trunk, with the elbow flexed at roughly 90 degrees and the forearm in pronation. There is no visible swelling or deformity, neurovascular exam is normal, and there is no tenderness or palpable abnormality of the wrist, distal forearm, upper arm, shoulder, or clavicle. Which of the following statements is correct?

   (A) Imaging may not be needed at this time.
   (B) These findings suggest supracondylar fracture.
   (C) This injury is common up to puberty.
   (D) This type of injury is commonly associated with child abuse.
   (E) Definitive treatment of this injury usually requires conscious sedation.

34. A felon is anatomically located in the

   (A) cuticle area
   (B) nail matrix
   (C) volar interphalangeal (IP) joint
   (D) palmar along flexor tendon sheath
   (E) distal digital pulp

35. Oral intubation in a patient with Down syndrome is potentially problematic for what reason?

   (A) mandibular retrusion
   (B) laxity of atlanto-axial joint
   (C) tubular (omega-shaped) epiglottis
   (D) oral trismus
   (E) frequent presence of Arnold–Chiari malformation

Items 36–37

A 47-year-old diabetic presents with floaters of the eye. Retinal examination reveals the findings demonstrated in Figure 6.3.

36. These findings are compatible with

   (A) vitreous hemorrhage
   (B) proliferative diabetic retinopathy
   (C) retinal detachment
   (D) cataract formation
   (E) central retinal vein occlusion

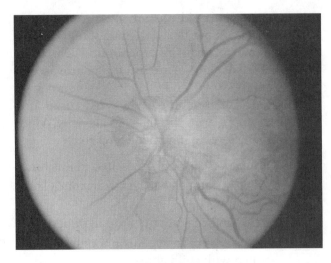

Figure 6.3

37. The appropriate therapy for this patient would be

(A) strict diabetic control
(B) immediate vitrectomy
(C) cataract surgery
(D) antihypertensive medications
(E) laser photocoagulation surgery

END OF SET

Items 38–41

A 32-year-old woman presents to your office complaining of a 6-week history of difficulty with intiation of urination, weakness of both legs, and a "beltlike" tightness around her upper abdomen. She has had marked improvement of all symptoms over the past week. At age 22, she had a decrease in vision in her right eye with improvement over the next several weeks. At age 25, she noted paresthesias of the right face, arm, and leg with partial resolution over a 3-month period of time. She had not sought medical care until this time. You obtain an MRI of her brain (Figure 6.4A, B).

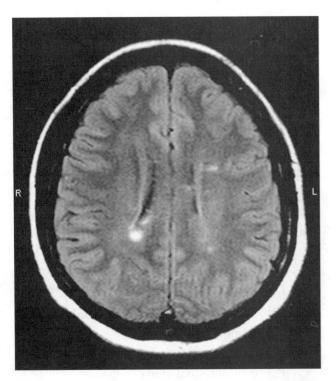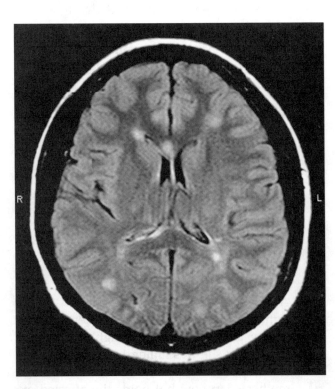

Figure 6.4 A and B

38. The most likely diagnosis is

   (A) Lyme disease
   (B) neurosyphilis
   (C) multiple sclerosis
   (D) multiple cerebral infarctions
   (E) vitamin B_{12} deficiency

39. Your next therapeutic course of action should be

   (A) IV methylprednisolone
   (B) oral prednisone
   (C) urology consultation
   (D) beta-interferon
   (E) observe for further symptoms

40. The patient complains of painful spasms in both legs with flexor spasms nocturnally. All of the following agents may be appropriate recommendations EXCEPT

   (A) baclofen
   (B) diazepam
   (C) tizanidine
   (D) botulinum toxin injections
   (E) cyclobenzaprine

41. In the setting of an acute exacerbation of multiple sclerosis, IV methylprednisolone may

   (A) shorten the duration and lessen the severity of an attack
   (B) prevent further exacerbations for a limited time after treatment
   (C) improve long-term outcome of disability arising from an attack
   (D) decrease the number of MRI lesions
   (E) all of the above

END OF SET

42. A 57-year-old woman is placed on a medication for atrial fibrillation. She is brought to the ED after experiencing a syncopal episode at work. The ECG shown in Figure 6.5 was recorded. What drug is this patient likely taking?

   (A) procainamide hydrochloride
   (B) digoxin
   (C) captopril
   (D) flecainide

43. Longitudinal growth of a long bone occurs mainly by means of

   (A) remodeling of the diaphysis
   (B) metaphyseal remodeling
   (C) remodeling of the epiphysis
   (D) cell multiplication by the chondrocytes of the epiphyseal plate (physis)
   (E) membranous bone formation

44. A 60-year-old man with a history of alcoholism is brought to the ED by a friend because of confusion, unsteady gait, and gaze paralysis. The most appropriate initial pharmacotherapy is

   (A) lorazepam
   (B) naltrexone
   (C) glucose
   (D) folate
   (E) thiamine

45. Which statement about the risks of blood transfusion is true?

   (A) The risk of developing transfusion-related acute lung injury is 1/50 units of blood transfused.
   (B) The risk of transfusion-transmitted hepatitis C is 1/330 units of blood transfused.
   (C) The risk of developing melanoma is tenfold higher in patients who have received transfusions.
   (D) The risk of transfusion-transmitted Chagas' disease is 1/500 units of blood transfused.
   (E) The risk of transfusion-transmitted human immunodeficiency virus (HIV) is 1/3,300 units of blood transfused.

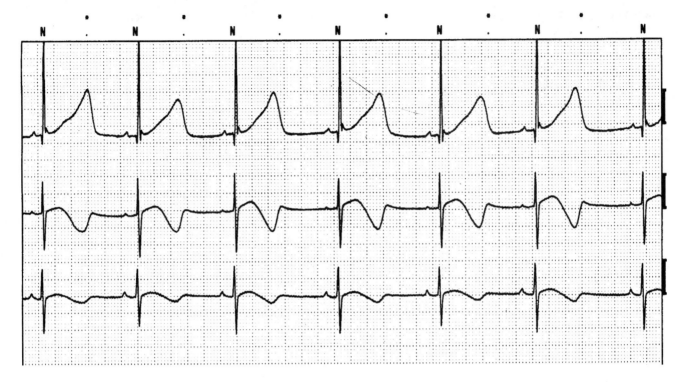

Figure 6.5

Items 46–50

A 26-year-old G5P1041 smoker, LMP last week, presents for routine annual gynecologic examination. She began having intercourse at age 14 and has three current sexual partners. Her only sexually transmitted infection (STI) was an outbreak of venereal warts about 2 years ago. Additionally, her mother underwent a hysterectomy at age 42 for cervical cancer. You perform routine cervical cultures as well as a Pap smear at this visit.

46. All of the following facts in her history are risk factors for the development of cervical neoplasia EXCEPT

    (A) maternal history of cervical cancer
    (B) early age of first intercourse
    (C) multiple sexual partners
    (D) smoking
    (E) venereal warts

47. The causative organism most closely associated with cervical neoplasia is

    (A) herpes simplex virus
    (B) human papillomavirus (HPV)
    (C) lymphogranuloma venereum
    (D) *Trichomonas vaginalis*
    (E) none has been identified

48. This patient's Pap smear comes back with a low-grade squamous intraepithelial lesion (LGSIL), favor mild to moderate dysplasia. The next most appropriate management would be

    (A) immediate hysterectomy
    (B) schedule for cone biopsy
    (C) colposcopy
    (D) cryotherapy of the cervix
    (E) LEEP procedure

49. Approximately what percentage of squamous intraepithelial neoplasia occurs in the squamocolumnar junction (or transformation zone) of the cervix?

(A) < 1%

(B) 10%

(C) 30%

(D) 75%

(E) 95%

50. Following appropriate management of LGSIL, the next Pap would

(A) be performed in 3 months

(B) be performed in 6 months

(C) be performed in 1 year

(D) be performed on the vaginal cuff only

(E) include an endometrial biopsy

END OF SET

Practice Test 6
Answers and Explanations

1. **(B)** In patients who have macroprolactinomas, serum levels of prolactin are at least 200 ng/mL. Lower serum levels can result from microprolactinomas or nonfunctioning pituitary macroadenomas (due to pituitary stalk compression and decreased prolactin-inhibiting factor or dopamine). Pregnancy is associated with increasing prolactin levels throughout the course of pregnancy owing to the stimulatory effect of estrogens that results in lactotroph hyperplasia and hypertrophy. Renal insufficiency leads to decreased clearance of prolactin as well as increased production as a result of disordered hypothalamic regulation of prolactin secretion. In primary hypothyroidism, levels of thyrotropin-releasing hormone (TRH) increase, resulting in stimulation of prolactin secretion.

2. **(A)** This patient's clinical picture is best explained by absence epilepsy. This genetic, generalized epilepsy is primarily limited to childhood and usually resolves by the time the patient reaches her third decade. School performance may be affected for some time before the diagnosis is confirmed. Other than valproic acid, both ethosuximide and lamotrigine have demonstrated effectiveness, while carbamazepine may worsen the condition.

3. **(E)** Through different mechanisms, all the drugs except lidocaine slow AV node conduction and can be used in the treatment of AV node–dependent tachyarrhythmias. Digoxin's effect is through increasing vagal tone. Diltiazem and amiodarone have direct effect on the AV node. Adenosine inhibits cyclic adenosine monophosphate–induced calcium influx.

4. **(C)** This presentation is consistent with HSV encephalitis. This is a rare complication of HSV-1 infection. It is most likely spread via neural routes to the brain during primary or recurrent infection. It has a predilection for the temporal lobes. Headache, seizures, and behavioral changes are often the presenting symptoms. Brain biopsy has historically been the gold standard for diagnosis; however, HSV polymerase chain reaction (PCR) currently is accepted for accurate diagnosis. Treatment is with intravenous acyclovir at 10 mg/kg every 8 hours for 2 weeks.

5. **(B)** This is the classic presentation of a nasal foreign body, particularly in this age group. This condition is often misdiagnosed as sinusitis and treated (ineffectively) with antibiotics.

6. **(D)** The ECG shown demonstrates diffuse ST-segment elevation with upright T waves. These findings are typical of early pericarditis. Over the next few days, the ST elevation will resolve, and diffuse T-wave inversion is likely to develop. The ECG and clinical findings in this case are most consistent with a diagnosis of acute pericarditis. An echocardiogram may be useful for detection of pericardial effusion and evaluation of the risk of possible pericardial tamponade. Treatment of pericarditis usually involves the administration of nonsteroidal anti-inflammatory drugs (NSAIDs). Heparin and thrombolytic agents are contraindicated.

7. **(A)** Soft tissue imaging with either a CT or MRI is rarely indicated in a man with clinically localized prostate cancer unless the serum PSA at the time of diagnosis is > 25 ng/mL. A bone scan, but not a CT or MRI, could be performed in the setting of chronic back pain to rule out bone metastases.

8. **(C)** Dopamine agonists (bromocriptine, cabergoline, and occasionally pergolide) are the primary treatment of choice for prolactinomas (90% success), even those with chiasmal compression and visual compromise. With medical treatment, significant changes in visual fields can be noted in 24 to 72 hours. Surgery is not indicated unless medial therapy is unsuccessful, because surgery is associated with significant morbidities (7%) and a high rate of relapse (20 to 30%). Radiotherapy has a low success rate and results in an unacceptably high incidence (50 to 70%) of hypopituitarism.

9. **(A)** *N. gonorrhoeae* should be suspected in any teenager presenting with the clinical appearance of septic arthritis. Intracellular gram-negative diplococci are not seen in 30 to 50% of samples. Joint fluid and samples from the cervix, urethra, pharynx, and skin lesions, if present, should be cultured. *N. gonorrhoeae* septic arthritis responds readily to IV antibiotics. In difficult cases, repeated aspiration may be necessary. Surgical irrigation is usually unnecessary.

10. **(B)** In restrictive cardiomyopathy, the left ventricular chamber size is typically normal. Diastolic dysfunction is fundamental to this disease. Restrictive cardiomyopathy can be either primary (idiopathic hypereosinophilic syndromes) or secondary. Secondary causes are either infiltrative (e.g., amyloidosis, sarcoidosis, malignancies, etc.) or noninfiltrative (e.g., carcinoid heart disease, scleroderma, radiation).

11. **(C)** Diabetic foot infections can be perplexing clinical problems. They are frequently chronic and polymicrobial. It is sometimes difficult to sort out which organisms are actu-

ally responsible for causing infection and which are contaminants. This is why a swab sample should never be sent for culture. Plain films may not reveal the true extent of the disease and a sedimentation rate is not very specific as a diagnostic tool. The only way to make a true diagnosis of a diabetic foot infection or osteomyelitis is to perform an intraoperative biopsy for culture and histological study.

12. **(A)** Because the patient has a definite intrauterine pregnancy on ultrasound and no tissue has been passed, the diagnosis of incomplete abortion or ectopic pregnancy is incorrect. The cervix must be dilated to make the diagnosis of inevitable abortion, and missed abortion is diagnosed when there is definite evidence of fetal demise on ultrasound (or classically, no uterine growth over a 4-week period without passage of products of conception). At 6 weeks from the last menstrual period, especially with a "quick" exam, a fetal heartbeat may not be definitely seen. One in four to five women has the vaginal bleeding in the first weeks of pregnancy that defines threatened abortion. About 50% of these women will eventually go on to miscarry.

13. **(D)** The history, exam, and beta hCG levels are all consistent with a completed spontaneous abortion. Surgical intervention is rarely needed when there is a history of passage of tissue with subsequent relief of cramps and decreased bleeding, as well as falling hCG levels. The history and exam and ED ultrasound also all make ectopic pregnancy (which would be diagnosed at laparoscopy or treated with methotrexate) a very unlikely diagnosis.

14. **(B)** If the mother is Rh negative, she should be given Anti-D immune globulin within 72 hours after miscarriage to decrease her chance of Rh sensitization. Up to 2% of Rh-negative women who have a spontaneous abortion become sensitized when Anti-D immune globulin is not administered. This sensitization is almost eliminated with adminis-

tration of Anti-D. While rubella antibody and HBsAg are part of initial prenatal testing, their results are unlikely to have immediate clinical impact. A 1-hour 50-g GTT is used to screen for gestational diabetes in later pregnancy and is not necessary in this setting.

15. **(D)** Society, as well as the medical profession, frequently minimizes the grief felt by parents, particularly mothers, when an early pregnancy is lost. It is important to anticipate and acknowledge the patient's grief and possible guilt in a supportive fashion and to reassure the patient that while the cause of many miscarriages is unknown, such things as intercourse, stress, anger, or prior elective abortion have *not* been shown to be associated with early pregnancy loss.

16. **(C)** Especially after the birth of two normal children, women between 20 and 30 have an 80 to 90% chance of delivering a viable baby with their next pregnancy after a spontaneous abortion.

17. **(A)** A prostate biopsy performed via transrectal ultrasound guidance is indicated in any adult male with an elevated serum PSA level or with the finding of an abnormal prostate nodule on DRE. The other options may represent signs of a urinary tract problem but would not be evaluated with a prostate biopsy, at least initially.

18. **(D)** Serum PSA levels have not been shown to change relative to the performance of a DRE. The other options include various methods for calculating and measuring PSA that have been demonstrated to improve the diagnostic accuracy of the test. Currently, the ratio of free to total PSA appears to offer improved diagnostic utility.

19. **(C)** A variety of genetic defects of ion channels lead to prolonged QT intervals. Penetrance is variable. Treatment includes beta blockers and implantable defibrillators. The latter should be done in this patient with syncope because of the history of syncope and the risk of death related to torsade de

pointes. The presentation of syncope with fright or exertion is consistent with long QT syndrome. Brugada syndrome and WPW syndrome can be associated with syncope and positive family histories for sudden death but have characteristic ECG patterns not seen here.

20. **(A)** The woman's symptoms are suggestive of bereavement, which is characterized by grief and sadness and may be accompanied by other symptoms of depression, including poor appetite, weight loss, and insomnia, following the death of a loved one. The diagnosis of major depression is not considered unless the symptoms have been present more than 2 months following the loss or in the presence of other symptoms that are not characteristic of normal grief.

21. **(B)** The patient has abnormalities consistent with vWF disease type I, which is the most common inherited bleeding disorder. It results from a qualitative or quantitative abnormality of vWF. The best therapy for mild vWF is to administer DDAVP, which stimulates the vascular endothelium to release larger multimers of vWF that are hemostatically effective. FFP is not used to treat vWF. Factor VIII is generally not used to treat vWF, although there are some new preparations rich in vWF (Humate-P). The cryoprecipitate fraction of plasma is often used for patients who are refractory to DDAVP or who have more severe disease. There is also a risk of viral infection with cryoprecipitate.

22. **(E)** It is very important to know what happens to this patient's glucose at 3:00 A.M., because he could have either Somogyi or Dawn phenomenon. In Somogyi phenomenon, hypoglycemia at 2:00 to 3:00 A.M. results in rebound hyperglycemia in the morning, due to counterregulatory hormone response. This will happen more if the evening NPH is taken at dinnertime, leading to a peak at 2:00 to 3:00 A.M. with resultant hypoglycemia. Moving NPH to bedtime will solve the problem. In Dawn phenomenon, morning hyperglycemia is not the consequence of 2:00 to

3:00 A.M. hypoglycemia. Glucose levels at 2:00 to 3:00 A.M. are normal. The treatment is to increase bedtime NPH. The best way to differentiate between both conditions is to ask your patient to check a 2:00 to 3:00 A.M. glucose (right answer in this case).

23. **(B)** He has chronic symptoms, which makes pulmonary embolus and pneumothorax unlikely. He also has no physical signs of CHF and no classic symptoms for angina. The most likely diagnosis is COPD.

24. **(C)** In patients with COPD, oxygen therapy and stopping smoking are the only treatments that have a survival benefit.

25. **(B)** Pulmonary function testing reveals a characteristic pattern in obstructive pulmonary diseases: decreased forced expiratory volume (FEV_1) and forced vital capacity (FVC) and decreased FEV_1/FVC ratio.

26. **(D)** Inhaled corticosteroids have shown no significant improvement in FEV_1 or survival in multiple large, randomized studies.

27. **(E)** This finding is almost pathognomic for necrotizing otitis externa, which is frequently seen in diabetics and immunocompromised patients. This condition is a medical emergency and should be treated with IV antibiotics and debridement.

28. **(A)** This clinical scenario represents a classic case of Guillain–Barré syndrome. When this diagnosis is suspected, neurology consultation is needed. Findings on LP help to support the diagnosis. Peripheral nerve conduction velocity (PNCV) testing is also very helpful but seldom available while the patient is in the ED. Progressive weakness of the respiratory muscles can lead to respiratory failure and death. Vital capacity (VC) measurements are far more sensitive than ABGs in the detection of respiratory failure associated with Guillain–Barré syndrome. As a rule of thumb, those patients with a measured VC of < 10 to 15 cc/kg need mechanical ventilatory assistance.

29. **(C)** Actinic keratoses are sun-induced precancerous lesions of the skin seen most comonly in elderly patients with fair skin. A small percentage of actinic keratoses progress to squamous cell carcinoma if left untreated.

30. **(D)** Treatment of arthritis patients with *more* than one NSAID or an NSAID plus corticosteroids, as well as treatment with a single NSAID in patients with a history of ulcers, constitutes higher-risk scenarios. Prednisone treatment without an NSAID, methotrexate, and history of a Mallory–Weiss tear are not risk factors.

31. **(E)** Persons with IgA deficiency and HLA-DR3 are at increased risk for celiac disease. Antigliadin and antiendomysial antibody levels usually are present and elevated in persons with celiac disease. Mild liver function test abnormalities are not unusual in persons with active celiac disease. An elevated serum gastrin level would very rarely be found in persons with celiac disease and pernicious anemia.

32. **(B)** Two or more of the following four criteria establish a diagnosis of Wegener's granulomatosis: (1) abnormal urinary sediment, (2) abnormal findings on chest x-ray, (3) oral ulcers or nasal discharge, (4) granulomatous inflammation on biopsy.

33. **(A)** The history and physical findings presented are most consistent with subluxation of the radial head, also known as "nursemaid's elbow," a common entity in children most often between the ages of 1 and 4 years. This is seldom seen beyond 7 years of age. Given a typical history and physical findings, reduction can be attempted without x-rays. If this is successful, radiography is not needed. This is a common childhood injury and by itself not commonly associated with child abuse. Reduction is usually very quick and minimally painful not requiring conscious sedation. Supracondylar fractures also occur commonly in childhood but in most cases are associated with significant edema, deformity,

and much more pain than radial head sub-luxation.

34. **(E)** Puncture wound to the distal digital pulp is the most common cause of a felon. Treatment is side-to-side, through-and-through incision and drainage of the abscess plus antibiotic treatment.

35. **(B)** This is a frequent problem in patients with Down syndrome, and aggressive extension of the neck can force the odontoid process into the spinal cord, with catastrophic neurologic complications.

36. **(B)** This illustrates typical neovascularization of the optic disc.

37. **(E)** Immediate laser photocoagulation surgery is indicated in patients with high-risk proliferative diabetic retinopathy. Laser photocoagulation surgery has been proven to be of benefit in reducing the risk of visual loss and blindness in patients with high-risk proliferative diabetic retinopathy such as disc neovascularization.

38–41. **(38-C, 39-D, 40-E, 41-A)** The patient described gives a classic description of multiple attacks separated by time and space (within the nervous system). These localize to the right optic nerve, left subcortical white matter, and a new lesion in the spinal cord. With the classic MRI appearance of subcortical white matter lesions oriented perpendicular to the ventricles and more peripherally oriented white matter lesions, a diagnosis of multiple sclerosis may be confirmed.

Early intervention with an immunomodulatory agent such as interferon or glutarimir acetate is now recommended to decrease the number of exacerbations and to decrease long-term disability due to disease progression. Steroid therapy will not have this effect and is of limited benefit when an individual attack is either mild or recovering.

Cyclobenzaprine is a muscle relaxant that will have no effect on the spasticity seen in upper motor neuron disease.

A short course of intravenous methyl-prednisolone will not change the eventual disability caused by an individual attack but can shorten duration and lessen the severity. It will have no effect on future attacks and will not decrease the number of MRI lesions (though it can resolve the gadolinium enhancement seen in more active MRI lesions).

42. **(A)** Procainamide is a class Ia antiarrhythmic that can be used to treat atrial or ventricular arrhythmias. It suppresses phase-4 depolarization in normal ventricular muscle and Purkinje fibers. It reduces the automaticity of ectopic pacemakers. Procainamide is useful in treatment of reentry since it slows intraventricular conduction. Because of its electrophysiologic effect, it prolongs the QT interval and may put the patient at risk for torsade de pointes. Because of this and its unfavorable side effect profile, it is not used often to treat atrial fibrillation.

43. **(D)** Growth of a particular bone ends when the chondrocytes of the physis cease dividing. A fracture across a physis can lead to the formation of a bony bar that will tether growth resulting in an angular deformity if occurring at a young age.

44. **(E)** This man has Wernicke's encephalopathy, which is characterized by delirium, ataxia, and ophthalmoplegia and can develop during alcohol withdrawal. It is due to the effects of thiamine deficiency. Therefore, it must be treated immediately with IM or IV thiamine to prevent persistent memory impairment. Glucose should not be given to a chronic alcoholic before the administration of thiamine because of the risk of precipitating an acute Wernicke's encephalopathy.

45. **(B)** The current risk of hepatitis C is 1/300 units of blood transfused. The risk of hepatitis B is 1/200,000 and HIV is 1/225,000. The major risk of HIV transmission is now limited to the "window" between initial viral exposure and the development of seropositivity averaging about 6 weeks. Blood transfusions are associated with long-term immunosuppressive effects, and because of this, a num-

ber of stuides have been done to determine whether there is an increased risk of developing tumors after transfusions. No association to date has been demonstrated. However, the tumors most strongly implicated are NHL and renal cell, melanoma not being one of these. *Trypanosoma cruzi*, the etiologic agent of Chagas' disease can be transmitted by blood transfusion by 15 to 20%. Transfusion related lung injury is rare and caused by the presence of antileukocyte antibodies in donor plasma.

46. **(A)** Cervical neoplasia is not familial in its pathophysiology, and thus the fact that her mother had cervical cancer is unrelated. It is a sexually transmitted infection and, as such, is related to risk factors for STIs. These include early age at first intercourse, multiple sexual partners, and venereal warts. Smoking has also been implicated as an associated factor in the development of cervical cancer. *(Beckmann, 514)*

47. **(B)** HPV is thought to be most closely associated with the process of cervical neoplasia, although it may not be a direct carcinogen itself. Although herpes simplex virus type 2 (HSV-2) was thought to be the associated pathogen in previous studies, it is not considered to be the direct cause of cervical neoplasia. The other pathogens are STIs but are not associated with the development of cervical neoplasia. *(Beckmann, 514)*

48. **(C)** Colposcopy would be the next most appropriate step in the workup of this patient. Although it is not immediately necessary as a result of the findings on colposcopy, a cone biopsy may be indicated for further diagnosis. Cryotherapy or the LEEP procedure may be used in the treatment of cervical dysplasia as well. Hysterectomy may be performed in the treatment of severe dysplasia or for carcinoma in situ. *(Beckmann, 519)*

49. **(E)** Approximately 95% of squamous intraepithelial neoplasia occurs within the transformation zone. *(Beckmann, 520)*

50. **(A)** Following colposcopy and appropriate treatment, if necessary, the patient should be advised to follow up with a repeat Pap smear in 3 months, and at 3-month intervals for the first year and 6-month intervals during the second year. The Pap should be done as usual on the endocervix and the exocervix. The vaginal cuff Pap is applicable only in women who have undergone a hysterectomy, which would not be the treatment in this case. Endometrial biopsy is the diagnostic test performed for endometrial cancer evaluation. *(Beckmann, 522)*

Practice Test 7
Questions

DIRECTIONS: (Questions 1 through 50): Each of the numbered items or incomplete statements in this section is followed by answers or by completions of the statement. Select the ONE lettered answer or completion that is BEST in each case.

1. A 23-year-old man with a previous history of mental illness states, "I am tormented by witches and I think they are spying on me. I couldn't sleep because they are watching me with a monitor." Which of the following is contraindicated?

   (A) olanzapine (Zyprexa)
   (B) risperidone (Risperdal)
   (C) ziprasidone (Geodon)
   (D) quetiapine (Seroquel)

2. All of the following are causes of chronic cough EXCEPT

   (A) angiotensin-converting enzyme (ACE) inhibitor
   (B) postnasal drip syndrome
   (C) asthma
   (D) gastroesophogeal reflux
   (E) all of the above

3. A common side effect of niacin is flushing related to vasodilation following the initial niacin dose. This response can be reduced by adding

   (A) naloxone
   (B) misoprostol
   (C) aspirin
   (D) cimetidine

4. Bone mineral density is graded according to T and Z scores, which describe the person under consideration in relation to peers. Which of the following statements is true?

   (A) Z scores describe the relationship of a given person to peak bone mass.
   (B) Z scores are used to define osteoporosis.
   (C) T scores describe the relationship of a given person to peak bone mass.
   (D) T scores of less than –3 define osteoporosis.
   (E) Z scores between –1 and –3 define osteopenia.

5. An immunocompromised patient admitted to the hospital with disseminated varicella-zoster should be placed in which type of isolation?

   (A) contact
   (B) airborne
   (C) standard precautions alone
   (D) droplet
   (E) airborne and contact

Items 6–8

A 33-year-old G2P1001 woman presents to your delivery room in active labor at 39 weeks. She has a history of genital herpes proven by culture prior to this pregnancy. She notes characteristic burning in her vulvar area for the last 24 hours, similar to that which she feels before a herpes outbreak. On vaginal exam her membranes are intact and her cervix is 6 cm dilated, with the fetal vertex at 0 station. You cannot see any lesions on her external genitalia or on speculum exam. Her pregnancy has been otherwise uncomplicated, and she has no medical problems.

6. Immediate management should include

   (A) intravenous (IV) maternal administration of acyclovir

   (B) preparations for vaginal delivery

   (C) amniocentesis to look for evidence of amniotic viral infection

   (D) cesarean section immediately

7. A few hours after her healthy baby is delivered, this patient develops her usual left vulvar lesions. She wants to know if she can safely breast feed her baby. You tell her that

   (A) she should be glad that she was lucky enough to have a healthy baby and she should not press her luck by breast feeding

   (B) she should be kept away from the baby completely until her lesions have healed

   (C) the herpesvirus is transmitted by direct contact with a lesion and that as long as they are limited to her vulvar lesions and she uses good hand washing after any personal contact with her lesions she can safely breast feed and otherwise bond with her baby

   (D) breast feeding is contraindicated for mothers who have genital herpes

8. The same patient returns to your care for her next pregnancy. She wants to know whether she should plan on having a cesarean section for her current pregnancy since she wants to be sure that this baby doesn't get herpes. You advise her that

   (A) since she has a history of herpes she may as well always have a cesarean section

   (B) she can take suppressive antiviral therapy throughout her pregnancy and this will eliminate all chance of recurrence

   (C) a cesarean section should not be performed based solely on the history of herpes in asymptomatic women

   (D) since her last baby didn't get herpes she does not need to worry about this problem in pregnancy again, no matter what her condition is at the time of labor

END OF SET

9. A 23-year-old woman is seen in the gynecology clinic complaining of left-sided lower abdominal pain for about 2 days. She is sexually active and admits to unprotected intercourse the week prior to presentation. On exam she appears ill and has a temperature of 40° C (104° F), heart rate of 125 bpm, and her abdomen is tender with rebound in the left lower quadrant (LLQ). On pelvic exam she has cervical motion tenderness, and discharge is seen in the cervical os. Her white blood count (WBC) is 18,000/mm^3. What is the most appropriate management plan for this patient?

   (A) Give her an injection of ceftriaxone and have her follow up in a week.

   (B) Give her an injection of ceftriaxone and oral doxycycline, and have her return in 7 days for an ultrasound.

   (C) Schedule her for an outpatient ultrasound and wait for the results before treating.

   (D) Admit her for IV antibiotics and ultrasound.

10. A 43-year-old woman comes to your office for preoperative evaluation before surgery with general anesthesia to remove a potentially malignant ovarian cyst. She tells you that she was in a car accident 4 months ago and had a major cerebral contusion, which was treated with dexamethasone 4 mg every 6 hours for 4 weeks, with subsequent taper. She has been off steroids for at least 2

months. What step would you take in treating this patient?

(A) Order an insulin tolerance test.

(B) Check cortisol and adrenocorticotropic hormone (ACTH) levels.

(C) Do a cosyntropin stimulation test.

(D) Test 24-hour urine free cortisol.

(E) Give stress-dose hydrocortisone perioperatively.

11. A 40-year-old man of Italian descent is seen for a routine physical and found to have a hematocrit of 35%, a mean corpuscular volume (MCV) of 63 fL, a WBC of 6,800/μL, a reticulocyte count of 0.4%, and a platelet count of 270,000/μL. His stool is negative for occult blood. What would be the most effective way of confirming the diagnosis?

(A) glucose-6-phosphate dehydrogenase (G6PD) screen

(B) measure iron, ferritin, total iron-binding capacity (TIBC)

(C) hemoglobin A_2 level

(D) peripheral smear

12. A 36-year-old African-American man with a history of human immunodeficiency virus (HIV) for 8 years and poor compliance with medications with a history of opportunistic infection presents to psych emergency service stating, "I need to find my apartment and I lost my address." The patient states that he just came here to get the address. He is alert, awake, and oriented to place and person, and his judgment is poor. He scored 22/33 on the Mini-Mental Status Exam (MMSE). Toxicology is normal including alcohol. What is the likely diagnosis?

(A) alcohol intoxication

(B) Pick's disease

(C) multivascular dementia

(D) HIV dementia

(E) Alzheimer's dementia

13. The history most suggestive of a malignant bone tumor is

(A) gradually increasing pain awakening the patient

(B) nocturnal pain relieved with ibuprofen

(C) intermittent pain of several years' duration

(D) leg pain at night relieved by sitting up and hanging the leg over the side of the bed

14. A 64-year-old smoker is admitted to the hospital with mental status changes. His physical exam is unremarkable other than a Glasgow Coma Scale (GCS) score of 9. His bloodwork reveals: Na 117, Cl 108, HCO$_3$ 26, and K 4.8. Chest radiograph reveals a 4 × 4-cm right suprahilar mass. Computed tomography (CT) of the abdomen reveals multiple lesions in the liver. What is the most likely diagnosis?

(A) carcinoid

(B) mesothelioma

(C) adenocarcinoma

(D) small cell carcinoma

(E) none of the above

15. A 23-year-old man comes to your office stating, "My parents are worried about my behavior. I don't want to be in a relationship, and I don't have any friends. I stay at home and watch television and surf the Internet. Also, I haven't had sex in my life and I don't have any desire. My parents are worried about me and they asked me to come see the psychiatrist. I feel like nothing's wrong with me and I don't know why they are worried." The most likely diagnosis is

(A) schizoid

(B) borderline

(C) narcissistic

(D) dependent

16. Honey should not be fed to infants for fear of

    (A) AIDS
    (B) botulism
    (C) diabetes
    (D) *Salmonella*
    (E) *Campylobacter*

17. A 37-year-old insulin-dependent diabetic woman sustained a nondisplaced fracture of the neck of the talus due to a twisting injury. She presents 6 months later with a rocker-bottom deformity of the foot, midfoot pain, and swelling. There is no history of skin ulcer, puncture wound, or any other trauma. Her latest lateral foot x-ray is shown in Figure 7.1. The most likely diagnosis is

    (A) osteomyelitis
    (B) missed fracture second metatarsal base with later dislocation of the forefoot
    (C) neuropathic arthropathy
    (D) none of the above

18. A 55-year-old male smoker presents to your office with progressive dyspnea over the past month. Physical exam reveals decreased breath sounds in the right base, dullness to percussion, no egophany, and decreased fremitus. Physical examination is consistent with

    (A) lobar consolidation
    (B) pneumothorax
    (C) pleural effusion

    (D) pulmonary fibrosis
    (E) none of the above

Items 19–21

19. A 32-year-old woman with infrequent migraine headaches that have not required therapy presents to the ED with a 12-hour history of her typical migraine characterized by right-sided throbbing pain, nausea, vomiting, and loss of peripheral vision bilaterally. Her neck is supple, CT scan of the head is normal, and a pregnancy test is negative. Your recommended therapeutic option is

    (A) meperidine
    (B) propranolol
    (C) verapamil
    (D) sumatriptan
    (E) diazepam

20. The patient returns to your office asking for therapy to prevent further migraines, which are now occurring twice per month. Which of the following medications will be useful for this purpose?

    (A) acetaminophen/caffeine/butalbital
    (B) propranolol
    (C) sumatriptan tablets
    (D) oxycodone
    (E) ergotamine

21. The patient has another severe migraine requiring a visit to the ED for parenteral therapy. She now asks you for suggestions for acute therapy she may use at home. All of the following medications may prove effective EXCEPT

    (A) rizatriptan sublingual therapy
    (B) zolmitriptan tablet
    (C) dihydroergotamine nasal spray
    (D) sumatriptan subcutaneous injection
    (E) acetaminophen/caffeine/butalbital

END OF SET

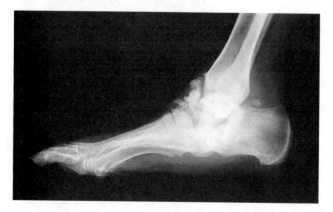

Figure 7.1

Items 22–25

A 58-year-old man with diabetes and hypertension presents to the ED with his first generalized seizure. The family tells you that the seizure lasted 1 minute and was preceded by a head turn to the left and eye deviation to the left. His exam currently demonstrates a mild left hemiparesis but normal mentation. He weighs 80 kg and is a long-time smoker. His blood glucose is 90, and all other routine laboratory values in the ED are normal. A CT scan with contrast is obtained (Figure 7.2A, B).

22. The most likely etiology of his seizure is

    (A) cerebral infarction
    (B) metastatic cancer
    (C) primary cerebral neoplasm
    (D) hypoglycemia
    (E) herpes simplex encephalitis

23. Your immediate management of his seizure in the ED should be

    (A) IV diazepam
    (B) 200 mg IV phenytoin
    (C) mechanical ventilation
    (D) A and C
    (E) none of the above

24. Of the following primary neoplasms, the one least likely to metastatize to the brain is

    (A) lung
    (B) breast
    (C) prostate
    (D) melanoma
    (E) renal cell

25. Assume that the 58-year-old patient described above is brought to the ED by his family after having intermittent seizures as above for the past 20 minutes without regaining consciousness. Your preferred immediate therapy should be

    (A) diazepam
    (B) lorazepam
    (C) phenytoin
    (D) phenobarbital
    (E) pancuronium

END OF SET

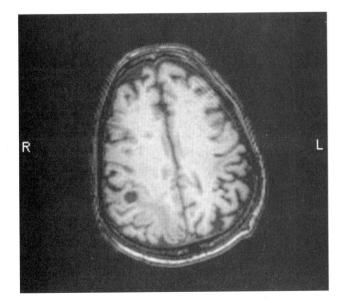 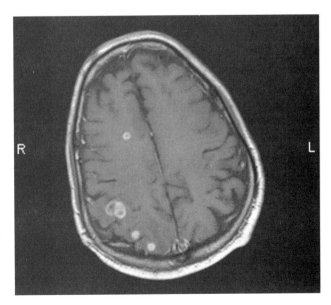

Figure 7.2 A and B

26. Which of the following antibiotics would be the safest to administer in someone with a previous anaphylactic reaction to penicillin?

    (A) cefazolin
    (B) aztreonam
    (C) imipenem
    (D) nafcillin

27. Which of the following is most characteristic of multiple endocrine neoplasia type 2B (MEN 2B) syndrome?

    (A) medullary thyroid carcinoma, thyroid carcinoma
    (B) medullary thyroid carcinoma, pheochromocytoma
    (C) parathyroid adenoma, thyroid carcinoma
    (D) parathyroid hyperplasia, thyroid carcinoma
    (E) medullary thyroid carcinoma, paraganglioma

28. A 24-year-old woman is seen for frequent urinary tract infections. The patient's symptoms improve following antibiotic therapy. However, she has become frustrated with the need for frequent courses of treatment. Her symptoms often occur following sexual intercourse. Appropriate recommendations now include

    (A) minimizing sexual activity
    (B) initiation of prophylactic antibiotic therapy, either postcoital or on a self-administered basis
    (C) radiologic evaluation of the urinary tract
    (D) administration of spermicidal jelly during intercourse

29. What percentage of men and women over the age of 65 have asymptomatic bacteriuria?

    (A) 5%
    (B) 10 to 20%
    (C) 30 to 40%
    (D) > 50%
    (E) there is no such entity as asymptomatic bacteriuria

30. Which of the following are the technique and pathophysiology of the Sestamibi scan for parathyroid localization?

    (A) The patient is given two radionuclide substances and scanned twice—once for initial uptake and once after "washout."
    (B) The patient is given two radionuclide substances and scanned twice; the results of the two scans are "subtracted" to identify the parathyroid tissue.
    (C) The patient is given a radionuclide that is taken up only by parathyroid tissue.
    (D) The patient is given radionuclide-labeled calcium, which concentrates in the parathyroid tissue.
    (E) The patient is given a radionuclide that is taken up by mitochrondria in both parathyroid and cardiac tissue.

31. A 30-year-old white man presents with no ocular complaints. His review of systems is negative. He denies any exposure to HIV. He is on no medications. His family history is negative. Ocular examination reveals retinal hemorrhages. Differential diagnosis includes

    (A) syphilis
    (B) HIV-associated retinopathy
    (C) Lyme disease
    (D) all of the above
    (E) none of the above

32. Each of the following statements regarding elderly patients presenting to the ED with abdominal pain is true EXCEPT

    (A) Approximately 10% of patients > 70 years of age presenting to the ED for evaluation of abdominal pain are ultimately found to have a vascular etiology (mesenteric ischemia, leaking/ruptured abdominal aortic aneurysm, or acute myocardial infarction).
    (B) Bloody diarrhea and pain out of proportion to tenderness in an elderly patient is most likely due to antibiotic-associated colitis associated with *Clostridium difficile*.

(C) Morbidity and mortality associated with acute abdominal pain is similar to that associated with acute chest pain in the elderly.

(D) The majority of elderly patients with acute cholecystitis and appendicitis are afebrile despite higher rates of perforation and sepsis compared to younger patients.

33. All of the following are true regarding alcoholic liver disease EXCEPT

(A) women are at greater risk compared to men

(B) chronic alcohol ingestion lessens the risk of acetaminophen toxicity

(C) Mallory bodies may be seen on liver biopsy

(D) aspartate transaminase (AST) levels and alanine transaminase (ALT) levels usually are < 300

(E) central vein fibrosis on liver biopsy carries a bad prognosis

34. A 22-year-old female student from Nigeria moves to Minnesota. Within weeks, she develops episodic, loose, multiple small stools as well as abdominal bloating. She denies fever, weight loss, gastrointestinal bleeding, abdominal pain, rash, joint symptomatology, or oral ulcers. Her physical exam, complete blood count, liver function tests, stool cultures for bacteria, stool exam for occult blood, stool for ova and parasites, and a flexible sigmoidoscopy are all normal or negative. Which of the following is the most likely diagnosis?

(A) diverticular disease

(B) endometriosis

(C) right-sided colon cancer

(D) lactose intolerance

(E) irritable bowel syndrome

35. What is the primary mechanism of action of retinoids in acne therapy?

(A) normalize follicular hyperkeratinization

(B) decrease sebaceous gland activity

(C) provide an anti-inflammatory effect

(D) reduce *Propionibacterium acnes* proliferation

36. Each of the following statements regarding thoracic trauma is correct EXCEPT

(A) the overall mortality rate due to thoracic trauma is about 10%

(B) thoracic trauma accounts for ~25% of all trauma-related deaths in North America

(C) < 10% of patients with blunt trauma to the chest will require thoracotomy

(D) most patients with penetrating chest trauma will require thoracotomy

37. A patient has a history of recurrent facial paralysis affecting both sides at different times, with associated recurrent edema of the face and lips, and a furrowed tongue. What is the most likely diagnosis?

(A) Mobius syndrome

(B) Heerfordt syndrome

(C) Guillain–Barré syndrome

(D) Melkersson–Rosenthal syndrome

(E) pseudobulbar palsy

38. A 23 month old is brought to the pediatricians office by the mother who is concerned about a rash on the child's face. The child has a temperature of 38.8° C (101.8° F), and the cheeks appear to have been slapped; there is also a lacy reticular rash that covers the back. You diagnose the child and tell the mother that she and other adults in the house are likely to develop what symptoms if infected also?

(A) the same rash as the child

(B) aplastic anemia

(C) aseptic meningitis

(D) transient arthralgias

39. A 52-year-old man is admitted with atypical pneumonia. He is dyspneic and has a non-productive cough. Chest x-ray reveals bilateral patchy infiltrates described as "ovoid densities." He tells you he is a hunter and has recently had an ulcerated lesion on his hand. You suspect

   (A) tuberculosis
   (B) tularemia
   (C) typhoid
   (D) tetanus

Items 40–41

40. A 24-year-old G1P1 nonsmoker is 2 days postpartum and complains of sudden-onset dyspnea and left pleuritic chest pain. What treatment would you recommend?

   (A) ceftriaxone IV
   (B) warm compresses
   (C) antidepressant
   (D) heparin
   (E) oral amoxicillin

41. What test should you order?

   (A) chest radiograph
   (B) electrocardiogram
   (C) echocardiogram
   (D) pulmonary angiogram
   (E) ventilation–perfusion scan

END OF SET

42. National Institutes of Health (NIH) consensus criteria for surgical intervention in the treatment of asymptomatic primary hyperparathyroidism include all the following EXCEPT

   (A) calcium more than 1.0 mg/dL greater than upper limit of normal
   (B) kidney stones
   (C) age < 50
   (D) 24-hour urine calcium > 200 mg/day
   (E) osteoporosis

43. A 25-year-old man falls on his outstretched hand, sustaining injury to the wrist as shown in Figure 7.3. These views were made 4 weeks postinjury. His injuries can be described as

   (A) fractures of the distal radius, ulna styloid, and lunate
   (B) fractures of the distal radius, ulna styloid, and hamate
   (C) fractures of the distal radius, ulna styloid, and scaphoid
   (D) fractures of the distal radius, ulna styloid, and lunate with avascular necrosis of the proximal pole of the lunate
   (E) fractures of the distal radius, ulna styloid, and scaphoid with avascular necrosis of the proximal pole of the scaphoid

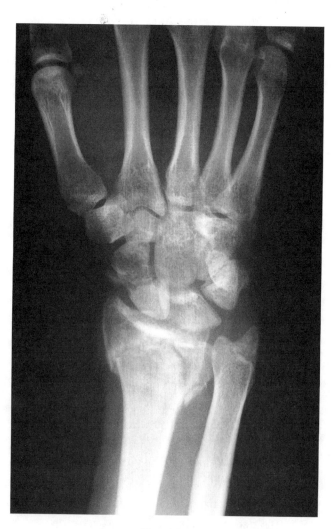

Figure 7.3

44. Patients with atrial fibrillation at risk for stroke should be anticoagulated. Which of the following statements is true?

   (A) Aspirin 325 mg daily is adequate protection in most patients.
   (B) Patients with atrial fibrillation should maintain an international normalized ratio (INR) of 1.5 to 2.5.
   (C) Patients with atrial fibrillation should maintain an INR of 2 to 3.
   (D) Patients with artificial heart valves may be advised to maintain an INR of 4 to 5.

45. Factors that impose a risk for stroke in patients with atrial fibrillation include all the following EXCEPT

   (A) chronic hypertension
   (B) recent history of heart failure
   (C) prior arterial thromboembolism
   (D) global left ventricular dysfunction
   (E) left atrial enlargement on echocardiogram
   (F) 50 years of age

46. A 68-year-old male smoker presents with recurrent pneumonia requiring multiple antibiotics. His lateral chest radiograph is shown in Figure 7.4 and is similar to multiple previous radiographs. What is the diagnosis?

   (A) pulmonary sequestration
   (B) mucoid impaction
   (C) bronchiectasis
   (D) right middle lobe syndrome
   (E) none of the above

Items 47–50

A 40-year-old G1P0010 woman presents to your office with a history of three years of gradually increasing chronic pelvic pain, which radiates to her back and down her anterior thigh, greater on the left than on the right. She denies fevers, chills, and vaginal discharge. She denies irregular menses and is not sexually active because of increasing dyspareunia on deep penetration. She has gotten no relief with nonsteroidal anti-inflammatory drugs

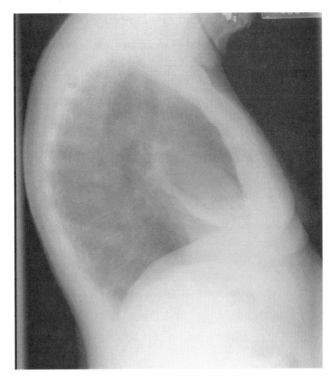

Figure 7.4

(NSAIDs) or oral contraceptives. Physical examination reveals a mildly tender, fixed, nonenlarged, retroverted uterus and slightly enlarged tender left adnexa. There is uterosacral nodularity on rectovaginal exam.

47. The next best step in the workup would be to

   (A) obtain a pelvic ultrasound
   (B) obtain a CA 125 level
   (C) perform an endometrial biopsy
   (D) obtain a serum beta hCG
   (E) do a Pap smear

48. The most likely pathophysiology here is

   (A) coelomic metaplasia
   (B) müllerian agenesis
   (C) bacterial dissemination
   (D) progesterone deficiency
   (E) retrograde menstruation

49. The gold standard of diagnosis would be

(A) endometrial glands, stroma, and hemo-siderin-laden macrophages on biopsy of peritoneal implants

(B) based on your physical exam findings

(C) secretory endometrium on endometrial biopsy

(D) demonstrated patency of the Fallopian tubes

(E) an elevated CA 125

50. The medical treatment of choice would be

(A) adriamycin

(B) gonadotropin-releasing hormone (GnRH) agonist therapy

(C) danazol therapy

(D) oral contraceptive therapy

(E) cisplatin

END OF SET

Practice Test 7
Answers and Explanations

1. **(C)** Geodon might cause QT interval prolongation.

2. **(E)** All are causes of chronic cough.

3. **(C)** Niacin (nicotinic acid) is a water-soluble vitamin. It can lower low-density lipoprotein (LDL) by 15 to 30% and raise high-density lipoprotein (HDL) by 10 to 30%. Flushing occurs in most patients, but most will accommodate to the drug. The use of aspirin 80 mg PO 30 minutes before the dose of niacin reduces flushing.

4. **(C)** Z scores define the patient in relation to age-matched controls; T scores define the relationship to peak bone mass. According to the World Health Organization, a T score of less than –2.5 defines osteoporosis; a T score between –1 and –2.5 defines osteopenia.

5. **(E)** Standard precautions with proper hand washing and personal protective equipment apply to all patients admitted to the hospital regardless of the diagnosis. Patients suspected of having tuberculosis are placed in respiratory isolation with negative pressure rooms and specially fitted respirator masks. Varicella may be spread via the airborne route in large droplets or by direct contact; therefore, these patients must be placed in contact as well as droplet isolation.

6. **(D)** The incidence of maternal to fetal transmission of herpes when the mother is having a recurrent infection is thought to be only about 3%. However, current management of a woman in labor with active genital herpes or prodrome of genital herpes is cesarean section to avoid direct fetal contact with the herpesvirus since fetal infection can be devastating.

7. **(C)** Unless the mother has lesions on her breast, she is unlikely to transmit the virus to her newborn as long as careful hand washing is observed.

8. **(C)** Antiviral therapy has not been shown to completely eliminate recurrence. There is no evidence that routine cesarean section for asymptomatic women with a history of herpes is of any benefit in the prevention of neonatal herpes infection. Outcome of a prior pregnancy has not been shown to affect future infection.

9. **(D)** The patient described in the vignette is presenting with pelvic inflammatory disease (PID). Some patients with mild PID may be treated as an outpatient with ceftriaxone and oral doxycycline or azithromycin. The initial event in PID is infection with *Neisseria gonorrhoeae* and or *Chlamydia trachomatis*. Any patient who is toxic appearing, pregnant, or cannot take oral medication must be admitted for inpatient parenteral antibiotics. Also, if there is any indication that the patient has an acute abdomen (e.g., tubo-ovarian abscess) or acute appendicitis cannot be ruled out, the patient must be admitted for further evaluation.

10. **(E)** Anyone who has received > 20 mg of prednisone a day (or > 2 mg of dexamethasone a day) for more than 3 weeks over the

past year should be assumed to have functional suppression of the hypothalamic–pituitary–adrenal (HPA) function; these patients do not need testing and should be treated with stress-dose steroids (100 mg of hydrocortisone intravenously every 8 hours) if exposed to a major stress, such as surgery. Patients who received between 10 and 20 mg of prednisone (or equivalent dose of other steroids) may have suppression of the HPA axis. There are two options to consider if these patients are scheduled to have surgery: Either give stress-dose steroids perioperatively or, if time permits, do a cosyntropin stimulation test (preferably low-dose: 1 μg. Cortisol, ACTH, and 24-hour urine free cortisol are not good tests of the HPA function. An insulin tolerance test is difficult to perform and carries some risk (e.g., hypoglycemia-induced seizures). After stopping steroids, the HPA axis can take up to 1 year to recover.

11. (C) The most likely cause of mild anemia in those of Mediterranean descent is beta-thalassemia trait. Assay of hemoglobin A_2 would show an increase in the level of this minor hemoglobin component. The peripheral smear would reveal microcytes with many target cells that are not pathognomonic of thalassemia. G6PD would be negative unless he inherited this disorder as well. Iron levels would rule out iron deficiency but would not necessarily help with the diagnosis.

12. (D) Development of acquired immune deficiency syndrome (AIDS) takes 8 to 10 years without treatment and noncompliance. Fifty percent of patients have neuropsychiatric complications. Alcohol is not the etiology because the toxicology is normal. Pick's disease presents with early behavioral changes. Alzheimer's and multivascular dementias are not likely due to his age.

13. (A) Night pain relieved with a nonsteroidal anti-inflammatory drug (NSAID) is common with an osteoid osteoma. Leg pain relieved by sitting up, and dangling the affected leg over the side of the bed is characteristic of peripheral vascular disease.

14. (D) Small cell carcinoma is a bronchogenic cancer and is the third most common. It is almost always associated with smoking, is often associated with paraneoplastic phenomena including the syndrome of inappropriate antidiuretic hormone (SIADH), and is commonly metastatic at presentation. Squamous cell carcinoma is the second most common lung cancer behind adenocarcinoma. Carcinoid and mesothelioma are both very rare tumors.

15. (A) Patients exhibit a pervasive pattern of development detachment from relationships. They lack a desire for relationships and prefer to be alone. They also don't enjoy bodily pleasure and sensory experiences, such as sexual relationships.

16. (B) Botulinal spores are found in raw honey and may germinate and produce toxin in a baby's immature intestine. Botulism is produced by toxins from *Clostridium botulinum,* resulting in descending paralysis, dysphagia, and diplopia.

17. (C) Neuropathic (Charcot) arthropathy often presents with severe joint destruction following a fairly minor injury. Insensitivity to pain is present, and electromyographic/nerve conduction velocity (EMG/NCV) studies often show a peripheral neuropathy. Periarticular calcifications are pathognomonic. The causes are multiple, with diabetes, spinal cord syrinx, and tertiary syphilis being the most common.

18. (C) Pleural effusion is associated with the above findings. Consolidation is also associated with decreased breath sounds and dullness to percussion; however, it usually has egophany and increased tactile fremitus. Pneumothorax and fibrosis are not associated with dullness to percussion.

19. (D) The ED provides an ideal setting for the first dose of subcutaneous sumatriptan, a serotonin inhibitor that may provide relief within 10 to 60 minutes of injection in 85% of patients. Hypertension and coronary artery vasospasm are potential side effects and

should be monitored for on initial injection. Opiates and benzodiazepines are useful only in promoting sleep, which in turn can relieve the migraine. Dihydroergotamine is a second parenteral medication that may quickly relieve the symptoms of migraine. An antiemetic such as metaclopramide should be coadministered to counteract its main side effect.

20. **(B)** Other than the beta blockers, the calcium channel blockers, selective serotonin reuptake inhibitor (SSRI) class of medications, and tricyclic antidepressants have shown efficacy in preventing migraine headaches. Meperidine is not an antimigraine medication and, along with opiates, has a potential for physical dependence. Both sumatriptan and ergotamine may be useful for acute treatment of migraine but should not be used as daily prophylactic therapy due to side effects.

21. **(E)** All of the other choices may have direct effect on the cause of migraine and may produce relief in minutes to a few hours. The medication marketed as Fioricet has no direct antimigraine action and can exert an effect via the barbiturate to produce drowsiness.

22–25. **(22-B, 23-E, 24-C, 25-B)** Cerebral neoplasm and cerebral infarction are the two most common etiologies of new-onset seizures in an older patient. The patient described here has had a focal seizure arising from the right hemisphere, and the new left hemiparesis is likely a postictal phenomenon (Todd's paralysis) and should resolve within 24 hours. The CT scan shown here is typical of metastatic brain cancer with other radiologic considerations, including multiple abcesses and other central nervous system (CNS) infections such as toxoplasmosis.

The loading dose of phenytoin is not 200 mg but rather 18 to 20 mg/kg. There is no role for the use of benzodiazapines or mechanical ventilation in a seizure patient who is not actively seizing or who is beginning to awaken.

Prostate cancer never (or almost never) spreads to brain parenchyma though it can cause neurologic symptoms by metastasizing to bone in the spine with secondary spinal cord compression. The other four primary neoplasms listed are also the four most common causes of metastatic brain cancer.

Status epilepticus is defined as either continuous seizure activity over more than 20 minutes or intermittent seizures without return of consciousness over the same time period. It is a medical emergency that requires immediate mechanical ventilation. Phenytoin may be effective but can be loaded no faster than 50 mg/min due to the risk of hypotension and bradycardia. Neuromuscular blockers should never be used in the treatment of seizures as they will mask the motor symptoms and not decrease the cerebral electrophysiologic seizure activity that causes the morbidity and mortality of status epilepticus. Lorazepam is preferred to diazepam because of its longer active half-life in the brain (6 to 8 hours compared to 15 to 20 minutes for diazepam).

26. **(B)** Cefazolin and nafcillin are both beta-lactam antibiotics that should be avoided. Cephalosporins may have up to a 20% chance of anaphylaxis in a patient with a history of penicillin allergy. Imipenem, a carbopenem, may also have a small chance of cross-reacting with beta-lactams. Aztreonam is a monobactem that will not cross-react and is safe to use in a penicillin-allergic patient.

27. **(B)** MEN 2B syndrome is characterized by pheochromocytoma, medullary carcinoma of the thyroid, and multiple mucosal neuromas.

28. **(B)** Postcoital therapy may reduce infections related to sexual intercourse, while the use of spermicidal jelly may actually increase the reinfection rates. Since urinary tract abnormalities are rare in women with routine bladder infections, a radiologic evaluation is unnecessary.

29. **(B)** Approximately 10 to 20% of men and women over the age of 65 have asymptomatic bacteriuria on routine urinalysis. This percentage may increase in nursing home patients, even in those without urethral catheters.

30. (E) The Sestamibi scan uses a technetium material, and scans are performed after cardiac uptake has already been washed out, leaving parathyroid tissue still concentrating the material.

31. (D) The presence of a single retinal hemorrhage in a young patient may be idiopathic in nature. However, the presence of multiple hemorrhages with no preceding history of any specific medical or physical problem requires that an appropriate workup be performed. This workup should include tests for syphilis, Lyme disease, and HIV. A negative history for HIV contact or venereal disease does not exclude these from the differential diagnosis. Obviously, the evaluation should include testing for hypertension, diabetes, and other systemic conditions that are associated with retinal hemorrhages.

32. (B) Elderly patients presenting to the ED for evaluation of abdominal pain should be approached with the same degree of concern we extend to patients being seen for chest pain. Absence of fever and minimal findings on exam do not exclude significant pathology. The combination of bloody diarrhea and pain out of proportion to physical findings in an elderly person indicates bowel ischemia until proven otherwise. Antibiotic-associated colitis may be a consideration among patients recently treated with antibiotics who present with diarrhea, but they usually do not have as much pain. "Constipation" should be considered as a final diagnosis of exclusion only after a careful workup.

33. (B) Chronic alcohol ingestion induces the cytochrome P-450 enzyme system and *increases* the risk of acetaminophen toxicity. Women are more prone to alcohol-related liver disease than men when matched for weight, body fat, and alcohol intake. Mallory bodies often are seen in alcohol-related hepatitis but can be seen in other conditions as well. AST often is greater than ALT, and both tend to be < 300 in alcohol-related liver disease. Central vein fibrosis does carry a poor prognosis.

34. (D) It is likely that her diet has changed, with more lactose and less fiber than in Nigeria. The intermittent nature of her symptomatology would favor lactose intolerance, common in persons from Africa, over irritable bowel syndrome. A trial of a lactose-free diet would most likely be helpful in confirming the clinical diagnosis. Her age, the evaluation to date, and her history do not suggest diverticulitis, endometriosis, or right-sided colon cancer.

35. (A) The principal pathogenic factor in acne vulgaris is an alteration from normal keratinization patterns, and retinoids are the most effective treatment modality targeting this abnormality.

36. (D) About 30% of patients who sustain penetrating trauma to the chest require thoracotomy. Generally accepted indications for thoracotomy following trauma to the chest include: (1) initial chest tube output > 20 cc/kg, (2) ongoing bleeding from the chest tube in excess of 7 cc/kg/hr, (3) increasing hemothorax seen on chest x-ray, (4) persistent hypotension despite blood transfusion after other causes of blood loss have been excluded, or (5) decompensation of the patient after initial response to resuscitation.

37. (D) This is the characteristic group of symptoms in Melkersson–Rosenthal syndrome.

38. (D) The classic presentation of parvovirus infection (fifth disease) in a child is a febrile illness with a lacy reticular rash on the trunk and limbs. The rash may also appear on the cheeks causing a "slapped cheek appearance." Adults are frequently asymptomatic with the exception of arthralgias and frank arthritis. Some patients (i.e., those with hematologic abnormalities) are at risk for developing aplastic anemia.

39. (D) Tularemia results from *Francisella tularensis,* usually found in animals. It is transmitted by insects or direct contact and results in an ulcerative lesion, lymphadenopathy, fever, or pneumonia.

40. (D) She has high pretest probability for pulmonary embolism, and empiric heparin should be started.

41. (E) A ventilation–perfusion (V/Q) scan is the most appropriate test with a high clinical pretest probability. A pulmonary angiogram is invasive and not indicated unless the less invasive tests are negative in the setting of intermediate V/Q scan with a medium to high clinical suspicion. A Doppler ultrasound of the legs, if positive, would obviate the need for any further testing.

42. (D) The consensus conference report recommends surgery if the patient meets all the criteria mentioned in the question, except 24-hour urine calcium, which should be > 400 mg/day (high risk of kidney stones); also included in the criteria is a declining renal function.

43. (E) Fractures of the scaphoid have a high incidence of avascular necrosis of the proximal fracture fragment. The major blood supply for the bone enters the distal pole or waist (middle) area in one third of patients. With disruption of the intraosseous supply to the proximal pole, avascular necrosis occurs. The distal pole is osteopenic on x-ray, indicating preservation of blood supply to that portion of the scaphoid. Calcium is absorbed from that portion of the bone in a response to disuse. The calcium content of the proximal pole is still normal, indicating a loss of blood supply.

44. (C) The INR is a measure of the time it takes for blood to clot. Blood clotting is caused by a series of over 13 chemical reactions that includes conversion of prothrombin to thrombin. A healthy person has an INR of 1.0. Aspirin alone for a patient with atrial fibrillation is inadequate protection. Warfarin therapy to maintain an INR of 2.0 to 3.0 is recommended in at-risk patients with atrial fibrillation.

45. (F) All the other factors are risk factors for stroke in patients with atrial fibrillation. Age alone does not become a risk factor for stroke until at least age 65. The recommendation for patients at risk of stroke with atrial fibrillation is an INR between 2.0 and 3.0.

46. (D) The chest radiograph is classic for right middle lobe syndrome, which is recurrent atelectasis of the right middle lobe frequently associated with adenopathy around the airway.

47. (A) This is a classic case presentation of endometriosis. There is increasing pelvic pain, with dyspareunia, and lack of relief with NSAIDs and oral contraceptives. As the disease progresses, there may be fixed uterine retroversion with uterosacral nodularity. Occasionally, there may be enlargement of one or both ovaries in the development of endometriomas. An ultrasound would be most helpful here to determine the presence of any ovarian pathology such as an endometrioma. A CA 125 level may be elevated in cases of moderate to severe endometriosis, although this is a nonspecific finding. An endometrial biopsy is not helpful to diagnose this disease. Finally, it is highly unlikely that this woman is pregnant given her history and the presence of endometriosis itself, which is often associated with infertility. A Pap smear should be done at all annual GYN exams, regardless of the symptomatology. *(Beckmann, 367–370)*

48. (E) Sampson's theory of retrograde menstruation is the most widely accepted theory of pathogenesis of endometriosis. Coelomic metaplasia, hematogenous dissemination, and lymphatic dissemination are the other less widely accepted theories. Bacterial dissemination is incorrect, as endometriosis is not an infectious process. Progesterone deficiency is the pathophysiology behind luteal phase defects and not directly associated with endometriosis. Müllerian agenesis is an extremely rare cause of endometriosis. *(Beckmann, 365–366)*

49. (A) The gold standard diagnosis of endometriosis lies in the histology of the implants themselves. The typical lesions are blue-black powder burn lesions characteristic of endometriosis. Histologically, the presence of endometrial glands, stroma, and hemosiderin-laden macrophages may be demonstrated. Although the disease can be suspected based on the findings from physical examination, it cannot be confirmed this way. Although CA 125 may be elevated in cases of advanced endometriosis, it may be elevated in other benign intra-abdominal gynecologic disease processes such as pelvic inflammatory disease (PID). Endometriosis cannot be demonstrated on routine uterine endometrial biopsy, but rather on biopsy of peritoneal implants. Fallopian tube patency does not indicate endometriosis. However, there may be tubal obstruction depending on the stage of the disease. *(Beckmann, 368–369)*

50. **(B)** Since endometriosis is classically an estrogen-dependent phenomenon, the drug treatment of choice is the GnRH agonists, which work by inducing a reversible menopausal state, thus resulting in low estrogen levels, causing the implants to shrivel up and become inactive. Although danazol has been used in the past, it is no longer used because of the masculinizing side effects. This particular patient was no longer responsive to the oral contraceptive (OC), and thus the OC would not be indicated in this case. Furthermore, there is a theoretical risk of worsening endometriosis, due to the estrogen component of the OC. Both cisplatin and adriamycin are chemotherapeutic agents used in the treatment of ovarian cancer and are not used in the treatment of benign disease such as endometriosis. *(Beckmann, 371–372)*

Practice Test 8
Questions

DIRECTIONS (Questions 1 through 50): Each of the numbered items or incomplete statements in this section is followed by answers or by completions of the statement. Select the ONE lettered answer or completion that is BEST in each case.

1. A patient is about to be started on topiramate. The patient should be warned about which of the following side effects?

    (A) eye pain and blurry vision
    (B) shortness of breath
    (C) rapid heartbeat
    (D) stiffness of joints
    (E) dysuria and frequent urination

2. A 72-year-old heavy smoker presents to the emergency department (ED) because of cough, shortness of breath, anorexia, and weight loss for the past few months. Physical examination shows a cachectic and lethargic man in mild respiratory distress and rhonchi in the right upper lobe. Laboratory studies show a serum calcium of 13 mg/dL (N: 8.5–10.5), serum phosphorus of 2.3 mg/dL (N: 2.5–4.5), serum creatinine of 1.8 mg/dL (N: 0.7–1.4), and blood urea nitrogen of 56 mg/dL (N: 10–26). A chest x-ray shows a 6-cm right hilar mass. Which of the following statements is true?

    (A) Patient's hypercalcemia is due to production of 1,25-hydroxyvitamin D by the lung mass.
    (B) The lung tumor is most likely small cell carcinoma.
    (C) Patient's hypercalcemia is due to bone resorption from metastases.

    (D) The immediate management should be pamidronate infusion.
    (E) Parathyroid hormone (PTH) levels should be suppressed.

3. A patient on clozapine should have his white blood count (WBC) checked

    (A) weekly for the first year only
    (B) weekly for the first 3 months only
    (C) weekly for the first 6 months and then monthly forever
    (D) weekly for the first 6 month and then every 2 weeks forever after 6 months

4. Clozapine needs to be discontinued when the WBC drops below

    (A) 3,000
    (B) 4,000
    (C) 5,000
    (D) 6,000

5. Plasmapheresis is indicated as management for

    (A) thrombotic stroke in sickle cell disease
    (B) asymptomatic patients with plasma cell dyscrasia and serum viscosity measurement greater than twice normal
    (C) dermatomyositis with an elevated creatine phosphokinase
    (D) myasthenia gravis in patients requiring ventilation

Items 6–7

A 49-year-old obese nonsmoking man presents to your office several days after a motor vehicle accident in which he fell asleep while driving home from work. You learn from his wife that he snores loudly at night. On examination he is 5'6", 280 lbs., has a blood pressure of 165/94, and has an S4; his lungs are clear, and there is 1+ pitting edema.

6. What is the most likely diagnosis?

    (A) restless legs syndrome

    (B) narcolepsy

    (C) obstructive sleep apnea (OSA)

    (D) common snoring

    (E) none of the above

7. What test would you perform next?

    (A) overnight oximetry

    (B) Epworth Sleepiness Scale

    (C) polysomnogram

    (D) arterial blood gas

    (E) echocardiogram

END OF SET

8. A 2-year-old female is brought to the ED with a 2-day history of fever and refusal to bear weight on her left leg. On examination, the left hip is extremely irritable. Peripheral WBC is 20,000/mm³, and an anteroposterior (AP) pelvic x-ray shows a slight widening of the left hip joint space. The left hip is aspirated under fluoroscopy, and the aspirate contains 100,000 WBC/mm³. No organisms are seen on Gram stain. The most appropriate treatment is

    (A) emergent open irrigation and gram-positive and gram-negative IV antibiotic coverage pending culture results

    (B) repeated hip joint aspiration and IV antibiotics pending culture results

    (C) light skin traction and observation assuming this is a viral synovitis of the hip

    (D) oral antibiotics and an appointment to be seen in the pediatrician's office the next day

Items 9–10

A 67-year-old man with a history of hypertension comes to the ED after an episode of searing chest pain radiating to his back. His blood pressure is 170/90 and his pulse is 90.

9. All of the following diagnostic tests may be of use in evaluating the patient with a suspected dissecting aortic aneurysm EXCEPT

    (A) electrocardiogram (ECG)

    (B) echocardiogram

    (C) magnetic resonance imaging (MRI)

    (D) computed tomography (CT)

    (E) cardiac catheterization

    (F) chest x-ray (CXR)

    (G) exercise stress test

10. Acute therapy for this patient might include all of the following EXCEPT

    (A) sodium nitroprusside

    (B) intravenous labetalol

    (C) trimethaphan camsylate

    (D) midodrine

END OF SET

11. A 28-year-old hospital nurse from Minnesota presents to your office with a positive purified protein derivative (PPD) found on his yearly test. He has no high-risk behavior and is known to be HIV negative. The area of induration is 12 mm, and three sputums are negative for acid-fast bacilli (AFB). He is asymptomatic. A chest radiograph is negative. What do you recommend?

    (A) no treatment needed because PPD is < 15 mm induration

    (B) isoniazid (INH), rifampin, ethambutol, and pyrazinamide (PZA) for a total of 6 months, stopping PZA at 2 months, and stopping ethambutol when cultures are negative

    (C) rifampin for 2 months

    (D) INH for 9 months

    (E) bronchoscopy

12. You are asked to evaluate a 56-year-old woman who has had diffuse and progressive bone pain for 3 years. Her past medical history is significant for a partial gastrectomy and gastrojejunostomy 15 years ago to manage a recurrence of peptic ulcer disease. On examination, the patient has tenderness to gentle pressure on the tibias. A bone scan shows multiple areas of increased uptake in the thoracic and lumbar spine, the right clavicle, both tibias, and the pelvic rami. Routine laboratory studies show a serum calcium of 8.1 mg/dL (N: 8.5–10.5) with normal albumin level, a serum phosphorus of 2 mg/dL (N: 2.5–4.5), and a serum creatinine of 0.8 mg/dL (N: 0.7–1.4). This condition is associated commonly with which of the following sets of laboratory results?

	25-hydroxy-vitamin D	Intact PTH	1,25-hydroxy-vitamin D	Alkaline Phosphatase
I	Low	Low	Low	Normal
II	Low	Normal	Low	High
III	Normal	Low	Low	High
IV	Low	High	Normal	High
V	Low	High	Low	Normal

(A) I
(B) II
(C) III
(D) IV
(E) V

13. A 25-year-old man is found to have hemolysis after taking a sulfa drug. He was also eating fava beans the night before and was found to have a hematocrit of 31%, a mean corpuscular volume (MCV) of 101, a WBC of 10,200/μL, a reticulocyte count of 4.5%, and a platelet count of 338,000/μL. Which of the following disorders is most consistent with this clinical scenario?

(A) beta-thalassemia
(B) sickle cell anemia
(C) autoimmune hemolysis
(D) glucose-6-phosphate dehydrogenase (G6PD) deficiency

Items 14–17

A 74-year-old man with hypertension is brought to see you because his family has concerns about his behavior over the past year. He has been getting lost while driving to the supermarket and on occasion has left the stove on several hours after cooking breakfast. The patient denies any of these problems and tells you in a conspiratory tone that he "feels fine and is here to humor his family." Mental status examination reveals an ability to recall 2 of 3 objects at 5 minutes, concrete abstraction, but normal orientation, general knowledge, calculation, and language function.

14. Your prime diagnostic consideration at this point should be

(A) depression
(B) dementia
(C) delirium
(D) right hemispheric cerebral infarction
(E) age-appropriate normal behavior

15. A CT scan of the head is obtained on this patient and demonstrates only atrophy. An electroencephalogram (EEG) shows mild slowing. Your working diagnosis at this point is dementia. All of the following diseases should now be considered as possible etiologies EXCEPT

(A) Creutzfeldt–Jakob disease (slow-virus)
(B) Alzheimer's disease
(C) vitamin B_{12} deficiency
(D) Lewy body disease
(E) hypothyroidism

16. A diagnosis of dementia of the Alzheimer's type is suspected on a clinical basis. Your therapeutic recommendation is to initiate

(A) anticholinergic therapy
(B) an acetylcholinesterase inhibitor
(C) dopaminergic therapy
(D) serotonergic therapy
(E) observation for further progression

17. The family informs you that the patient has not been sleeping at night. He has been walking around the house at night, and they are fearful that he will injure himself. When they tell him this, he becomes belligerent and will scream at them. On one occasion, he physically attacked a family member. Your therapeutic recommendation is to initiate

(A) benzodiazepine therapy
(B) diphenhydramine for sleep
(C) butyrophenone therapy
(D) family psychotherapy
(E) padded mechanical restraints

END OF SET

18. A 67-year-old woman presents to the ED complaining of a productive cough and fever for the past 24 hours. She had a shaking chill the night before. Her CXR reveals a dense consolidation of the right middle lobe. Her sputum Gram stain is shown in Figure 8.1. What is the bacterial etiology of her pneumonia?

(A) *Mycoplasma pneumoniae*
(B) *Streptococcus pneumoniae*
(C) *Staphylococcus aureus*
(D) *Legionella pneumophila*
(E) *Mycobacterium tuberculosis*

19. All of the following are predisposing causes of preterm labor EXCEPT

(A) fetal anomalies
(B) preterm rupture of the membranes

(C) abruptio placentae
(D) multiparity
(E) severe maternal infection

20. Maternal administration of glucocorticoids after 26 weeks to mothers at risk for preterm delivery is believed to reduce which neonatal complication of prematurity?

(A) respiratory distress syndrome
(B) necrotizing enterocolitis
(C) neonatal sepsis
(D) intraventricular hemorrhage
(E) visual impairment

21. Steady, episodic, aching pain in the upper face and forehead that lasts for at least 1 hour each episode is most consistent with

(A) giant cell arteritis
(B) geniculate neuralgia
(C) Sluder syndrome
(D) classical migraine
(E) trigeminal neuralgia

22. What is the most common pathogen in community-acquired urinary tract infections?

(A) *Chlamydia*
(B) *Enterococcus faecalis*
(C) *Escherichia coli*
(D) *Proteus* species
(E) *Staphylococcus saprophyticus*

23. A 20-year-old woman discovers a breast lump on self-examination. She is in the luteal phase of her cycle. The most reasonable suggestion would be to

(A) reexamine her in the follicular phase of her next menstrual cycle
(B) perform fine-needle aspiration of the lump
(C) order immediate mammography
(D) refer for excisional biopsy
(E) reassure her and observe for any changes over the next year

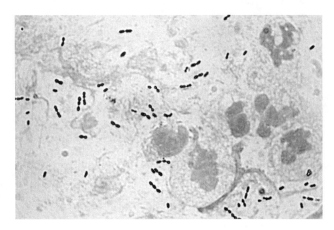

Figure 8.1

24. The diagnosis of fibrocystic breast disease is made, and all of the following recommendations are made EXCEPT

(A) restriction of caffeine
(B) wide local excision of cysts
(C) low-sodium diet
(D) low-dose danazol therapy
(E) mild diuretics

25. Which of the following statements is true about breast cancer?

(A) Multiparity is a risk factor.
(B) Breast cancer is the second most common malignancy in women.
(C) The incidence of breast cancer is 1 in 50 women.
(D) Eighty percent of breast cancers are of the infiltrating intraductal type.
(E) The most common presentation is bloody nipple discharge.

26. All of the following types of pneumonia are likely to cavitate EXCEPT

(A) *Streptococcus pneumoniae*
(B) *Staphylococcus aureus*
(C) *Pseudomonas aeruginosa*
(D) *Klebsiella pneumoniae*

27. What is the most common location of congenital head and neck teratomas?

(A) nasopharynx
(B) neck
(C) oropharynx
(D) hypopharynx
(E) tongue

28. A 21-year-old woman presents to your office with her third episode of cystitis including dysuria, frequency, and urgency in the past 12 months. What is the optimal therapy for her acute infection?

(A) empiric antibiotic therapy for 3 days
(B) empiric antibiotic therapy for 7 days

(C) urine culture with delayed therapy based on results
(D) radiologic evaluation of urinary tract

29. Upon awakening from cardiac surgery, a 42-year-old patient described painless loss of vision in one eye. The patient's surgical procedure was mitral valve surgery. The differential diagnosis includes all of the following EXCEPT

(A) central retinal artery occlusion
(B) occipital lobe stroke
(C) retinal hemorrhage
(D) anterior ischemic optic neuropathy
(E) postoperative exposure keratopathy

30. What is the causative agent of hot tub folliculitis?

(A) *Streptococcus bovis*
(B) *Staphylococcus aureus*
(C) *Klebsiella pneumoniae*
(D) *Pseudomonas aeruginosa*
(E) *Sporotrichosis schenkii*

31. A 70-year-old man is brought to the hospital with fever, mild hypotension, jaundice, right upper quadrant pain, and slight confusion, all recent in onset. A leukocytosis is found on peripheral blood smear with a shift to the left. Emergency ultrasound of the abdomen reveals dilated intrahepatic and extrahepatic bile ducts. All of the following are acceptable treatment options EXCEPT

(A) blood cultures, then metronidazole, ampicillin, and gentamicin intravenous therapy
(B) same as A, plus endoscopic retrograde cholangiography and pancreatography
(C) same as A, plus percutaneous transhepatic cholangiography
(D) same as B, but ceftazidime instead of gentamicin and ampicillin

32. A 55-year-old man with a long history of heartburn undergoes an upper endoscopy. Several tongues of orange-colored mucosa extend 6 cm upward from the gastroesophageal junction. Biopsies of this orange mucosa would be diagnostic of Barrett's esophagus, and would be premalignant with which of the following epithelia?

    (A) gastric fundic type
    (B) colonic type
    (C) specialized columnar type
    (D) gastric cardia–like

33. The best marker for procainamide-induced lupus is

    (A) antinuclear antibody (ANA)
    (B) anti-Ro Ab
    (C) anti-Sm Ab
    (D) anti-nRMP Ab
    (E) antihistone Ab

34. A patient returning from a tour of the American Southwest has a fever, cough, and painful lesion on her right anterior lower leg. What would be the most likely cause for her illness?

    (A) *Blastomyces dermatitidis*
    (B) *Histoplasma capsulatum*
    (C) *Penicillium marfenii*
    (D) *Coccidioides immitis*

35. What is the most common organism cultured from the paranasal sinuses in patients with cystic fibrosis?

    (A) *Staphylococcus aureus*
    (B) *Streptococcus pneumoniae*
    (C) *Pseudomonas maltophila*
    (D) *Pseudomonas aeruginosa*
    (E) *Haemophilus influenzae*

36. The development of a bladder infection is related to all of the following factors EXCEPT

    (A) bacterial ascent from fecal flora
    (B) presence of urethral catheters

    (C) bacterial adhesion proteins
    (D) low fluid intake
    (E) alkaline vaginal fluid in women

37. A 36-year-old woman has a recurrent vesicular eruption on her buttock associated with a burning sensation. It first occurred five years ago and recurs every few months. What disorder do you suspect?

    (A) herpes simplex
    (B) contact dermatitis
    (C) dermatitis herpetiformis
    (D) bullous pemphigoid
    (E) porphyria cutanea tarda

Items 38–39

A 20-year-old college student originally from South America develops recent epigastric pain 2 hours after meals, which is relieved by eating or antacids. She is on no medications and does not smoke, drink, or use nonsteroidal anti-inflammatory drugs (NSAIDs). On exam, her weight is up 5 pounds, and a stool specimen is guaiac negative. A complete blood count (CBC) and upper gastrointestinal (GI) series are normal. She says she was told she had an ulcer 2 or 3 years ago.

38. Which of the following would be the best test to perform next?

    (A) repeat upper GI series
    (B) urea breath test
    (C) upper endoscopy
    (D) serology for *Helicobacter pylori*
    (E) fasting serum gastrin

39. This patient has the test, and you are mildly surprised to find out the result is unremarkable/negative. Which of the following treatments is best for this patient at this time?

    (A) antacid, 60 cc, 1 and 3 hours after meals and before bed for 4 to 8 weeks
    (B) proton pump inhibitor, before breakfast, for 4 to 8 weeks

(C) H$_2$-receptor blocker, twice a day, for 4 to 8 weeks

(D) misoprostol, 200 μg, four times a day, for 4 to 8 weeks

(E) metoclopramide, 10 mg, 30 minutes before meals and before bed, for 4 to 8 weeks

END OF SET

40. The most common side effect of dapsone is

(A) peripheral neuropathy

(B) agranulocytosis

(C) renal failure

(D) hemolysis

(E) hepatotoxicity

41. You are in the ED of a small community hospital. The town's only orthopedic surgeon is 12 hours away. A patient arrives with an open fracture of the tibia with a 3 × 4-cm dirty wound occurring in a fall from a 6-foot ladder. There are no other injuries. The best course of action would be to

(A) apply a sterile dressing to the wound, administer IV antibiotics, and admit the patient for the local orthopedist to treat when he returns

(B) irrigate the wound, splint the tibia fracture, and admit the patient for the local orthopedist to treat tomorrow

(C) leave the extremity as is and immediately transfer the patient to a hospital with an orthopedist on duty

(D) apply a sterile dressing, splint the tibia fracture, administer IV antibiotics, and transfer to a hospital with an orthopedist on duty

(E) perform emergent debridement and irrigation

42. Which of the following is the mechanism of action of low-molecular-weight heparin?

(A) inhibition of gamma carboxylation of glutamic acid residues of factors II, VII, IX, and X

(B) inhibition of adenosine diphosphate–mediated platelet activation

(C) antithrombin III–independent inhibition of thrombin

(D) antithrombin III–dependent inhibition of factor Xa

(E) platelet production of biologically inactive thromboxane A$_3$

43. A 24-year-old woman in her seventh month of pregnancy is brought to the ED complaining of headache, nausea, and right-sided weakness. Your exam confirms a right hemiparesis, and deep tendon reflexes are not overactive. Fundoscopic exam reveals the following (see Figure 8.2): As you are evaluating her, she has a witnessed seizure with clear focal onset in the right arm. CT scan of the head without contrast is normal. The most likely diagnosis is

(A) pseudotumor cerebri

(B) eclampsia

(C) cortical vein thrombosis

(D) choriocarcinoma

(E) enlargement of a left hemisphere meningioma

44. A 24-year-old construction worker is brought to the ED after an injury on a job site. He nearly severed his right foot with a saw, passed out, and fell into a muddy hole. He also has a head injury and cannot answer any questions. His coworkers think he was born in Honduras. In addition to treating his other injuries, what are you going to do regarding treatment for possible tetanus?

(A) administer tetanus toxoid

(B) administer tetanus immune globulin

(C) administer both tetanus toxoid and tetanus immune globulin at different sites

(D) do nothing

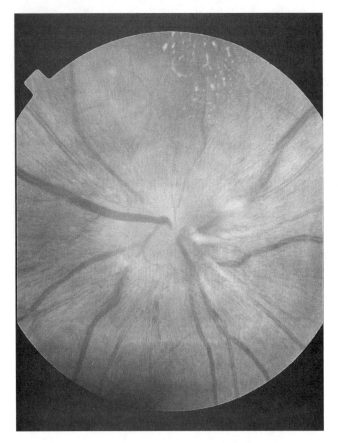

Figure 8.2

45. A 30-year-old teacher with a history of asthma normally well controlled with use of an albuterol inhaler on an "as-needed" basis presents with increased wheezing over the past 48 hours associated with nasal congestion that has responded poorly to her inhaler. She is a nonsmoker with no other significant medical problems and has never required hospitalization for her asthma. Initial exam shows mild tachypnea and diffuse wheezes. Her pulse is 110, and she is afebrile with a room air O_2 saturation of 95% by pulse oximetry. After three treatments with nebulized albuterol in the ED, wheezing is minimal, tachypnea has resolved, and she feels better. Peak expiratory flow is ~75% of her predicted value and room air pulse oximetry shows 97% saturation. The most appropriate management at this time is to

(A) prescribe a macrolide antibiotic and continue using the albuterol metered-dose inhaler at home

(B) prescribe a 3- to 5-day nontapering course of oral prednisone and continue the albuterol metered-dose inhaler at home

(C) arrange for a home nebulizer unit for the patient

(D) suggest that the patient be kept overnight for observation

(E) add oral theophylline to her current regimen and discharge home

46. Atypical presentations of acute myocardial infarction (MI) are most frequently encountered in each of the following groups of patients EXCEPT

(A) diabetics
(B) the elderly
(C) younger female patients
(D) young males infected with HIV

47. Contraindications to beta blocker therapy include all of the following EXCEPT

(A) resting heart rate of 50 on therapy
(B) systolic blood pressure < 90 systolic off therapy
(C) PR interval of 280 msec off therapy
(D) wheezing on physical exam

48. All of the following are complications of obstructive sleep apnea EXCEPT

(A) pulmonary hypertension
(B) systemic hypertension
(C) left ventricular hypertrophy
(D) hypercapnic respiratory failure
(E) peripheral edema
(F) all of the above

49. An example of a truly benign bone tumor is

(A) giant cell tumor
(B) osteoid osteoma
(C) myeloma
(D) low-grade chondrosarcoma

50. A 49-year-old man has had 4 months of left flank pain, intermittent gross hematuria, weight loss, and a hematocrit of 64% (N: 42–52%)

	Calcium	Phosphorus	Intact PTH
I	High	Low	High
II	High	Low	Low
III	High	High	Low
IV	Low	High	Low
V	Low	Low	High

(A) I
(B) II
(C) III
(D) IV
(E) V

Practice Test 8
Answers and Explanations

1. **(A)** A recent study found cases of eye pain and blurry vision in patients on Topamax. Patients should be asked about these symptoms.

2. **(E)** This patient most likely has a squamous cell carcinoma secreting PTH-rp (related peptide), which, like PTH, will give hypercalcemia and hypophosphatemia. The hypercalcemia will inhibit PTH secretion. Diagnosis is made by measuring PTH-rp levels. The immediate treatment is saline infusion because the patient is dehydrated. Pamidronate can also be given to lower calcium levels, but should be done after fluids have been started.

3. **(D)** According to current guidelines, the WBC should be checked weekly for the first 6 months, and thereafter it should be checked every 2 weeks.

4. **(A)** Clozapine needs to be discontinued when the WBC drops below 3,000, according to recent suggestions.

5. **(D)** Plasmapheresis is effective for the removal of pathologic plasma components such as myasthenia gravis particularly if ventilated. It is also used in thrombotic thrombocytopenic purpura (TTP) and acute Guillain–Barré syndrome. Controlled trials of plasmapheresis have failed to show efficacy in dermatomyositis and systemic lupus erythematosus (SLE). There is no rationale for its use in sickle cell disease. Patients with Waldenstrom's macroglobulinemia or myeloma with symptoms of hyperviscosity should be emergently treated with plasmapheresis to lower the monoclonal (M) component.

6. **(C)** The most likely diagnosis is OSA, with his history of loud snoring, obesity, and daytime sleepiness. Restless legs and narcolepsy are both sleep disorders but usually are not associated with obesity and snoring.

7. **(B)** All of the above tests would be important in the workup of this patient. However, the Epworth Sleepiness Scale is a noninvasive, easy test to administer that is very sensitive for pathologic sleep disorders. If positive, he should have a polysomnogram. If negative, the screening overnight oximetry should be done.

8. **(A)** Viral synovitis of the hip is frequently seen in children following an upper respiratory tract infection. The peripheral WBC count is usually only mildly elevated or even normal. A hip joint aspirate will be normal. Light skin traction and observation is all that is needed. Bacterial septic arthritis is generally due to *Staphylococcus aureus*, which is very chondrolytic. Repeated aspiration of the hip is not sufficient in removing organisms from the joint. Open irrigation is the only acceptable treatment in the case.

9. **(G)** A stress test in the setting of a potential dissection could lead to a clinical catastrophe. The ECG may help detect disruption of the coronary arteries in a proximal dissection. The echocardiogram may show a proximal dissection or abnormality in the ascending aorta. It may also reveal disruption and re-

gurgitation of the aortic valve. MRI is a non-invasive imaging procedure that uses magnetic fields and a computer to produce high-resolution cross-sectional or three-dimensional images. This is a reliable way of detecting dissections. CT is a radiographic imaging technique whereby x-ray pictures of tissues from various angles are obtained and a computer is used to consolidate the pictures to create a detailed, three-dimensional, cross-sectional image. Cardiac catheterization may be done to evaluate the aorta and to determine whether the coronary arteries have been disrupted. The chest x-ray may show widening of the mediastinum, suggesting aortic aneurysm or dissection.

10. **(D)** Sodium nitroprusside is the first-line treatment to acutely lower blood pressure and should be titrated to a systolic blood pressure of 100 to 120 mm Hg. Since nitroprusside increases left ventricular stroke volume and cardiac output, it should be used in combination with a beta-adrenergic antagonist such as labetalol. Trimethaphan camsylate is a ganglionic blocking agent. It can be used if nitroprusside or labetalol is not effective or is not tolerated. Midodrine is used in the treatment of orthostatic hypotension to raise blood pressure. It has no role here.

11. **(D)** This patient has latent tuberculosis infection (LTBI), so the terms *chemoprophylaxis* and *preventive therapy* should no longer be used. Current approved treatment regimens for all adults are INH for 9 months, INH and PZA for 2 months, or rifampin for 4 months in patients who cannot tolerate PZA. He is a hospital worker, and a PPD > 10 mm is positive. Bronchoscopy is not indicated.

12. **(D)** This is a typical case of osteomalacia, due to hypovitaminosis D from the gastrectomy. The common findings are:

- Low 25-hydroxyvitamin D reflecting vitamin D stores in the body
- High intact PTH reflecting secondary hyperparathyroidism from hypocalcemia
- Normal 1,25-hydroxyvitamin D, synthesis of which is strongly stimulated by high

levels of PTH, so 1,25-hydroxyvitamin D may be normal even in patients with severe vitamin D deficiency
- High alkaline phosphatase reflecting the activity of the osteoblasts

13. **(D)** The hemolysis in the above man on both a sulfa agent and fava beans was due to G6PD deficiency. The coalescence of the hemoglobin within the cells produces Heinz bodies that attach to the cell membrane. When these aggregates are removed from cells by the reticuloendothelial system, the surviving cells have pieces of membrane removed consistent with "bite" cells. An unstable enzyme decays before the end of the life cycle of the red cell and the result is an inadequate production of NADPH to combat oxidant stress to older erythrocytes. This is sex linked, and full expression is in males. Hemoglobin oxidation produced by natural products such as fava beans and certain drugs with a sulfur moiety can produce acute intravascular hemolysis that ranges in severity from mild to fulminant.

14–17. **(14-B, 15-A, 16-B, 17-C)** The clear sensorium exhibited by this patient excludes a delirium (or encephalopathy) and the progression over a 1-year period without focal neurologic symptoms makes a cerebral infarction unlikely. The decreased concentration exhibited while driving a car and cooking meals along with the reduced immediate memory function and concrete abstraction are more in favor of a dementia rather than depression. This clinical picture is not consistent with normal behavior in the elderly of whatever age.

Multi-infarct dementia has been excluded by the CT scan and lack of a stepwise progression of focal neurologic signs and symptoms. The next most common cause of dementia apart from Alzheimer's disease is Lewy body disease, which may be characterized by prominent psychotic symptoms that worsen when treated with phenothiazines. Both B_{12} deficiency and hypothyroidism are among the few treatable metabolic conditions associated with a dementing illness. Creutzfeldt–Jakob disease due to slow-virus infection is a rapidly progressive dementia over months and is always associated with myoclonic movements and a characteristic periodic EEG.

Alzheimer's disease has been associated with decreased activity of central nervous system choline acetyltransferase found within cholinergic neurons. Increasing cholinergic activity in the brain by inhibiting the enzyme responsible for breakdown of acetylcholine has been shown to have modest benefits in slowing progression of the disease. Medications such as haloperidol and risperidone are useful in controlling the psychiatric symptoms most common in these patients nocturnally (sundowning) or when in an unfamiliar environment (e.g., a hospital). The latter drug has some dopaminergic qualities to lessen the parkinsonian signs often caused by this class of medication. Benzodiazepine therapy will often worsen the cognitive changes, and mechanical restraints should be limited as they can further agitate the patient.

18. **(B)** Pneumococcal pneumonia often presents with a sudden onset of fever and chills. The Gram stain is still a useful diagnostic tool if a predominant organism along with neutrophils can be identified. In contrast, an "atypical" pneumonia will not have bacteria present on a Gram stain. Lobar consolidation is very typical for pneumococcal pneumonia.

19. **(D)** Unless a mother has a prior history of preterm delivery, having had prior children does not increase her risk for preterm delivery.

20. **(A)** Maternal administration of glucocorticoids is felt to decrease the chance of an infant born prematurely developing respiratory distress syndrome.

21. **(A)** The time course and area of pain are most consistent with giant cell arteritis. Neuralgias usually present as sharp, lancinating pain that lasts only seconds or minutes; Sluder syndrome is sphenopalatine neuralgia and causes pain in the lower half of the face. Classical migraine usually causes diffuse

headache lasting several hours, with associated aura and other symptoms.

22. **(C)** *E. coli* is responsible for 85% of community-acquired infections and approximately 50% of hospital-acquired infections.

23. **(A)** This is a classic presentation of benign fibrocystic breast disease. In addition, the woman is in the luteal phase of her cycle, which is the least accurate time to examine the breasts. It would be most appropriate to reexamine her in the follicular phase of her next cycle. If the discrete mass is still present, a mammogram is probably the next step, but is not accurate in younger women because of the denseness of the breast tissue. Eventually, fine-needle aspiration may be indicated, unless it is solid, in which case an excisional biopsy may be necessary. Observation is not the correct answer, because this mass cannot be dismissed. *(Beckmann, 392–394)*

24. **(B)** Wide local excision is not appropriate for benign fibrocystic breast disease. There is nothing to widely locally excise, since the fibrocystic nature is diffuse throughout both breasts. All of the other choices are helpful in the management of the condition. *(Beckmann, 388)*

25. **(D)** Most breast cancers are of the infiltrating intraductal type. Nulliparity or first child after age 35 is a risk factor. Breast cancer is the most common malignancy of women; roughly one in nine women will have breast cancer in her lifetime. The most common presentation is a mass. *(Beckmann, 386–391)*

26. **(A)** Many bacterial pneumonias cavitate, especially those that involve anaerobes or gram-negative organisms. Pneumonias caused by *Pseudomonas aeruginosa, Klebsiella pneumoniae,* and *Staphylococcus aureus* all can cavitate. *Streptococcus pneumoniae* is not likely to cavitate. Also one must remember that mycobacteria, fungal infections, and several noninfectious disorders all can present as a cavitary pneumonia.

27. **(B)** These lesions usually present as a complex neck mass in infancy. CT scan is helpful in the diagnosis.

28. **(A)** In the absence of unusual symptoms such as fever or flank pain, this patient may be treated for the acute infection with a 3-day course of antibiotics such as trimethoprim–sulfamethoxazole, nitrofurantoin, or a fluoroquinolone.

29. **(B)** Occipital lobe stroke is almost always associated with bilateral visual impairment. Central retinal artery occlusion, retinal hemorrhages, ischemic optic neuropathy, and postoperative keratopathy can occur unilaterally and cause decreased vision in patients following surgery. The unilaterality of this patient's symptoms helps to eliminate occipital lobe infarct from the differential diagnosis.

30. **(D)** *Pseudomonas aeruginosa* is the causative agent of hot tub folliculitis. It is characterized by pruritic, follicular papules, vesicles, or pustules occurring within a few days of bathing in a hot tub, whirlpool, or swimming pool that is not adequately disinfected.

31. **(A)** This patient has biliary obstruction with cholangitis and will die without biliary drainage. Antibiotics alone will not be enough. All the other options can be lifesaving because they can relieve pus under pressure.

32. **(C)** Barrett's esophagus is, by definition, metaplastic specialized columnar–type epithelium, and it is premalignant.

33. **(E)** Drug-induced lupus is generally milder than idiopathic systemic lupus erythematosus (SLE). Common culprits include procainamide, hydralazine, and isoniazid. The ANA in SLE is antihistone. Drug-induced lupus usually resolves with discontinuation of the drug.

34. **(D)** *Coccidioides immitis* is a dimorphic fungus that is found in arid regions such as the American Southwest, Mexico, and parts of South and Central America. Most cases go unrecognized or are thought to be a mild respiratory tract infection. Some patients presenting with acute pulmonary infection may also complain of erythema nodosum. This occurs more often in females and also may be associated with multiple arthralgias.

35. **(D)** These patients are often also colonized with *Staphylococcus aureus;* the second most common organism is *H. influenzae.*

36. **(D)** Both host and bacterial factors are associated with the development of a symptomatic infection. However, dietary factors such as fluid intake, herbal additives, and cranberry juice are not associated with prevention or development of infections.

37. **(A)** Recurrent vesicular eruption associated with burning sensation of the sun-protected buttock skin is most consistent with herpes simplex infection.

38. **(D)** This patient has a history of a probable ulcer, and although she is young, she is from an area of the world where *H. pylori* infection is common. It would be cost effective and important to check her serology for *H. pylori.* If it were positive, with her history of a probable ulcer in the past, she would need to be treated. The upper GI is reasonable in excluding a current ulcer. The urea breath test is more expensive; fasting serum gastrin is unlikely to be abnormal (Zollinger–Ellison syndrome); upper endoscopy is expensive, invasive, and unnecessary given the upper GI series; and a repeat upper GI series is unlikely to be helpful.

39. **(C)** There is no evidence for a motility disorder, so metoclopramide, which has a lot of side effects, is not indicated. Misoprostol also has a lot of side effects, and its use in a reproductive-age woman requires extreme caution. This patient, given the negative test results, most likely has dyspepsia, for which misoprostol is not indicated. Proton pump inhibitors are more expensive than H$_2$ blockers,

and antacids seven times a day are not indicated for dyspepsia and also have more side effects than H$_2$ blockers, which are the best initial treatment in this situation.

40. **(D)** Hemolysis is the most common side effect of dapsone.

41. **(E)** This patient has a Type IIIB open tibia fracture in need of emergent debridement and irrigation. This should be performed within 12 hours. After 12 hours, an open fracture is considered to be one grade higher in severity. After 12 hours of delay in treatment, a Type III open fracture is considered an infected fracture. IV antibiotics should be started as soon as possible after injury.

42. **(D)** Low-molecular-weight heparin is produced from conventional heparin by enzymatic cleavage of unfractionated heparin. Like fractionated heparin, it enhances the inhibitory action of antithrombin III on factor Xa but has a relatively reduced ability to catalyze antithrombin III inhibition of thrombin in contrast to conventional heparin.

43. **(C)** Papilledema may be seen in all of the conditions listed, which may occur during pregnancy with the exception of meningioma. The presence of a seizure excludes pseudotumor cerebri, and the focal nature of the seizure and the exam makes eclampsia unlikely. She is too late in her pregnancy for metastatic choriocarcinoma. Cortical vein thrombosis is the likely diagnosis, which may be confirmed by observing a filling defect in the venous sinus (delta sign) on contrast head CT scan or by magnetic resonance venogram.

44. **(C)** A patient without any known tetanus vaccination should receive both tetanus toxoid (active immunity) and tetanus immune globulin (passive immunity) if the injury is severe and the wound is contaminated. The patient must receive passive immunization because it will take greater than a week for the patient to develop antibodies from the active immunization.

45. **(B)** Viral respiratory infections, inhaled allergens, dust, smoke, and fumes are often responsible for acute exacerbation of asthma. Asthma is now recognized as primarily an inflammatory condition. Unless a patient seen in the ED with wheezing immediately clears with a nebulized bronchodilator such as albuterol, treatment with steroids should be initiated. Antibiotics are generally not appropriate for an acute asthma flare unless there is evidence of a bacterial infection. Home nebulizer units add substantial cost to the care of asthma, but for most patients, they are no more effective than a metered-dose inhaler with a spacer. Observation units are sometimes appropriate for patients who appear to be gradually improving but not ready for discharge. Theophylline is no longer considered a primary agent in the management of asthma due to its narrow therapeutic index.

46. **(D)** Ischemic heart disease is an uncommon problem among young males with HIV infection. Silent ischemia and atypical presentation of MI are encountered relatively often among diabetics and the elderly. Ischemic heart disease is relatively uncommon in younger women, but when women in the 30- to 50-year age range suffer MI, their presentation is often atypical. Women in this age group represent a significant portion of missed MIs in the ED, and we should carefully evaluate such patients.

47. **(A)** A drop in the resting heart rate is expected, and dosage is titrated until a decrease in heart rate is seen. A rate of 50 to 55 bpm would be appropriate in therapy. A resting heart rate of 50 off therapy would be cause for concern.

48. **(F)** All of the above are complications of obstructive sleep apnea.

49. **(B)** Osteoid osteoma is a benign bone tumor characterized by a small central vascular nidus and surrounding thick, reactive bone that is very "hot" on technetium bone scan. The lesion has a predilection for the femoral

neck and posterior elements of the spine. It characteristically produces night pain that responds well to aspirin in a significant number of patients. The cure is excision. Giant cell tumor can be an aggressive lesion and has the potential for malignant degeneration, especially if treated with radiation therapy.

50. **(B)** The patient has a renal carcinoma, which produces PTH-rp (related peptide), leading to hypercalcemia and hypophosphatemia, a picture very similar to primary hyperparathyroidism, except that PTH is low from the hypercalcemia. If measured, PTH-rp will be high. The elevated hematocrit is due to secretion of erythropoietin by the cancer.

Practice Test 9
Questions

DIRECTIONS (Questions 1 through 50): Each of the numbered items or incomplete statements in this section is followed by answers or by completions of the statement. Select the ONE lettered answer or completion that is BEST in each case.

1. An 8-year-old girl is admitted to the hospital with fever and lethargy. An examination of the cerebrospinal fluid (CSF) reveals a white blood count (WBC) of 1,800/mm^3, glucose 12 mg/dL, and protein 120 mg/dL. The Gram stain shows numerous gram-positive diplococci. What antibiotics would you empirically initiate while awaiting the culture and susceptibility results?

   (A) ampicillin and gentamicin
   (B) cefazolin
   (C) ceftriaxone
   (D) vancomycin
   (E) ceftriaxone and vancomycin

Items 2–3

2. What is the finding on the sinus x-ray shown in Figure 9.1?

   (A) unilateral maxillary sinus opacification
   (B) bilateral maxillary sinus opacification
   (C) unilateral maxillary sinus air–fluid level
   (D) bilateral maxillary sinus air–fluid level
   (E) septal deformity

3. Which view is shown on the sinus x-ray in Figure 9.1?

   (A) Caldwell view
   (B) submental–vertex view
   (C) Waters view
   (D) lateral view
   (E) Townes view

END OF SET

4. With respect to a patient with renal stone disease, a thorough evaluation for metabolic abnormalities is required in

   (A) all children
   (B) family history of urolithiasis
   (C) osteoporosis
   (D) cystine stones
   (E) all of the above

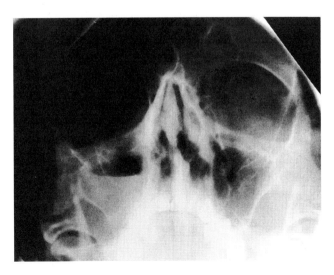

Figure 9.1

5. A 78-year-old patient complains of acute loss of vision in the left eye. Fundus photography shows a lesion present (see Figure 9.2). The most likely diagnosis is that of

(A) toxoplasmosis
(B) papilledema
(C) central retinal vein occlusion
(D) sarcoidosis
(E) HIV-associated retinopathy

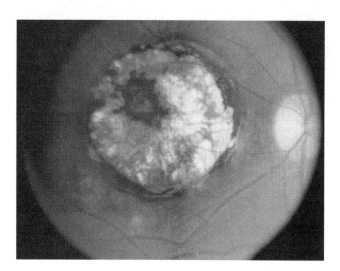

Figure 9.2

6. A previously healthy 28-year-old man is bitten by a spider while cleaning out a backyard toolshed. He subsequently develops sudden onset of severe abdominal cramping with associated nausea and vomiting. Exam shows tachycardia to 130, BP 180/95, temperature of 38° C (100.4° F), and abdominal rigidity with hyperactive bowel sounds. Which of the following represents the most appropriate immediate intervention?

(A) Administer IV methylprednisolone.
(B) Request an abdominal ultrasound.
(C) Administer a benzodiazepine IV.
(D) Give subcutaneous epinephrine 1:1,000 0.3 to 0.5 mg.
(E) Insert a nasogastric (NG) tube.

7. A healthy 35-year-old man falls on his outstretched hand while playing basketball and complains of pain on the radial side of the wrist. Exam shows mild swelling and tenderness between the distal radius and the base of the thumb in the area of the anatomical snuffbox. Anteroposterior (AP), lateral, and oblique x-rays of the wrist as well as a scaphoid view demonstrate mild soft tissue edema with no obvious fracture or dislocation. Which of the following choices represents the most appropriate management?

(A) Recommend ice pack, elevation, and oral nonsteroidal anti-inflammatory drug (NSAID).
(B) Refer the patient to a physical therapist.
(C) Place the patient in a thumb spica splint.
(D) Apply an elastic bandage to the wrist.
(E) Immobilize the forearm with sugar tong splint.

8. A mildly obese 38-year-old woman stumbles while walking down a flight of steps wearing high heels. She grasps the handrail to avoid falling but twists the foot and ankle and feels a pop in the ankle with onset of severe pain over the entire foot and ankle. She is unable to bear weight. Your careful exam includes the Thompson test in which you gently squeeze the calf muscle of the affected extremity while the patient is in a kneeling position. Failure to observe movement of the foot during this maneuver suggests

(A) talar fracture
(B) grade III disruption of the deltoid ligament
(C) disruption of the Achilles tendon
(D) fracture of the fibula
(E) calcaneo–metatarsal dislocation (Lisfranc injury)

9. Possible target dose range of ziprasidone as a maintenance dose in remission is

(A) 40 to 80 mg
(B) 80 to 120 mg
(C) 120 to 160 mg
(D) 80 to 160 mg

10. A 56-year-old woman has primary hyperparathyroidism. What signs and symptoms would you expect to see?

(A) hypocalcemia

(B) hyperthyroidism and dementia

(C) goiter and renal failure

(D) positive urine nitrate

(E) bilateral flank pain, microscopic hematuria, and polyuria

11. Suggestive of bipolar disorder rather than major depression are all of the following EXCEPT

(A) early age of onset

(B) late age of onset

(C) high frequency of depression episodes

(D) greater proportion of time ill

12. All of the following have restrictive patterns on spirometry EXCEPT

(A) idiopathic pulmonary fibrosis

(B) sarcoidosis

(C) obesity

(D) asthma

(E) neuromuscular weakness

13. A patient is seen in a walk-in clinic with the chest radiograph seen in Figure 9.3. He is from India and just moved to New York City 6 months ago. He has a productive cough with blood-tinged sputum and has lost more than 15 lbs. in 2 months. Sputum is obtained for acid-fast bacilli (AFB) smear and culture. You choose to start medications for tuberculosis. Which of the following regimens would be the most appropriate?

(A) rifampin, isoniazid, pyrazinamide, and ethambutol

(B) rifampin and isoniazid

(C) rifampin, isoniazid, and pyrazinamide

(D) rifampin and pyrazinamide

14. Both serum and urine pregnancy tests currently used involve assays of the beta subunit of human chorionic gonadotropin (hCG). This is to avoid cross-reaction with

(A) prolactin

(B) dehydroepiandrosterone (DHEA)

(C) luteinizing hormone (LH)

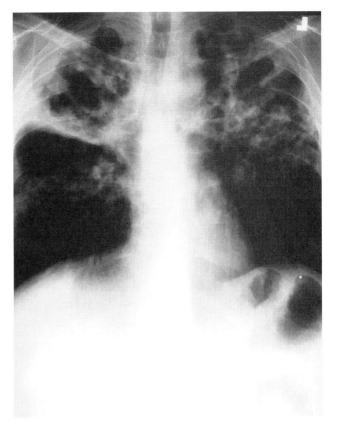

Figure 9.3

(D) estradiol

(E) progesterone

15. In a primiparous patient, quickening is usually felt by

(A) 12 weeks after the last menstrual period (LMP)

(B) 16 weeks after the LMP

(C) 20 weeks after the LMP

(D) 24 weeks after the LMP

<u>Items 16–17</u>

A 40-year-old man is seen with a 2-week history of right leg pain that began insidiously. He has a history of mild, nagging, early morning low back pain for the past 3 years that has suddenly resolved. He has pain when sitting that is relieved by standing or walking. He has not had any changes in bowel or bladder function. A magnetic resonance imaging (MRI) scan of his lumbar spine is shown in Figure 9.4.

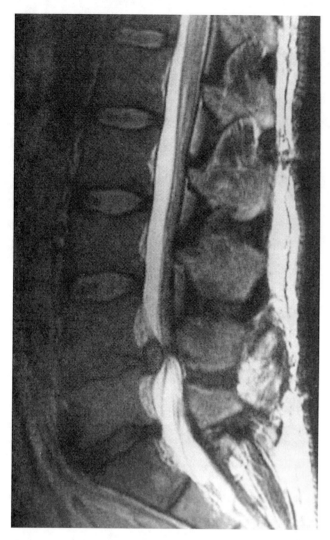

Figure 9.4
(Reproduced, with permission, from Witte D: Magnetic resonance imaging in orthopaedics. In Canale ST (ed.). *Campbell's Operative Orthopaedics*, 9th ed. St. Louis, MO: Mosby, 1998.)

16. On physical examination, what would you expect to find?

(A) leg pain with straight leg raising
(B) pain with sciatic stretch testing
(C) extensor hallucis longus weakness
(D) decreased sensation on the dorsum of the foot
(E) all of the above

17. The patient presents to the emergency department (ED) with sudden inability to void. The appropriate treatment is

(A) Foley catheter
(B) Foley catheter and IV steroids

(C) Foley catheter and emergency decompression
(D) none of the above

END OF SET

18. A 34-year-old man with chronic cough productive of copious, foul-smelling, mucopurulent sputum presents to your office. Physical examination reveals clubbing of the digits. Which therapy will most decrease exacerbations of his lung disease?

(A) inhaled ipratropium
(B) chest physiotherapy
(C) oral doxycycline for 10 days
(D) oral steroids
(E) none of the above

19. A 72-year-old man presents to your office complaining of tremor. Your exam reveals a rapid, bilateral tremor of both outstretched hands and in his head. His tremor resolves at rest. The rest of his neurologic exam is normal. An effective medical therapy may include

(A) phenobarbital
(B) carbamazepine
(C) valproic acid
(D) verapamil
(E) propranolol

20. A 35-year-old woman is witnessed to lose consciousness and fall to the ground. A well-meaning bystander lifts her up in his arms. She immediately becomes pale, perspires, is incontinent of urine, and develops clonic movements of both arms. She is returned to the supine position and immediately stops shaking, regains normal consciousness, and in a few minutes is able to get up to get help for herself. The most likely diagnosis is

(A) seizure
(B) syncope
(C) transient ischemic attack (TIA)
(D) cerebrovascular accident (CVA)
(E) conversion disorder

21. The major advantage of allogeneic bone marrow transplantation over autologous bone

marrow transplantation in patients with acute myelocytic leukemia (AML) is

(A) less likelihood of infection
(B) wider eligibility for the procedure
(C) less relapse due to graft versus leukemia effect
(D) greater graft versus leukemia effect
(E) less likelihood of graft versus host disease

22. A 34-year-old woman comes to the ED with a swollen right hand. Her cat had bitten her on the volar surface of the hand the day before. She thinks her last tetanus booster was 9 years ago. She now has a great deal of pain that extends above her wrist. On examination she is febrile and has marked limitation of range of motion of her wrist and fingers. All of the following interventions are necessary EXCEPT

(A) elevation of the hand
(B) tetanus toxoid
(C) ampicillin–sulbactam
(D) cefazolin
(E) orthopedic consult for possible debridement and irrigation

23. An 18-year-old man is being treated for acute lymphoblastic leukemia. Eight days after induction chemotherapy, he has a shaking chill and fever of 40° C (104° F). His WBC is 230/mm^3 with 100% lymphocytes. On exam he has severe mucositis, and his Hickman catheter site is extremely tender to touch, with some surrounding erythema. What antimicrobial therapy will you initiate in this patient?

(A) ceftazidime
(B) ceftazidime and tobramycin
(C) vancomycin
(D) vancomycin and ceftazidime

24. The most common treatable cause of anosmia is

(A) allergic rhinitis
(B) cribriform plate fracture
(C) esthesioneuroblastoma

(D) post–viral neuropathy
(E) sinusitis

25. The metabolic abnormalities associated with urinary tract stones include all of the following EXCEPT

(A) increased intestinal absorption of calcium
(B) increased renal excretion of calcium
(C) decreased renal absorption of phosphate
(D) decreased renal excretion of citrate
(E) hyperparathyroidism

26. What type of stones is most often associated with urinary tract infections?

(A) calcium oxalate
(B) cystine
(C) struvite
(D) staghorn
(E) uric acid

27. A 37-year-old patient presents in the office with the progressive onset of blurred vision in both eyes at distance. The patient has not been seen by a medical doctor for many years. He has no systemic complaints. His review of systems is negative. He states that he has not had to change his eyeglasses over the last several years. Ocular examination reveals, through undilated pupils, the disc and macula to be grossly normal in both eyes. The most likely diagnosis is

(A) sarcoidosis
(B) syphilis
(C) tuberculosis
(D) diabetes mellitus
(E) all of the above

28. Which of the following is most closely associated with the development of porphyria cutanea tarda?

(A) cocaine
(B) ethanol
(C) heroin
(D) marijuana
(E) tobacco

29. Which virus is the most common causative agent of hand, foot, and mouth disease?

   (A) coxsackievirus
   (B) poxvirus
   (C) papovavirus
   (D) echovirus
   (E) herpesvirus

30. A 47-year-old previously healthy man comes to your office after a 10-day trip to Haiti with "really bad watery diarrhea." All of the following are likely to be found on laboratory testing EXCEPT

   (A) fecal osmotic gap < 50
   (B) positive stool examination for *Isospora belli*
   (C) fecal polymorphonuclear leukocytes
   (D) Charcot–Leyden crystals in stool
   (E) fasting stool volume > 500 g/d

31. Which of the following viral infections is of importance to pregnant women because of risk of hydrops fetalis?

   (A) parvovirus
   (B) poxvirus
   (C) hepatitis A virus
   (D) herpes simplex virus
   (E) coxsackievirus

32. An 8-year-old boy develops guttate psoriasis. What infection is most likely to coexist?

   (A) *Staphylococcus*
   (B) *Pseudomonas*
   (C) *Candida*
   (D) *Streptococcus*
   (E) *Helicobacter*

33. A 32-year-old woman presents with a history of severe, recurrent gastric and duodenal ulcers, erosive esophagitis, diarrhea, and weight loss. Each of the following laboratory tests would be consistent with her history EXCEPT

   (A) basal acid output 12 mEq/hr, maximal acid output 130 mEq/hr

   (B) fasting serum gastrin 950 pg/mL
   (C) personal history of kidney stones
   (D) sister with amenorrhea and galactorrhea
   (E) personal history of hypercalcemia

34. A 76-year-old man with a long history of benign prostatic hypertrophy (BPH) and voiding symptoms presents to the office with a complaint of 1 week of a dribbling urinary stream and a sense of lower abdominal fullness. What is the most likely diagnosis?

   (A) urinary tract infection
   (B) CVA with a neurogenic bladder
   (C) urinary retention
   (D) prostate cancer
   (E) constipation

35. A patient with end-stage renal disease due to severe hypertension presents after missing his last two scheduled hemodialysis sessions. He is weak and hypotensive with a thready radial pulse. His electrocardiogram (ECG) is shown in Figure 9.5. Which of the following is the most appropriate choice for initial treatment?

   (A) calcium chloride IV
   (B) atropine IV
   (C) isoproterenol IV
   (D) magnesium sulfate IV
   (E) transcutaneous pacing

36. When treating diabetic ketoacidosis (DKA) using IV insulin infusion, failure of serum glucose to decline may be attributed to each of the following EXCEPT

   (A) renal failure
   (B) acute myocardial infarction (MI)
   (C) occult infection
   (D) circulating insulin antibodies

Items 37–38

A patient is seen in the ED with palpitations. Symptoms began when she bent down to tie her shoe. The ECG recording shown in Figure 9.6 was taken in the ED.

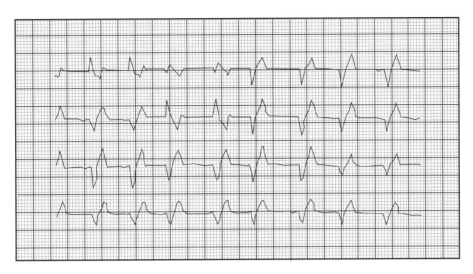

Figure 9.5

37. What is the rhythm?

    (A) atrioventricular (AV) node reentry
    (B) atrial fibrillation
    (C) sinus tachycardia
    (D) ventricular tachycardia

38. The patient responds to treatment and is seen in the office to discuss management. She is a young, healthy person with no other medical problems. After initial treatment for her arrhythmia, all of the following therapies might be considered EXCEPT

    (A) digoxin
    (B) atenolol
    (C) diltiazem
    (D) mexiletine
    (E) flecainide

    END OF SET

39. A 55-year-old woman with metastatic breast cancer to bone presents with fever of 38.7° C (101.8° F). She received chemotherapy 10 days ago. Her only symptom is a vesicular rash along the right thorax. She appears acutely ill, with a normal oropharynx, clear chest, and negative cardiac and abdominal exams. She has a vesicular rash along the right T11 dermatome. Her hemoglobin is 10 g/dL, and her WBC is 300/μL with a platelet count of 20,000/μL. Blood and urine cultures are sent, and a chest x-ray is obtained, which is without pneumonia. What is the next intervention?

    (A) platelet transfusion
    (B) parenteral acyclovir and ceftazidime
    (C) granulocyte colony-stimulating factor (G-CSF)
    (D) all of the above

40. A 16-year-old girl is brought by her mother on the advice of the school nurse following a positive scoliosis school screening test. Menarche was at age 12. On examination she has a slight right rib hump on forward bending when viewed from behind. Standing AP and lateral thoracolumbar x-rays show a midthoracic curve of 10 degrees. Her iliac apophyses have closed. Leg lengths are equal. The best treatment is

    (A) bracing program as the curve will increase
    (B) refer for surgery
    (C) reassurance as this curve will not increase
    (D) physical therapy for electric muscle stimulation to the spine

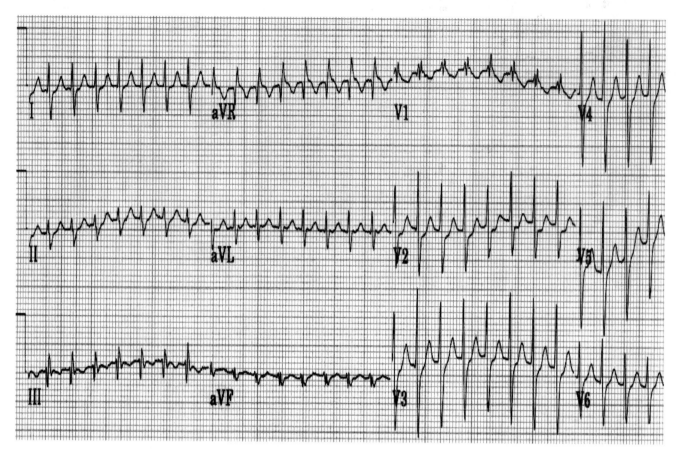

Figure 9.6

41. Which of the following diagnoses is consistent with primary amenorrhea in a 46,XY individual?

    (A) imperforate hymen
    (B) androgen insensitivity
    (C) müllerian agenesis
    (D) Turner syndrome
    (E) transverse vaginal septum

42. A 25-year-old man is seen with a painful, swollen erythematous right hand 4 days after a fight in a bar. There is a 1-cm laceration over the metacarpophalangeal (MCP) joint of the little finger. The most likely diagnosis is

    (A) *Staphylococcus* infection
    (B) *Streptococcus* infection
    (C) *Escherichia coli* infection
    (D) *Pseudomonas* infection
    (E) *Eikenella corrodens* infection

43. A 24-year-old man presents to your office with a sharp substernal chest pain. Physical exam is normal except for some diplopia on prolonged upward gaze. Chest radiograph reveals an anterior mediastinal mass. What is the most likely diagnosis?

    (A) substernal thyroid
    (B) lymphoma
    (C) teratoma
    (D) thymoma
    (E) none of the above

44. All of the following are causes of hypoxemic respiratory failure with a high A-a gradient EXCEPT

    (A) ventilation perfusion mismatch
    (B) shunt
    (C) hypoventilation

(D) diffusion impairment

(E) all of the above

45. Which of the following is not part of Cluster B personality disorder?

(A) antisocial

(B) borderline

(C) avoidant

(D) histrionic

(E) narcissistic

46. Which of the following is correct regarding Graves' disease?

(A) The disorder received its name due to the high death rate.

(B) It is most common in ages 30 to 50.

(C) It is more common in men.

(D) There is no familial predisposition.

(E) The disorder is viral.

47. A 51-year-old patient presents with increased fatigue and shortness of breath. A complete blood count (CBC) is obtained, revealing a hemoglobin of 7.3 g/dL. What diagnostic test would be considered most useful?

(A) bleeding time

(B) reticulocyte count

(C) Coombs' test

(D) bone marrow evaluation

(E) mean corpuscuar hemoglobin concentration

48. A 39-year-old woman has had 2 months of hypercalcemia, fever, joint aches, and hilar adenopathies. What condition do you suspect?

(A) rheumatoid arthritis

(B) erythema nodosum

(C) sarcoidosis

(D) scleroderma

(E) vasculitis

49. A 70-year-old woman with a history of resected stage I lung cancer 20 years ago comes into your office complaining of low back pain. Initially, she described the pain as dull, aching discomfort that has now progressed to chronic, severe pain. Over the past several days, the pain is exacerbated by movement, and she has worsening discomfort in the supine position. On exam, she has unremarkable point tenderness, mostly in the lumbar spine. On neurological exam, diffuse weakness is noted. Spinal x-rays are unrevealing. What is the next course of action?

(A) lumbar puncture

(B) nerve conduction velocity

(C) MRI

(D) bone scan

(E) computed tomography (CT) scan of the brain

50. A 36-year-old previously healthy man presents with facial swelling over 1 week. He acknowledges that he has been a three-pack-a-day smoker for 20 years. He also complains of dyspnea and swelling in his right arm. On exam, he has bilateral facial swelling and upper extremity edema. A chest x-ray is obtained, revealing a right mediastinal mass. You do all of the following EXCEPT

(A) call radiation oncology

(B) CT scan of the chest

(C) schedule a biopsy of the mass

(D) call medical oncology

(E) emergency surgery to remove the mass

Practice Test 9
Answers and Explanations

1. **(E)** The patient's presentation and Gram stain are consistent with bacterial meningitis caused by *Streptococcus pneumoniae.* This is the most common etiology of bacterial meningitis in most age groups. Treatment consists of either ceftriaxone or cefotaxime—both third-generation cephalosporins with pneumococcal coverage and good CSF penetration. Because of the increasing concern for resistance of *S. pneumoniae* to penicillin and cephalosporins, vancomycin must be added pending susceptibility results.

2. **(C)** This is a clear example of a unilateral air–fluid level in the maxillary sinus.

3. **(C)** The head is tilted back slightly (as if drinking a glass of "water") to show the maxillary sinus clearly. If the x-ray is taken with the head straight, the maxillary sinuses will overlap the temporal bones; that would be a Caldwell view. Submental–vertex view is taken from the chin to the top of the head; a lateral view is obviously lateral; a Townes view demonstrates the mandibular condyles with the mouth open.

4. **(E)** Each of these clinical situations may signal the presence of an underlying metabolic abnormality, which is responsible for the development of renal stone disease.

5. **(A)** Toxoplasmosis causes a retinitis with secondary choroidal involvement and scarring. This chorioretinitis results in a scar that is often associated with satellite lesions and significant hyperplasia of the pigment epithelium surrounding the active lesion. Reacti-

vation is not uncommon, and old scars with pigmentation are often present.

6. **(C)** The history suggests envenomation by a black widow spider (*Lactrodectus mactans*). History is very important since the clinical presentation can be quite dramatic, suggesting a surgical abdomen. Given an appropriate history, abdominal ultrasound and NG suction are not indicated. Since the patient's symptoms are the result of a toxic venom and not an allergic phenomenon, epinephrine and steroids are not indicated. Most adults do well with symptomatic treatment. Usually, the most effective treatment is to administer IV benzodiazepines to relax the spasm of the muscles of the abdominal wall. While specific antivenin is available, it carries a substantial risk of adverse effects and is usually reserved for young children, pregnant women, and the elderly, who may be more susceptible to the toxic effects of the spider's venom and are statistically at a greater risk of death.

7. **(C)** About 10% of fractures of the scaphoid (carpal navicular) fail to initially show up on plain films. Unfortunately, missing a fracture of the scaphoid lays the groundwork for subsequent avascular necrosis of the proximal fragment of the fractured bone and a bad long-term outcome for the patient. The safest course of action is to immobilize the patient with a thumb spica splint if there is tenderness of the snuffbox area following trauma to the hand or wrist even if the x-ray appears normal. These patients are then kept in immobilization for 10 to 14 days and then re-x-rayed looking for callus formation. Another

option would be to immediately obtain an MRI scan of the scaphoid. This is usually not practical in terms of the cost as well as the lack of "stat" availability of such a study in most emergency departments.

8. **(C)** The Thompson test is used to detect disruption of the Achilles tendon. It is wise to routinely include this maneuver whenever a patient with an ankle injury is examined. The other physical findings commonly associated with disruption of the Achilles tendon include tenderness over the posterior aspect of the ankle and a palpable discontinuity of the tendon.

9. **(A)** Forty to 80 mg is used as a maintenance dose once in remission.

10. **(E)** The patient has primary hyperparathyroidism. Her flank pain and hematuria are due to kidney stones. Her polyuria is due to hypercalcemia, which can induce nephrogenic diabetes insipidus.

11. **(B)** Late age of onset.

12. **(D)** Asthma has an obstructive pattern on spirometry.

13. **(A)** Patients from foreign countries are at risk for the development of drug-resistant tuberculosis (TB) infection. Patients from areas that have a > 4% drug-resistant rate must be started on a four-drug antituberculosis regimen while awaiting susceptibility results. After the susceptibility results, the regimen may be tapered down. Multidrug-resistant TB (MDR TB) is very difficult and costly to treat and it carries much greater mortality than drug-susceptible TB.

14. **(C)** While LH and hCG both share the same alpha subunit, the beta subunits of LH and hCG differ enough for antibody testing to distinguish between the two.

15. **(C)** Maternal recognition of fetal movements (quickening) usually occurs by 20 weeks' ges-

tation with the first pregnancy. With subsequent pregnancies, the mother often senses movement by 16 to 18 weeks.

16. **(E)** The MRI scan shows a frank herniation of the L4–5 disk. The L5 nerve root is usually compressed. This patient gives a classic history for a ruptured lumbar disk. A degenerative disk will cause nagging back pain that may be suddenly relieved when the disk herniates.

17. **(C)** Cauda equina syndrome results from a sudden massive disk herniation compressing the sacral roots. Emergent decompression is necessary.

18. **(B)** Recognize bronchiectasis and the role of chest physiotherapy and postural drainage in the management of this disease.

19. **(E)** This patient most likely has essential tremor, which is usually familial. Other etiologies include hyperthyroidism and medication toxicity (valproic acid, caffeine, lithium). Mysoline may also be an effective first-line therapy.

20. **(B)** The alteration is skin color but especially the rapid return to normal function is highly suggestive of syncope. The clonic movements reflect persistent cerebral hypoxia brought on by lifting the patient up before blood flow could be returned to the brain. The urinary incontinence is likely due to increased parasympathetic tone associated with the syncopal attack. Alteration in consciousness is unusual in cerebrovascular disease and is seen only when the brain stem (including the reticular-activating system, which controls wakefulness) is involved.

21. **(C)** Patients with AML who undergo allogeneic bone marrow transplant may have acute or chronic graft versus host disease (GVHD). Thus, they react to donor T lymphocytes, whereas in autologous transplant the patients receive their own T lymphocytes. Immunosuppressive agents such as methotrexate and cyclosporine attempt to reduce

this GVHD. Those who undergo autologous transplant do not need immunosuppressives, and thus their risk of infection is far less. Those patients who undergo allogeneic transplant relapse less from their leukemia due to graft versus leukemia effect.

22. **(E)** Cat bites may be very serious and must never be underestimated. The sharp teeth of cats make for deep puncture wounds, often into the hand where tendons and bones are near the surface. They are often associated with *Pasturella multocida*. This organism is not susceptible to cephalosporins, and the drug of choice is ampicillin–sulbactam or ampicillin–clavulanic acid, and in the penicillin-allergic patient doxycycline. As with any bite, a tetanus booster is often indicated. The deep nature of cat bites often requires surgical exploration.

23. **(D)** Empiric therapy for neutropenic fever often can be managed by ceftazidime alone, as has been demonstrated in multiple studies. However, when there is evidence of a central venous catheter infection, the regimen must include vancomycin to cover for gram-positive infections such as *Staphylococcus aureus* or *Staphylococcus epidermidis*. The catheter often has to be removed if the blood cultures cannot be cleared or the catheter is infected with *Candida* species or *Pseudomonas*.

24. **(A)** Allergic rhinitis is common and treatable, and is a common cause of anosmia. Cribriform plate fracture and post–viral neuropathy both cause anosmia but are not treatable; esthesioneuroblastoma is treatable but is very rare; sinusitis is rarely a cause of anosmia.

25. **(C)** Aberrations in urinary calcium levels as a result of increased intestinal absorption or increased renal excretion of calcium are the most common metabolic causes of urolithiasis. Additionally, a reduction in the urinary level of citrate, a known inhibitor of stone formation, is associated with stone disease.

26. **(C)** Struvite calculi are most commonly associated with urinary tract infections by urea-splitting organisms such as *Proteus* and *Klebsiella* species.

27. **(D)** Diabetes mellitus may present with an acute change in refractive error. While the patient's ocular examination may appear to be normal, the presence of hyperglycemia changes the shape of the patient's normal crystalline lens and thus the refractive error. The patient then complains of blurred vision. Immediate blood glucose evaluation is essential in patients with this constellation of findings. It is not uncommon for an ophthalmologist to be the first to make a diagnosis of diabetes mellitus in this setting.

28. **(B)** Ethanol and estrogens are the two most common agents to exacerbate porphyria cutanea tarda (PCT). PCT is due to a deficiency of the heme biosynthetic pathway enzyme, uroporphyrinogen decarboxylase, and presents clinically as skin fragility following sun exposure.

29. **(A)** Hand, foot, and mouth disease is usually seen in infants or young children. It is caused by one of several enteroviruses, most commonly coxsackievirus.

30. **(C)** *Isospora belli* is endemic in Haiti, and typically presents as massive, watery diarrhea in healthy as well as immunocompromised (HIV-infected) persons. It causes a secretory diarrhea (no osmotic gap, high fasting stool volumes) and can be accompanied by eosinophilia as well as Charcot–Leyden crystals in the stool. Typical fecal leukocytes (polymorphonuclear leukocytes) are not found, as there is no cytotoxic colitis.

31. **(A)** Human parvovirus, the etiologic agent of erythema infectiosum, readily infects erythroblasts and may result in hydrops fetalis and fetal death.

32. **(D)** Guttate psoriasis is most often associated with streptococcal pharyngitis but may also

be seen following perianal streptococccal infections.

33. **(A)** The patient's history of erosive and ulcerative disease of the esophagus, stomach, and duodenum, as well as diarrhea and weight loss (i.e., malabsorption and/or maldigestion) is consistent with the Zollinger–Ellison syndrome. Twenty-five percent of patients with this syndrome have multiple endocrine neoplasia type I (MEN I) syndrome, with a personal or family history of hyperparathyroidism, pancreatic tumors, and/or pituitary tumors. Fasting gastrin levels usually are elevated with gastrinomas, and both the basal (BAO) and maximal (MAO) acid outputs often are elevated, typically with a BAO/MAO ratio > 0.6 (i.e., A (12/130) would not be likely).

34. **(C)** The most likely diagnosis is acute urinary retention with a distended bladder. A urinary tract infection could produce urinary frequency and a weak stream but not a lower abdominal mass. Constipation could result in a mass and a weak urinary stream, but this would likely be secondary to urinary retention associated with the constipation.

35. **(A)** Patients with end-stage renal disease who miss dialysis are hyperkalemic until proven otherwise. Cardiac dysrhythmias, especially those associated with bizarre wide ventricular complexes and poorly defined or lost p-waves, are often seen with hyperkalemia. The patient presented is in shock due to his cardiac dysrhythmia caused by hyperkalemia. Calcium chloride IV is the primary drug of choice for treatment in this case. In the scenario presented, immediate treatment is indicated on the basis of history, exam, and findings on the ECG monitor before the result of a serum potassium can be obtained. Other agents that may be used subsequently include glucose and insulin, sodium bicarbonate, nebulized albuterol, and sodium polystyrene sulfonate resin. Atropine, isoproterenol, and pacing are not appropriate interventions in this situation. Magnesium sulfate is also inappropriate and is contraindicated in the setting of renal failure.

36. **(A)** Continuous low-dose IV insulin infusion has become the most commonly used routine for treatment of DKA. Ideally, treatment with an infusion at a rate of 0.1 U of regular insulin per hour should result in a decline in the glucose level of about 50 to 100 mg/dL per hour. If the glucose level fails to significantly decline or actually rises during insulin infusion, the likely cause is insulin resistance. Common causes of insulin resistance include occult infection, circulating insulin antibodies, and acute MI. The importance of a thorough history and physical, ECG, chest x-ray, urinalysis, and WBC for patients with DKA should be readily evident. Renal failure results in prolonged insulin effect rather than insulin resistance.

37. **(A)** AV node reentry typically is of abrupt onset and may be triggered by minimal triggers such as described in the question. Bending likely results in minor changes in the vagal tone, which permits unidirectional block and makes the patient vulnerable to reentry.

38. **(D)** Digoxin, atenolol, and diltiazem all are potential agents to treat AV node reentry. Flecainide, a class Ic antiarrhythmic, is contraindicated in patients with structural heart disease. However, it is safe and effective in young, healthy patients but is generally reserved until after other more benign drugs have failed. Mexiletine, a class Ib antiarrhythmic, plays no role in the management of supraventricular tachycardia.

39. **(B)** The patient has neutropenic fever from prior chemotherapy 10 days ago. She also has an exam relevant for herpes zoster in the T11 dermatomal distribution. Thus, acyclovir is appropriate. In addition, she has a WBC count of 300/μL and, with an absolute neutrophil count < 500/μL, there is a high risk of bacterial infection, which needs to be treated with broad-spectrum antibiotics until the leukocyte count recovers. Therapy with G-CSF at this time would be of little benefit. Studies show that the role of G-CSF is to prevent febrile neutropenia. Platelet transfusions are not needed in a patient with no symp-

toms of bleeding, even at a platelet count of 20,000/μL.

40. **(C)** This girl has probably reached skeletal maturity, and her curve will not progress. Curves of > 40 degrees in skeletally immature or mature teenage girls should be considered for fusion. Curves of 20 to 40 degrees in skeletally immature girls should be braced and followed closely for progression. In skeletally mature girls, repeat x-rays are needed in one year to document nonprogression of the curve.

41. **(B)** Testicular feminization, or androgen insensitivity syndrome, is characterized by female external genitalia, a blind vaginal pouch, normal breast development, and scant or absent pubic hair in a 46,XY individual. Imperforate hymen, müllerian agenesis (Rokitansky syndrome), and transverse vaginal septum are all anomalies of the müllerian system in otherwise phenotypically and genotypically normal 46,XX individuals. Turner syndrome is associated with a 45,XO karyotype, sexual infantilism, webbed neck, shield chest, and many other stigmata. *(DeCherney, 1010–1013)*

42. **(E)** The 1-cm laceration over the MCP joint is from a human tooth. *Eikenella* is found in normal human mouth flora and is the usual pathogen in such infections. The appropriate treatment is IV antibiotics and operative debridement and irrigation of the intra-articular laceration.

43. **(D)** All of these are associated with anterior mediastinal masses; however, the diplopia suggests a neurological process, and thymoma is often associated with myasthenia gravis.

44. **(C)** All of the options are causes of hypoxemia; however, only hypoventilation has a normal A-a gradient as there is no pulmonary parenchymal or vascular disorder.

45. **(C)** Cluster B includes borderline, histrionic, antisocial, and narcissistic personality disorders. *(Kaplan & Sadock, 775)*

46. **(B)** Graves' disease is a common disorder of unknown cause, resulting in thyrotoxicosis. Symptoms include tremor, insomnia, anxiety, sweating, and heat intolerance.

47. **(B)** In the initial presentation of anemia, the first test that should be considered is a reticulocyte count. This allows one to rule out the possibility of an underlying bone marrow process; a low reticulocyte count would suggest diminished bone marrow production of erythrocytes. A high reticulocyte count might suggest erythrocyte destruction.

48. **(C)** The patient has sarcoidosis with hypercalcemia due to production of 1,25-hydroxyvitamin D by the granulomas.

49. **(C)** The major issue is the location and extent of the probable spinal cord lesion. A bone scan may reveal some bony disease, but there was no evidence of lytic lesions on the x-rays. CT scan of the brain could demonstrate a cause for weakness, but point tenderness makes this less likely to be in the brain rather than the cord. Lumbar puncture could rule out carcinomatous meningitis, but it is less likely with this presentation. The differential really includes cord compression or brain metastases, and thus MRI would be the most definitive test. Nerve conduction tests have little utility.

50. **(E)** This scenario represents superior vena cava (SVC) syndrome. A CT of the chest is clearly needed to define the lesion and allow an approach to biopsy, which is needed to rule out non–small cell lung cancer versus small cell lung cancer since chemotherapeutic interventions are clearly different. Superior vena cava syndrome is not necessarily a medical emergency as previously thought, yet radiation oncology as well as medical oncology should be involved as soon as possible to determine a course of action. Thus, emergency surgery to remove the mass has no role.

Practice Test 10
Questions

DIRECTIONS (Questions 1 through 50): Each of the numbered items or incomplete statements in this section is followed by answers or by completions of the statement. Select the ONE lettered answer or completion that is BEST in each case.

1. Thrombolytics are contraindicated in all of the following patients presenting with an acute myocardial infarction (MI) EXCEPT

   (A) a 59-year-old man with chronic mild hypertension
   (B) a 70-year-old woman with a hemorrhagic stroke 3 weeks prior to presentation with an MI
   (C) a 49-year-old man who received thrombolytics for pulmonary embolism and had a serious allergic reaction
   (D) a 36-year-old woman who gave birth 4 weeks prior to an MI
   (E) a 60-year-old man whose infarct presented as a cardiac arrest, who was brought to the emergency department (ED) in full cardiac arrest and is receiving cardiopulmonary resuscitation

2. A patient with a history of alcohol abuse is given a prescription for an infection and comes in the next day with severe nausea and vomiting. What was the likely antibiotic prescribed?

   (A) penicillin
   (B) metronidazole
   (C) levofloxacin
   (D) azithromycin

3. Which of the following is the most likely cause of a mass on the right side of the neck on a computed tomography (CT) scan that was taken with intravenous contrast?

   (A) branchial cleft cyst
   (B) parotid gland carcinoma
   (C) tonsil hypertrophy
   (D) carotid artery aneurysm
   (E) thyroglossal duct cyst

4. A 36-year-old woman presents with a breast mass. Her mother died of some type of cancer at age 50, and her grandmother had breast cancer and died at 42. Which of the following is the most likely genetic cause?

   (A) p53 suppressor gene mutation
   (B) RET autosomal dominant gene mutation
   (C) 14,18 translocation involving bcl-2
   (D) the Philadelphia chromosome, t9,22
   (E) BRCA 1 mutation

Items 5–9

A 35-year-old woman who has delivered three full-term pregnancies and had one first-trimester elective abortion presents to the ED with a 3-day history of spotting accompanied by right lower quadrant pain. Although she is uncertain of the exact date, her last normal menstrual period was 4 to 6 weeks ago. She is currently sexually active with one male partner and has been inconsistently using condoms. She is ambivalent about becoming pregnant.

5. All of the following historical factors would increase this woman's risk of having an ectopic pregnancy EXCEPT

   (A) history of pelvic inflammatory disease (PID)
   (B) history of prior appendectomy for a ruptured appendix
   (C) history of diagnostic laparoscopy showing endometriosis with subsequent tubal reconstruction
   (D) history of gestational diabetes with her prior pregnancies

6. The concept of the "discriminatory zone" of human chorionic gonadotropin (hCG) means

   (A) the level of hCG above which an ectopic pregnancy cannot exist
   (B) the amount of increase expected in hCG in an early normal pregnancy over 48 hours
   (C) the range of serum hCG concentration above which an early intrauterine pregnancy (IUP) can be consistently visualized on transvaginal ultrasound
   (D) the level of hCG that must be present in the serum for a urine hCG test to be positive

7. The use of the discriminatory zone to aid in the diagnosis of early ectopic pregnancy can be compromised by all of the following EXCEPT

   (A) maternal obesity
   (B) uterine fibroids
   (C) multiple gestation
   (D) uncertain last menstrual period (LMP)
   (E) operator inexperience with transvaginal ultrasound

8. Assuming that the patient's urine pregnancy test is positive, what single test is most likely to exclude the diagnosis of ectopic pregnancy in this patient?

   (A) complete blood count (CBC)
   (B) abdominal and pelvic CT scan
   (C) transvaginal ultrasound

   (D) serum beta hCG level
   (E) culdecentesis

9. Assume that the patient has mild right adnexal tenderness on exam and no peritoneal signs. Her vital signs are stable. Her serum hCG level is 3,500 IU, and an empty, normal-sized uterus is seen on adequate transvaginal ultrasound by an experienced examiner. No adnexal masses are seen, and normal ovaries are visualized bilaterally. There is a small amount of fluid seen in her cul-de-sac. She has no significant medical history, and her hemoglobin is 12 g. She is able to return for follow-up care and wants to avoid an operation if at all possible. Which of the following pharmacological agents is appropriate to offer the patient?

   (A) methotrexate
   (B) adriamycin
   (C) norethindrone
   (D) diethylstilbestrol
   (E) medroxyprogesterone acetate

   END OF SET

10. All of the following are associated with the diagnosis of preeclampsia EXCEPT

   (A) hypertension
   (B) edema
   (C) proteinuria
   (D) fetus small for gestational age (SGA)
   (E) elevated blood sugar

11. A patient presents with idiopathic unilateral facial nerve paralysis for 3 days. What is the probability that, if no active treatment or intervention is initiated, facial nerve function will return to normal or near normal within 6 months?

   (A) 20%
   (B) 50%
   (C) 60%
   (D) 80%
   (E) 95%

12. A 17-year-old high school football player is brought to the ED with severe knee pain after being tackled. The knee has a 2+ effusion, and he will not allow much in the way of an examination due to pain. X-rays of the knee are normal. The most appropriate treatment is

   (A) compression dressing, knee immobilizer, and crutches with repeat examination in 3 to 4 days

   (B) compression dressing, knee immobilizer, crutches, and a magnetic resonance imaging (MRI) scan

   (C) compression dressing and crutches and return to school to work with the athletic trainer

   (D) compression dressing and crutches and outpatient physical therapy

13. All of the following are true EXCEPT

   (A) nonsteroidal anti-inflammatory drugs (NSAIDs) affect platelet function

   (B) aspirin effects on platelet function can last for more than 2 days

   (C) the long bleeding time in aspirin-treated patients can be corrected by vitamin K

   (D) sodium salicylate does not prolong the bleeding time when used for arthritis pain

   (E) when patients who have taken aspirin have emergency surgery, platelet transfusions are rarely required to control excessive bleeding

14. A 43-year-old man has had 10 years of postprandial abdominal bloating, loose stools, and vague discomfort in the bones of the lower extremities. Which do you suspect?

   (A) severe GERD
   (B) enteritis
   (C) rheumatoid arthritis
   (D) laxative abuse
   (E) celiac disease

15. A 42-year-old man presents for a routine physical. He was treated in the past with combination chemotherapy, including bleomycin, etoposide, and cisplatin, for metastatic testicular cancer 14 years prior. Potential treatment complications include all of the following EXCEPT

   (A) hypomagnesmia
   (B) hypertension
   (C) acute myeloid leukemia
   (D) hyperuricemia
   (E) hepatic fibrosis

16. Which defense mechanism would you most likely find in obsessive–compulsive personality disorder (OCPD)?

   (A) fantasy
   (B) isolation
   (C) projection
   (D) sublimation

17. A 55-year-old man is admitted to the intensive care unit (ICU) with acute hypoxemic respiratory failure. His wife states he had been completely asymptomatic prior to going to work today. Chest radiograph reveals diffuse, bilateral, fluffy infiltrates. His ventilator settings are tidal volume 700 mL (7 cc/kg), 18 breaths per minute, positive end-expiratory pressure (PEEP) of 7, and 100% FiO_2 that maintains his SaO_2 at 89%. His complete blood count (CBC) and metabolic panel are normal, initial electrocardiogram (ECG) shows no acute changes, and troponin T is negative. What should you do next?

   (A) Obtain a transthoracic echocardiogram to assess left ventricular function.

   (B) Place a pulmonary artery catheter.

   (C) Begin broad-spectrum antibiotics.

   (D) Place him in the prone position.

   (E) none of the above

18. A 65-year-old former smoker with severe emphysema presents to the ED with acute-onset dyspnea after a coughing spell. Physical exam shows BP 85/55, pulse 132 (sinus), and respirations 36, with severe respiratory distress, trachea slightly deviated to the left, and decreased breath sounds on the right. What should you do?

  (A) Decompress the left side with an 18-gauge needle in the sixth intercostal space (ICS) in the midaxillary line.
  (B) Decompress the right side with an 18-gauge needle in the sixth ICS in the midaxillary line.
  (C) Decompress the left side with an 18-gauge needle in the second ICS in the midclavicular line.
  (D) Decompress the right side with an 18-gauge needle in the second ICS in the midclavicular line.
  (E) Place a chest tube in the sixth ICS in the right midaxillary line.

19. A 31-year-old woman presents for evaluation after 6 months of amenorrhea. She tells you that she has been pregnant three times and she has delivered two living children. A pregnancy test is negative. She has no withdrawal bleeding after therapy with medroxyprogesterone 10 mg for 5 days. Her physical exam is unremarkable, including pelvic exam. Prolactin and thyroid-stimulating hormone (TSH) are normal. What should be the next step?

  (A) MRI of the pituitary gland
  (B) estradiol level
  (C) follicle-stimulating hormone (FSH) level
  (D) pelvic ultrasound
  (E) trial of oral contraceptives

20. A 39-year-old African-American man is seen in the office for a routine exam. He is found to have a blood pressure of 160/90. In considering hypertension in this patient, which of the following statements is correct?

  (A) The prevalence is lower in African-Americans than in whites.

  (B) Compared to whites, African-Americans receiving adequate treatment will have less overall decline in blood pressure.
  (C) Cardiovascular risk factors are more common in the African-American population.
  (D) Diuretics are of limited use in African-Americans.

21. A patient with acquired immune deficiency syndrome (AIDS) is admitted to the medicine service with weight loss and severe pain with swallowing. On exam he is thin, afebrile, and orthostatic. His oropharynx is without evidence of thrush. The most appropriate management of this patient would include

  (A) IV acyclovir empirically for herpes simplex virus esophagitis
  (B) IV fluconazole empirically for esophageal candidiasis
  (C) steroids for presumed apthous ulcer in the esophagus
  (D) sending urine for *Histoplasma* antigen
  (E) scheduling for esophagoscopy with biopsies

22. Which of the following groups of symptoms is most consistent with Ménière's disease (endolymphatic hydrops)?

  (A) vertigo, ear pain, cranial nerve (CN) VI palsy
  (B) ear pain, otorrhea, CN VII palsy
  (C) vertigo, tinnitus, hearing loss
  (D) aural pressure, headache, tinnitus
  (E) vertigo, oscillopsia, nausea

23. What is the most common cause of erectile dysfunction in men?

  (A) psychological causes
  (B) premature ejaculation
  (C) pelvic nerve injury
  (D) arterial disease
  (E) venous leak syndrome

24. All of the following statements regarding use of the ECG for evaluation of myocardial ischemia are true EXCEPT

(A) about 50% of patients experiencing angina show ischemic changes on the ECG while experiencing pain

(B) up to 40% of patients presenting with acute MI fail to show diagnostic changes on the initial ECG

(C) a patient presenting in shock with no acute ST-segment or T-wave changes is unlikely to have cardiogenic shock

(D) the combination of a normal ECG and normal troponin T level rules out myocardial ischemia

25. Potential causes of metabolic acidosis associated with an increase in the anion gap include each of the following EXCEPT

(A) methanol ingestion
(B) uremia
(C) ethylene glycol toxicity
(D) lactic acidosis
(E) renal tubular acidosis

26. A 60-year-old man with a history of Type 2 diabetes mellitus presents with a 2-hour history of nausea, vomiting, and epigastric discomfort. Bedside glucose by fingerstick is 195 mg/dL. He is afebrile with a BP of 110/70 and a pulse of 50. His abdomen is nontender. Based on the information provided, which of the following represents the most appropriate initial plan of management?

(A) Administer IM promethazine and send the patient to radiology for an ultrasound study of the gallbladder.

(B) Send the patient to radiology for flat and upright abdominal x-rays.

(C) Order an ECG.

(D) Obtain an arterial blood gas with co-oximetry.

(E) Order an enema.

27. The most characteristic change noted after division of one recurrent laryngeal nerve is

(A) harsh, strangled voice
(B) inspiratory stridor
(C) niphasic stridor

(D) normal voice with inability to sing high notes or project the voice

(E) weak, breathy voice

28. What is the preferred pharmacologic agent for the treatment of voiding symptoms secondary to an enlarged prostate estimated to be > 50 g in size?

(A) terazosin
(B) oxybutinin
(C) baclofen
(D) finasteride
(E) tamulosin

Items 29–33

A 70-year-old patient presents for routine evaluation. Ocular examination reveals normal visual acuities. Slit lamp examination is normal. Fundoscopic examination reveals the optic disc to have an enlarged cup-to-disc ratio in both eyes.

29. Which of the following must be considered the most likely diagnosis?

(A) central retina artery occlusion
(B) glaucoma
(C) papilledema
(D) anterior segment optic neuropathy
(E) optic disc drusen

30. Which of the following would be an appropriate test to perform?

(A) visual field testing
(B) intraocular pressure testing
(C) gonioscopy
(D) all of the above
(E) none of the above

31. If the visual fields were normal, this would rule out

(A) glaucoma
(B) anterior ischemic optic neuropathy
(C) optic disc drusen
(D) all of the above
(E) none of the above

32. Which of the following statements is correct?

(A) All patients with glaucoma must have elevated intraocular pressures.

(B) Patients with glaucoma must have visual field defects.

(C) All patients with glaucoma must have a family history of glaucoma.

(D) Patients with glaucoma may have normal pressures.

(E) Patients with glaucoma must have loss of visual acuity.

33. Which of the following statements is correct?

(A) All patients with anterior ischemic optic neuropathy have abnormal cups.

(B) All patients with optic disc edema have red swollen discs.

(C) All patients with large cups have glaucoma.

(D) all of the above

(E) none of the above

END OF SET

34. What is the age-specific prostate-specific antigen (PSA) level for a 50-year-old man?

(A) 0 to 2.5 ng/mL

(B) 0 to 4.0 ng/mL

(C) 2.5 to 5.0 ng/mL

(D) < 10 ng/mL

35. A 20-year-old male college student with a 2-day history of mild flulike symptoms is now brought in with confusion, fever, and a widespread confluent petechial skin rash. Which of the following is the most appropriate order of interventions for optimal management of this patient?

(A) Obtain a head CT, perform a lumbar puncture (LP), and give antibiotics if cerebrospinal fluid (CSF) findings are consistent with a bacterial infection.

(B) Give acetaminophen, draw blood cultures, perform an LP, and give antibiotics as soon as the CSF results are reported.

(C) Draw blood cultures, give IV antibiotics, obtain a head CT, and then perform an LP.

(D) Draw an arterial blood gas (ABG), order a urine toxicity screen, give naloxone, and obtain a head CT.

36. Alpha-1-antitrypsin deficiency has been associated with which skin condition?

(A) acne

(B) panniculitis

(C) erythema multiforme

(D) psoriasis

(E) alopecia areata

37. Which of the following types of alopecia are nonscarring?

(A) alopecia areata

(B) discoid lupus erythematosus

(C) lichen planopilaris

(D) tufted folliculitis

38. All of the following conditions associated with chronic hepatitis C virus (HCV) infection should NOT be treated with interferon and ribavirin therapy EXCEPT

(A) renal failure

(B) manic depression

(C) alcoholism

(D) genotype I infection

(E) hemolytic anemia

(F) pregnancy

(G) advanced cirrhosis

39. Which of the following drugs has a category X rating due to high risk of teratogenicity?

(A) isotretinoin

(B) cyclosporine

(C) methotrexate

(D) acyclovir

(E) tetracycline

40. A 35-year-old man with AIDS who has taken no prescription medications in the past 3 months now presents with nonproductive cough and dyspnea on exertion, which has developed gradually over the past 2 weeks. Review of old records show a CD4 count of 150 6 months ago. ABG shows a room air PO_2 of 60. Chest x-ray shows minimal interstitial infiltrates bilaterally. Which of the following choices is most appropriate?

(A) Start oral trimethoprim–sulfamethoxazole (TMP-SMZ) and discharge home.
(B) Admit this man to an ICU.
(C) Give supplemental O_2 and IV steroids, start doxycycline, and admit.
(D) Administer clarithromycin and IM dexamethasone and admit.
(E) Give supplemental O_2, administer steroids, start TMP/SMZ, and admit.

41. Which of the following is true concerning monoclonal gammopathies of unknown significance (MGUS)?

(A) It is present in about 3% of the population > 70 years of age.
(B) It is associated with a decrease in polyclonal immunoglobulins in the serum.
(C) It is usually associated with plasmacytosis (more than 10% plasma cells) of the bone marrow.
(D) It often evolves into a malignant process.
(E) The concentration of monoclonal protein in the serum usually increases with time.

Items 42–43

42. A 42-year-old laborer feels a "pop" in his lower back while at work. After 1 week of bed rest, he is seen in your office, where his neurologic exam demonstrates 4/5 power of the left extensor hallucis longus, tibialis anterior, peroneus longus, and tibialis posterior muscles. Deep tendon reflexes in the legs are normal. Sensory exam reveals loss of sensation over the dorsal great toe. Your diagnosis is

(A) left peroneal neuropathy
(B) left sciatic neuropathy
(C) left lumbar plexopathy
(D) left L5 radiculopathy
(E) right spinal cord compression

43. An appropriate first therapy for this patient may include

(A) bed rest, moist heat, and anti-inflammatory agents
(B) physical therapy
(C) epidural steroid injection
(D) lumbar laminectomy
(E) immediate return to work at full duty

END OF SET

44. Which of the following antibiotics must be renally adjusted in a hemodialysis patient in order not to precipitate seizures?

(A) imipenem
(B) cefazolin
(C) ceftriaxone
(D) doxycycline

45. A young adult presents after blunt trauma to the head with a swollen, tender auricle. After evacuation of the hematoma, what is the most important next step in management?

(A) intravenous antibiotics
(B) placement of a drain
(C) oral antibiotics
(D) CT scan of temporal bone
(E) pressure dressing

46. A 65-year-old man presents to the ED with a 4-hour history of severe right side flank pain, gross hematuria, nausea, and vomiting. A plain radiograph of the abdomen fails to reveal the presence of a calculus. A subsequent renal ultrasound demonstrates a right renal hydronephrosis and a hyperechoic mass in the proximal ureter consistent with a stone. What is the presumptive diagnosis?

(A) acute renal infarction
(B) a calcium stone that is too small to visualize on the radiograph
(C) a uric acid calculus
(D) a calcified ureteral cancer
(E) acute pyelonephritis with abscess formation

47. A 56-year-old man presents with sexual dys-function over the past year. Libido is normal, but erections have been difficult and rare. There is no galactorrhea. His medical history is significant for 10 years of diabetes mellitus, hypertension, and hypercholesterolemia. His medications include metformin, glipizide, quinapril, and atorvastatin. On physical ex-amination, the patient is 5'7", 325 lbs. Vitals are normal. Virilization is normal, and the testes are normal at 4 cm in length bilaterally. Laboratory tests show a serum total testos-terone of 224 ng/dL (N: 270–1070), FSH of 9 μ/mL (N: 1–14), and LH of 12 μ/mL (N: 2.3–13). Which of the following most likely explains the laboratory findings?

    (A) prolactinoma
    (B) nonfunctioning pituitary adenoma
    (C) hypothyroidism
    (D) obesity
    (E) diabetes

48. Regarding their maladaptive behavior, peo-ple with personality disorders feel

    (A) no anxiety
    (B) some anxiety

    (C) very anxious
    (D) often suicidal
    (E) none of the above

49. A 36-year-old rancher who has never smoked presents to the ED in March with 3 weeks of waxing and waning symptoms of fever, as well as cough and dyspnea that seem to oc-cur about 4 hours after putting out hay for his cattle. His chest radiograph reveals dif-fuse bilateral alveolar infiltrates. What is the most likely diagnosis?

    (A) asthma
    (B) community-acquired pneumonia
    (C) silo filler's lung
    (D) farmer's lung
    (E) sarcoidosis

50. A 64-year-old male smoker presents to your office with 3 weeks of hemoptysis. Which of the following is the most appropriate test?

    (A) bronchoscopy
    (B) sputum cytology
    (C) chest radiograph
    (D) bronchial artery angiogram
    (E) CT scan of the chest

Practice Test 10
Answers and Explanations

1. **(A)** Thrombolytics are contraindicated in all the listed conditions except mild hypertension. They are contraindicated in severe hypertension.

2. **(B)** Metronidazole is an antibiotic that possesses excellent anaerobic and some parasitic activity. It is generally well tolerated. Patients should be advised not to drink alcohol while taking metronidazole because a disulfiram-like reaction may occur.

3. **(A)** This is clearly a cystic mass, lateral in the neck. A parotid carcinoma would appear solid. The tonsils are medial in the neck and would protrude into the airspace of the pharynx. The carotid artery is clearly seen (it takes up contrast) and is normal. Thyroglossal duct cysts are in the midline of the neck.

4. **(E)** This woman is considerably younger than the usual presentation of breast cancer. Sixty-six percent of patients are over the age of 50. Three generations of affected women suggests an autosomal dominant inheritance pattern. This is consistent with a mutation in the BRCA 1 gene on chromosome 17. The relatives of carriers have an 85% lifetime risk of developing the disease plus a 20 to 60% risk of developing ovarian cancer. The p53 suppressor mutation is seen in Li–Fraumeni syndrome. The 14,18t is consistent with follicular lymphoma and the t9,22 is consistent with chronic myelocytic leukemia (CML). The RET gene is seen in multiple endocrine neoplasia (MEN) type IIA syndrome.

5. **(D)** All of the other historical factors put the patient at risk for tubal damage and subsequent ectopic pregnancy. A history of gestational diabetes is not associated with any increased risk of ectopic pregnancy.

6. **(C)** While first defined using transabdominal ultrasound, currently the discriminatory zone describes the level of hCG above which an intrauterine gestational sac can be reliably visualized on transvaginal ultrasound in a normal uterus. Once an intrauterine gestation is confirmed, the diagnosis of ectopic pregnancy becomes very unlikely, except when assisted reproductive technology (ART) has been used.

7. **(D)** All of the other factors can interfere with the reliability of transvaginal ultrasound in the detection of early intrauterine gestation and therefore decrease the reliability of the discriminatory zone.

8. **(C)** Once an intrauterine pregnancy is confirmed on ultrasound, the diagnosis of ectopic pregnancy becomes very unlikely. While serum hCG levels can be helpful as serial measurements to confirm appropriate doubling and to see if the patient's level is in the discriminatory zone, a single hCG level in isolation only confirms pregnancy if positive. It does not exclude or confirm the diagnosis of ectopic pregnancy. Ultrasound is more sensitive than CT scan in the diagnosis of early intrauterine pregnancy. While a low hemoglobin or hematocrit may raise suspicion of intra-abdominal bleeding and therefore ec-

topic pregnancy, there are many other potential causes for anemia. In addition, the CBC is frequently normal in women with ectopic pregnancies. Finally, while a culdecentesis may diagnose intra-abdominal bleeding, false-positive testing can occur, and a negative result does not exclude the diagnosis of ectopic pregnancy.

9. **(A)** The patient has a very high likelihood of an ectopic pregnancy with an hCG over 2,000 and no IUP on an adequate transvaginal ultrasound. She is hemodynamically stable and is able to return for follow-up care. She is an excellent candidate for the medical management of ectopic pregnancy with methotrexate, which has a median success rate of approximately 90% in resolving the ectopic pregnancy without surgical intervention. The other agents mentioned have not been used in the treatment of ectopic pregnancy.

10. **(E)** The classical triad of symptoms and signs associated with eclampsia are hypertension, edema, and proteinuria. Fetal growth restriction leading to SGA infants is seen with preeclampsia and is felt to be secondary to placental insufficiency caused by vascular changes at the placental level. While elevation of blood sugar is associated with gestational diabetes, it is not associated with preeclampsia, especially as an isolated finding.

11. **(E)** Large prospective studies have shown that even without treatment, facial nerve function returns to normal or near normal in Bell's palsy 95% of the time.

12. **(A)** Often following a significant injury, the knee is much too painful to allow an adequate examination. The best early treatment is splinting, rest, and ice. A good examination once the knee has "cooled off" may easily reveal the true extent of the injury.

13. **(C)** The prolonged bleeding time in aspirin-treated patients is not a vitamin K–dependent phenomenon as with coagulation factors II, VII, IX, and X. This can be corrected

with DDAVP (desmopressin) if this is needed during a bleeding episode. NSAIDs do affect platelet function, and the effects of aspirin on platelet function last through the life span of the platelet, which is 10 to 14 days.

14. **(E)** The patient has vitamin D deficiency due to malabsorption from celiac disease and secondary hyperparathyroidism.

15. **(E)** The cure rate for metastatic testicular cancer is greater than 80%, with toxicities noted in less than 10% of patients. However, side effects can be chronic and need to be evaluated. Those most notable include acute myeloid leukemia, melanoma, hypercholesterolemia, Raynaud's phenomenon, pulmonary fibrosis, hearing loss, hypomagnesemia, hyperuricemia, hypertension, mild renal insufficiency, and peripheral neuropathy.

16. **(B)** Isolation is a characteristic of the orderly, controlled people who are often labeled OCPD. (*Kaplan & Sadock, 780*)

17. **(A)** In the setting of hypoxemic respiratory failure and diffuse pulmonary infiltrates, it is essential to know whether the pulmonary edema is cardiogenic or noncardiogenic. Knowing what the left ventricular function is will determine the treatment. If low, this could be cardiogenic pulmonary edema; if normal, then it is likely adult respiratory distress syndrome (ARDS). A pulmonary artery catheter could be used if an echo was not readily available.

18. **(D)** Recognize a tension pneumothorax with hemodynamic compromise and the appropriate initial therapy. The first thing to do is to relieve the pressure. This is rapidly and easily accomplished by placing an 18-gauge Angiocath into the second ICS in the midclavicular line. This will ease the hemodynamic compromise and allow you to gather equipment needed for more definitive therapy (i.e., tube thoracostomy).

19. **(C)** After ruling out pregnancy and hyperprolactinemia, a negative medroxyprogesterone trial means that the patient is hypoestrogenic. It is therefore important to know if the hypoestrogenic state is due to ovarian or pituitary failure. FSH will help distinguish between both etiologies. If it is high, then premature ovarian failure is the diagnosis. If it is normal or low, then pituitary imaging is indicated. There is no need to measure estradiol, since we know that the patient is hypoestrogenic.

20. **(D)** The prevalence of hypertension in African-Americans is among the highest in the world. Hypertension develops at earlier ages and there are a greater number with stage 3 hypertension. Complications of hypertension are higher in African-Americans. On adequate therapy, hypertension responds similarly. There is a higher prevalence of cardiovascular risk factors such as obesity, smoking, and Type 2 diabetes in African-Americans. In both African-Americans and whites, diuretics have been proven to reduce morbidity and mortality from hypertension. It should be given as the initial drug of choice in the absence of a specific contraindication.

21. **(E)** The differential diagnosis for odynophagia, not just dysphagia, in a patient with AIDS includes apthous ulcers, esophageal candidiasis, herpes simplex virus, and cytomegalovirus as well as multiple other infections. One could pick a number of agents to empirically treat with while potentially missing the correct diagnosis. An endoscopic examination will provide the diagnosis so that the appropriate regimen may be prescribed.

22. **(C)** This is the classic "triad" of Ménière's disease, which typically occur together as a paroxysm or "spell." Patients will often have aural pressure with the classic triad as well.

23. **(E)** Although each of the areas identified may result in erectile dysfunction in men, it is the venous leak syndrome, which is the most common abnormality in men. This syndrome results in the inability to store blood in the corpora cavernosum with a secondary weak erection, which is lost quickly.

24. **(D)** The ECG and serum markers such as CK-MB, troponin T, and troponin I are very helpful in the identification of patients who have sustained myocardial injury. Currently, however, no combination of serum markers and ECG findings can reliably exclude myocardial ischemia. Clinical judgment and appropriate use of chest pain observation unit protocols involving serial ECGs and cardiac enzymes, as well as other testing, are necessary to evaluate patients with chest pain who are felt to be at risk for cardiac ischemia.

25. **(E)** The "MUDPILES" mnemonic is a useful way to remember common causes of metabolic acidosis associated with an increased anion gap. These include **m**ethanol ingestion, **u**remia, **d**iabetic ketoacidosis, **p**araldehyde ingestion, **i**ron and **i**soniazid ingestion, **l**actic acidosis, **e**thylene glycol ingestion, and **s**alicylate intoxication. Renal tubular acidosis causes a metabolic acidosis with a normal anion gap.

26. **(C)** The patient has at least three of the traditional risk factors for myocardial infarction: diabetes mellitus, male sex, and age. Diabetes mellitus is a major risk factor for MI. MI represents the major cause of death among diabetics. Also, diabetic patients appear to be more likely to have "silent" MI, in which infarction is not accompanied by chest pain. Nausea and vomiting is frequently the presenting complaint in such cases. An immediate ECG is essential to appropriately evaluate this patient.

27. **(E)** Division of the recurrent laryngeal nerve causes the vocal cord to be paralyzed in an off-midline position, causing a weak, breathy voice. Unilateral vocal cord paralysis almost never causes stridor. Inability to sing high notes or project the voice is caused by injury to the external branch of the superior laryngeal nerve.

28. (D) Finasteride (Proscar) is an inhibitor of 5-alpha reductase and leads to a reduction in dihydrotestosterone levels in the prostate. This results in a reduction in the size of the prostate over 6 to 12 months with an improvement in voiding symptoms. The drug is most efficacious in men with large prostate glands > 40 to 50 g in size. Alpha blockers such as terazosin (Hytrin) and tamulosin (Flomax) may be helpful as well.

29. (B) Glaucoma is a major cause of painless loss of vision. Patients are asymptomatic initially. Their visual acuities remain stable until severe loss of vision occurs. Enlargement of the optic cup relative to the optic disc is characteristic of patients with glaucoma.

30. (D) Glaucoma is a diagnosis made based on clinical findings. These include an optic disc with an enlarged cup-to-disc ratio, elevated intraocular pressure, and abnormal visual fields. The intraocular pressure is tested routinely. Visual field testing may show an abnormality to the field if elevated intraocular pressure causes damage to the optic nerve. Elevated intraocular pressure is a leading risk factor for optic disc damage. The grading of the anterior chamber angle to determine if the patient has open-angle glaucoma, narrow-angle glaucoma, or trauma-associated glaucoma is done using the technique of gonioscopy.

31. (B) Anterior ischemic optic neuropathy, whether caused by nonarteritic or arteritic vasculopathy, is associated with visual field abnormalities. Glaucoma may be associated with normal visual fields early in the course of the disease. The patient may have had elevated intraocular pressure, which may have been treated before visual field defects occurred. Optic disc drusen may also be associated with visual field defects, but a normal visual field does not rule out the presence of optic disc drusen.

32. (D) While glaucoma is usually associated with elevated intraocular pressures, abnormal cupping of the disc, and visual field ab-

normalities, not all patients have these findings. Normal tension glaucoma does exist. These patients experience damage to their nerve head even though their pressures are normal by the definition of normal. For this reason, the findings of severe cupping of the nerve head may lead to the diagnosis of glaucoma in spite of normal intraocular pressures.

33. (E) Patients with anterior ischemic optic neuropathy may have pale or atrophic-looking nerve heads but the cup-to-disc ratios may be normal. Patients with optic disc edema may have pale swelling as is seen in diabetic optic disc edema. Large cup-to-disc ratios may be indicative of glaucoma. On the other hand, there are patients who have large cup-to-disc ratios that may represent normal variations. Glaucoma is usually a constellation of findings including increased cup-to-disc ratio, elevated intraocular pressure, and visual field defects. Independent and isolated findings should not be taken out of context.

34. (B) The general range for men of all ages is 0 to 4.0 ng/mL. However, younger men tend to have smaller prostate glands in general and therefore the most sensitive cutoff level is 0 to 2.5 ng/mL.

35. (C) When dealing with the possibility of bacterial meningitis, it is generally best to "shoot first and ask questions later." The correct order of intervention is to first assess and stabilize ABCs (airway, breathing, circulation), collect blood cultures, and administer empiric antibiotic therapy. CT of the head and LP can be done *after* initial stabilization and antibiotics.

36. (B) Alpha-1-antitrypsin deficiency may result in a necrotizing panniculitis.

37. (A) Alopecia areata is a common form of nonscarring hair loss that most likely has an autoimmune etiology. It frequently presents as well-circumscribed oval or round patches of hair loss on the scalp. It has a variable, unpredictable course.

38. **(D)** Age at initial HCV infection, viral load, genotype, gender, presence of fibrosis, and weight may help predict response to therapy and length of treatment, but they do not contraindicate therapy. Pregnancy is a contraindication to either medication. Hemolysis is a side effect of ribavirin therapy, and hemolytic anemia a contraindication. Renal failure precludes ribavirin due to dosing/toxicity concerns. Manic depression and advanced liver disease preclude interferon therapy (i.e., risk of worsening mania or depression, suicide, liver failure). Alcoholism should be treated before antiviral therapy is given.

39. **(A)** Teratogenicity is the most important adverse effect of the retinoid isotretinoin. The putative mechanism involves toxic effects on cephalic neural crest development.

40. **(E)** The patient has findings most consistent with *Pneumocystis carinii* pneumonia (PCP). The chest x-ray shows very minimal interstitial infiltrates at both bases. The "typical" chest x-ray in PCP shows diffuse bilateral infiltrates, but the appearance of the film can range from essentially normal to focal consolidation. The antibiotic of choice for PCP is TMP-SMZ. Because of his hypoxemia, he also needs admission for supplemental oxygen and steroids.

41. **(A)** The finding of a low level (< 3.5 g/dL) paraprotein and anemia is becoming quite common in older individuals. In general, MGUS does not progress to a malignant disorder, most commonly multiple myeloma, although if followed for 20 years, 2.2% can develop myeloma, amyloidosis, or macroglobulinemia. Features that distinguish MGUS from myeloma are the presence of no lytic lesions on skeletal survey, < 20% plasma cells in the bone marrow, and monoclonal spike < 3.5 g/dL immunoglobulin G (IgG) or < 2.0 g/dL immunoglobulin A (IgA). In general, the monoclonal protein of MGUS does not change much over time, again suggestive of a benign disorder.

42–43. **(42-D, 43-A)** This patient has had the acute onset of left L5 radiculopathy. The sudden onset makes herniation of an intervertebral disk most likely. The weakness of tibialis posterior (tibial nerve supplied) excludes peroneal neuropathy. The motor weakness suggests a more severe axonal injury and may allow for more aggressive therapies such as laminectomy, but first-line therapy should always be conservative. Surgery may be appropriate at a later date if the weakness persists, pain becomes intractable, or neuroimaging demonstrates a more severe structural lesion unlikely to respond to conservative management.

44. **(A)** Imipenem is a very broad-spectrum antibiotic. Seizures have been reported when it is used in patients with underlying seizure disorders or patients with renal failure when the dose was not adjusted. It is metabolized renally.

45. **(E)** The largest risk after auricular hematoma is re-formation of the hematoma in the potential space between the perichondrium and the cartilage. To minimize this risk, a pressure dressing of some type must be placed to hold the perichondrium against the cartilage; suturing the dressing in place can be particularly helpful.

46. **(C)** A uric acid calculus will be radiolucent on radiographic studies but will appear hyperechoic on ultrasound. Although a small calcium stone is possible, it would be unlikely to cause hydronephrosis and gross hematuria.

47. **(D)** Morbid obesity is associated with diminished levels of sex hormone–binding globulin (SHBG), resulting in low levels of total testosterone, but free testosterone is normal. Low levels of SHBG may be an effect of high levels of insulin on hepatic expression of this protein. The cause of this patient's erectile dysfunction is most likely diabetes.

48. **(A)** Patients with personality disorder do not feel anxiety about their maladaptive behavior. Personality disorder symptoms are alloplastic and ego syntonic. *(Kaplan & Sadock, 775)*

49. **(D)** Recognize the symptoms of hypersensitivity pneumonitis, which characteristically occur 4 to 8 hours after each exposure to the offending agent. Farmer's lung is due to thermophilic actinomycetes in moldy hay.

50. **(C)** The next best test is the chest radiograph. This will locate an obvious lesion and help direct bronchoscopy or surgery. In this patient at high risk for cancer, sputum cytology can also be helpful. In the presence of a negative chest radiograph, both CT and bronchoscopy are appropriate tests. Bronchial artery angiogram is not indicated this early in the workup.

Practice Test 11
Questions

DIRECTIONS (Questions 1 through 50): Each of the numbered items or incomplete statements in this section is followed by answers or by completions of the statement. Select the ONE lettered answer or completion that is BEST in each case.

1. A 32-year-old woman comes to your office complaining of a 2-month history of episodes of shortness of breath, racing heart, tingling fingers, dizziness, and an overwhelming fear that she is having a heart attack and is dying. These episodes last only a few minutes, but she is afraid they will happen unexpectedly, so she has restricted her usual activities. She has no significant past medical history and no history of substance abuse. Her medical workup is negative. She most likely suffers from

   (A) hypochondriasis
   (B) malingering
   (C) panic disorder
   (D) social phobia
   (E) histrionic personality disorder

2. Regarding valvular aortic stenosis, which of the following statements is true?

   (A) The most common cause of aortic stenosis in North America is rheumatic heart disease.
   (B) Degenerative aortic stenosis is associated with changes similar to those seen in coronary artery disease.
   (C) The overwhelming majority of patients with bicuspid aortic valves develop aortic stenosis.
   (D) Angina is a rare symptom of aortic stenosis.

3. A 55-year-old woman was started on captopril 3 weeks ago and presents to the emergency department (ED) with a feeling of swelling in her throat with no pain or fever. Examination of the mouth and oropharynx are unremarkable. What is the most appropriate next course of action?

   (A) subcutaneous epinephrine
   (B) consultation for airway evaluation
   (C) lateral neck soft tissue x-ray
   (D) cricothyroidotomy
   (E) discontinuation of captopril

4. A man presents with low back pain, urinary frequency, and a tender prostate. A urine sample is obtained for microscopic analysis. What is the most convincing sign of prostatic inflammation?

   (A) > 10 leukocytes per high-power field
   (B) presence of macrophages containing fat (oval bodies)
   (C) hematuria
   (D) nitrites on dipstick analysis
   (E) urinary crystals

Items 5–7

An 82-year-old patient is evaluated with a chief complaint of double vision. The patient is found to have ptosis and limited movement of the right eye. The pupil is normal. The patient's medical history is notable for diabetes mellitus. There were no other neurology signs or symptoms.

5. The most likely cranial nerve to be involved is

   (A) I
   (B) III
   (C) V
   (D) IV
   (E) VI

6. The most likely cause for this problem is

   (A) aneurysm
   (B) trauma
   (C) apex lesion of the lung
   (D) vasculopathic cranial nerve palsy
   (E) none of the above

7. All of the following tests should be obtained EXCEPT

   (A) magnetic resonance imaging (MRI)
   (B) chest x-ray
   (C) glucose evaluation
   (D) blood pressure
   (E) sedimentation rate

END OF SET

Items 8–12

A 38-year-old G3P2012 woman, last menstrual period (LMP) 3 weeks ago, presents to your office for her annual gynecologic exam. Her last Pap smear was 1 year ago, and it was normal. She is not sexually active currently. On further questioning, she admits to a 6-month history of increasing menorrhagia and abdominal pain. She also admits to urinary urgency and a feeling of pressure on her bladder. Physical examination reveals an enlarged, 12-week-size uterus that is irregular and firm. Her adnexa are nontender and not enlarged.

8. The next test that you would obtain at this time would be

   (A) serum beta human chorionic gonadotropin (hCG)
   (B) complete blood count (CBC) with differential
   (C) MRI
   (D) serum CA 125
   (E) pelvic ultrasound

9. You suggest all of the following options for treatment EXCEPT

   (A) myomectomy
   (B) gonadotropin-releasing hormone (GnRH) agonist therapy
   (C) hysterectomy with node sampling
   (D) observation
   (E) uterine artery embolization

10. You explain to her that the incidence of sarcomatous change in such cases is

   (A) < 1%
   (B) 10%
   (C) 30%
   (D) 75%
   (E) > 99%

11. The growth of uterine fibroids is most closely associated with

   (A) progesterone
   (B) growth hormone
   (C) human placental lactogen
   (D) estrogen
   (E) androstenedione

12. Which of the following types of uterine fibroids is most likely to be associated with menorrhagia and recurrent pregnancy loss?

   (A) pedunculated
   (B) intramural
   (C) subserosal
   (D) intraligamentary
   (E) submucosal

END OF SET

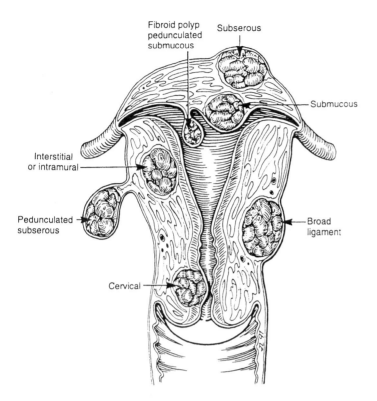

Figure 11.1 Uterine fibroid types

13. In regard to medullary carcinoma of the thyroid (MCT), which of the following statements is NOT true?

    (A) It can be associated with adrenal tumors.
    (B) It can be associated with pituitary and pancreatic tumors.
    (C) When MCT is familial, it has an autosomal dominant inheritance.
    (D) The biochemical marker is calcitonin.
    (E) When familial, the best screening test for family members is Ret oncogene analysis for mutations.

14. A 55-year-old man is seen in the ED with left upper quadrant pain and has a white blood count (WBC) of 280,000/μL. On exam, he has an enlarged spleen and a friction rub in the left upper quadrant. Other hematologic data include a platelet count of 850,000/μL, hemoglobin of 12.5 gm/dL, and differential with 61% segs, 110% bands, 55 metamyelocytes,

4% myelocytes, 3% promyelocytes, 2% myeloblasts, 4% monocytes, 5% eosinophils, 3% basophils, and 3% lymphocytes. What is the most likely diagnosis?

    (A) Leukemoid reaction to splenic infarct.
    (B) Interferon is contraindicated.
    (C) The eosinophilia and basophilia are unexpected findings.
    (D) The most likely molecular genetic correlate for this clinical presentation is the finding of t(9,22) involving bcr-abl (Philadelphia chromosome).
    (E) There is no role for allogeneic stem cell transplant in this disease.

15. Which of the following is consistent with sulfonylurea use in a patient with hypoglycemia (plasma glucose of 35 mg/dL)?

	Insulin	C-Peptide	Proinsulin
I	High	Low	High
II	High	High	High
III	High	High	Normal
IV	High	Low	Normal

    (A) I
    (B) II
    (C) III
    (D) IV

16. Police stopped a 35-year-old successful lawyer after a traffic accident. In the ED, he was observed to be extremely agitated and talkative. He was profusely sweating, with a rapid heart rate and dilated pupils. He stated that he felt like insects were crawling on his arms and legs. The most likely diagnosis is

    (A) phencyclidine (PCP) intoxication
    (B) bipolar disorder, manic
    (C) cocaine intoxication
    (D) amphetamine intoxication
    (E) all of the above

17. Following a closed fracture of the humeral shaft at the junction of the middle and distal thirds, the radial nerve is viewed not to function. All of the following are true EXCEPT

(A) wrist extension is present but not metacarpophalangeal (MCP) extension
(B) neither wrist nor MCP extension is present
(C) wrist and MCP extension are absent but the patient can extend the interphalangeal (IP) joints
(D) there is diminished sensibility in the anatomic snuffbox

Items 18–19

A 64-year-old woman with hypertension presents to your office with a complaint of two separate episodes of a loss of vision to the superior aspect of her left eye over the past few weeks. She denied headache or other neurologic symptoms and has no past history of similar episodes. She takes aspirin at a dose of 81 mg/day. Her neurologic examination is normal though a loud bruit is auscultated over the left carotid artery.

18. Diagnostic considerations at this point may include

(A) amaurosis fugax
(B) temporal arteritis
(C) migraine
(D) A and C
(E) A, B, and C

19. The patient has a normal computed tomography (CT) scan of the brain, normal echocardiogram, and a normal sedimentation rate. A carotid ultrasound suggests 70% stenosis of the left carotid artery and an arteriogram confirms this result. Your management at this point should be to

(A) increase the dose of aspirin
(B) switch to a different antiplatelet agent
(C) switch to warfarin
(D) suggest carotid endarterectomy
(E) wait for further symptoms

END OF SET

20. Rheumatic heart disease occurs as a late consequence of rheumatic heart disease. The valve most frequently involved is the

(A) aortic
(B) mitral
(C) pulmonic
(D) tricuspid

21. Which of the following is NOT a risk factor for developmental (congenital) dislocation of the hip?

(A) breech presentation
(B) Caucasian
(C) male
(D) first born
(E) other congenital anomalies

22. A 60-year-old woman from a developing country comes to the office complaining of difficulty lying flat because of shortness of breath. She has been awakened at night several times by shortness of breath that is not relieved until she sits or stands at the bedside. On physical exam, a III/VI diastolic rumble is heard at the lower left sternal border. There is a loud opening snap heard in diastole. Her chest x-ray shows left atrial prominence and elevation of the left mainstem bronchus. The most likely diagnosis is

(A) aortic stenosis
(B) mitral stenosis
(C) aortic regurgitation
(D) mitral regurgitation

23. An 18-year-old college student who was born in India has a 12-mm reaction to an intradermal (purified protein derivative [PPD]) TB test. He has proof of a bacillus Calmette–Guérin (BCG) vaccination as an infant in India. He has a negative chest radiograph and denies any fever or cough. How should you counsel him?

(A) Tell him the positive PPD is a result of the BCG vaccination and he should receive no further treatment.

(B) He is protected from pulmonary tuberculosis with the history of the BCG vaccine.

(C) He needs 9 months of therapy with isoniazid because it is impossible to tell if the positive reaction is secondary to the BCG.

(D) He is at no risk for the development of tuberculosis, so he should not receive any therapy.

24. The most critical aspect of the management of severe preeclampsia at or near term is

(A) medical management of blood pressure elevations

(B) bed rest

(C) careful fluid management

(D) delivery

(E) close monitoring of platelets and liver function

(F) seizure precautions at the bedside

25. A 40-year-old woman presents with a large nasal septal perforation with crusting and submucosal inflammation elsewhere in the nasal cavity. Chest x-ray reveals some discrete lesions in the lung parenchyma. Which of the following is the most appropriate next diagnostic test?

(A) C1 esterase level

(B) erythrocyte sedimentation rate (ESR)

(C) antineutrophil cytoplasmic antibody (ANCA)

(D) antinuclear antibody (ANA)

(E) angiotensin-converting enzyme (ACE) level

26. What is the definition of chronic bacterial prostatitis?

(A) pelvic pain of > 4 weeks' duration

(B) recurrent fever after adequate treatment with antibiotics

(C) recurrent urinary tract infections with persistence of bacteria in the prostatic secretions

(D) persistent urinary urgency and frequency after antibiotic therapy

27. An 80-year-old man with a history of hypertension, for which he takes a diuretic, slips on a throw rug, striking his head on the corner of a table while at home. He sustains a 3.5-cm forehead laceration but does not lose consciousness. Bleeding is controlled with direct pressure by his son, who witnessed his fall and has driven him to the hospital. He complains only of soreness of the forehead area but has no nausea or vomiting and generally feels well. His son indicates that his only reason for bringing him was to have the wound sutured. He is appropriately oriented, with a nonfocal neurological exam. His pulse is 80 and regular with a BP of 140/74. The remainder of his exam is remarkable only for a superficial forehead laceration. Which of the following is most appropriate?

(A) Order a skull series.

(B) Order a serum magnesium level.

(C) Order a head CT scan.

(D) Suture his laceration and send him home.

(E) Order an electrocardiogram (ECG) before making a final disposition.

28. A 50-year-old man with a history of chronic gastroesophageal reflux presents at 11 P.M. with a complaint of a piece of steak stuck in the throat since eating dinner around 6 P.M. He is having no difficulty breathing or speaking but has not been able to swallow liquids and complains of a sensation of something "hung" in the upper midchest area anteriorly. He is spitting his saliva into a cup. Which of the following actions is most appropriate?

(A) Order a barium swallow.

(B) Have the patient attempt to slowly sip a mixture of meat tenderizer (papain) and warm water.

(C) Give the patient an IM injection of a benzodiazepine for anxiolysis and advise him to see his primary care doctor tomorrow.

(D) Establish an IV line, start IV fluids, and order a chest x-ray.

(E) Order a CT scan of the chest.

29. What is the most appropriate treatment for scabies?

    (A) mupirocin
    (B) terbinafine
    (C) corticosteroids
    (D) acyclovir
    (E) permethrin

30. An otherwise healthy 15-year-old boy presents with a 2-hour history of cramping lower abdominal pain radiating to the right groin, which began while he was at soccer practice. He has subsequently developed nausea with two episodes of vomiting. Exam reveals a nontender abdomen with active bowel sounds. There is no hernia and no urethral discharge. There is mild testicular swelling and associated tenderness on the right. The right testicle is oriented in a horizontal axis, and there is absence of the cremasteric reflex on the right side. Each of the following statements is true EXCEPT

    (A) these findings are most consistent with acute epididymitis
    (B) immediate urology consultation is appropriate
    (C) Doppler ultrasound may be helpful in confirming your clinical impression but must not delay definitive treatment
    (D) IV fluids and parenteral analgesics are appropriate, and the patient should be kept NPO

31. Sézary syndrome is a subtype of

    (A) multiple myeloma
    (B) systemic lupus erythematosus (SLE)
    (C) dermatomyositis
    (D) cutaneous T-cell lymphoma
    (E) sarcoidosis

32. All of the following laboratory tests are consistent with a diagnosis of genetic hemochromatosis in a 65-year-old white man with cirrhosis EXCEPT

    (A) serum alanine transaminase (ALT) 312 U/L
    (B) C282Y/C282Y

    (C) serum ferritin 1,190 ng/mL
    (D) transferrin saturation 73%
    (E) hepatic iron index 2.3 μmol/g/year

33. All of the following persons should be given the hepatitis B virus (HBV) vaccination series EXCEPT

    (A) intravenous drug abuser, anti-HCV positive, HBsAg negative, anti-HBc positive, anti-HBs negative
    (B) alcoholic cirrhotic, anti-HCV negative, HBsAg negative, anti-HBc negative, anti-HBs negative
    (C) newborn premature baby, mother anti-HCV negative, HBsAg positive, anti-HBc positive, anti-HBs negative
    (D) predental student with no history of risk factors for hepatitis, who promises to be compliant with universal precautions
    (E) 60-year-old diabetic, anti-HCV negative, HBsAg negative, anti-HBc negative, anti-HBs negative

34. A 20-year-old woman is transported to the ED by EMS in a stuporous state after drinking some wine and ingesting "some pills" within the past hour. The patient is tachycardic, flushed, and warm to touch, with dry oral mucosa and dilated pupils. A 12-lead ECG obtained during transport by the EMS crew is shown in Figure 11.2. Based on the available information, which of the following toxins has most likely been ingested?

    (A) lorazepam
    (B) amphetamines
    (C) phenobarbital
    (D) amitriptyline
    (E) oxycodone

35. Untreated infantile scoliosis can lead to which of the following problems in later life?

    (A) bowel obstruction
    (B) pulmonary failure
    (C) cardiac problems
    (D) back pain
    (E) spinal stenosis

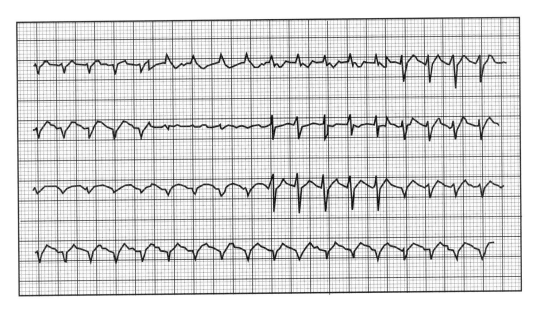

Figure 11.2

Items 36–40

A 29-year-old G3P1011 African-American woman presents to the delivery room at 35 weeks' gestation complaining of acute onset of moderate vaginal bleeding accompanied by crampy abdominal pain for the last 3 hours. Recent ultrasound on her chart shows that her placenta is fundal with no evidence of previa. Repeat ultrasound in the delivery room confirms fundal placental location. Speculum exam shows dark blood slowly oozing from the patient's cervical os, which is found to be 3 cm dilated and 80% effaced with the fetal vertex at –1 station on exam. Maternal vital signs show a BP of 130/90, pulse 80, respirations 16, and temperature 37° C (98.6° F). Maternal abdomen is soft, with estimated fetal weight of 5 lb. 8 oz. The fundus is mildly tender. The fetal monitor strip is shown in Figure 11.3.

36. What is the most likely cause for this patient's bleeding?

(A) placenta previa
(B) placental abruption
(C) cervical laceration
(D) bloody show

37. Immediate management of this mother and fetus should include all of the following EXCEPT

(A) urgent cesarean section
(B) intravenous fluids
(C) obtaining CBC and platelet count
(D) continuous fetal monitoring

38. All of the following are associated with placental abruption EXCEPT

(A) maternal age
(B) increased parity
(C) chronic hypertension
(D) personal history of abruption with a prior pregnancy
(E) multifetal pregnancy

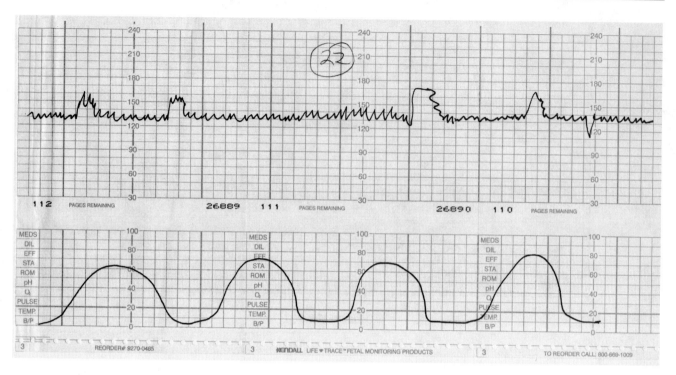

Figure 11.3

39. One hour after admission, maternal blood pressure is 160/110, and urine dipstick shows 2+ proteinuria after negative testing of urine for protein on admission. Cervical exam is 6 cm, 100% with the vertex at 0 to +1. The patient has had only spotting since admission, and the rest of her vital signs are stable. CBC on admission was normal, with a hemoglobin of 12 g and a platelet count of 200,000. Fetal monitor tracing is shown in Figure 11.4. Immediate management should include

(A) urgent cesarean section
(B) IV diazepam
(C) subcutaneous terbutaline to stop contraction
(D) initiation of IV magnesium sulfate
(E) fetal scalp pH

40. While the loading dose of magnesium sulfate is being administered, the patient's nurse confides in you that she thinks she has mixed 40 g instead of the usual 4 g into the IV solution and roughly one fourth of the solution has been administered. The patient acutely complains of shortness of breath, and a quick check of her patellar reflexes (after stopping the IV magnesium sulfate infusion) shows them to be absent. In addition to calling anesthesia STAT for possible intubation and respiratory support, what should you immediately administer intravenously?

(A) a 50% dextrose solution
(B) calcium gluconate
(C) potassium chloride
(D) terbutaline
(E) pitocin

END OF SET

41. A 37-year-old white man is brought to the ED after he was found unconscious in an alley. He has shallow respirations and pinpoint pupils and responds only to deep pain. The substance most likely to produce these symptoms is

(A) alcohol
(B) heroin
(C) PCP
(D) cocaine
(E) marijuana

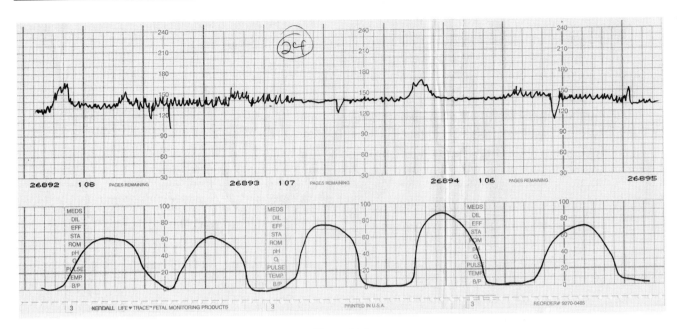

Figure 11.4

42. A 19-year-old man with Type 1 diabetes for 6 years presents to the ED with nausea, vomiting, and abdominal pain for 12 hours. He is on an NPH/regular insulin regimen. On physical examination, he is afebrile, orthostatic, and has a mildly tender abdomen.

    Laboratory studies show a plasma glucose of 562 mg/dL, sodium 121 mEq/L, potassium 3.1 mEq/L, chloride 92 mEq/L, bicarbonate 12 mEq/L, and pH 7.13. He is given an insulin infusion at a rate of 7 U/hr, following a loading dose of 7 U. A saline infusion is also running at 500 mL/hr. With therapy, the glucose level falls progressively, and at 7:00 A.M., his glucose is 84 mg/dL. Dextrose is added to the fluids. Anion gap is now 10, and ketones are negative. Breakfast will be ready in about 30 to 45 minutes. What would you do?

    (A) Decrease the rate of insulin infusion to 2 U/hr.

    (B) Stop insulin infusion.

    (C) Stop insulin infusion and give him his usual insulin dose (NPH/regular).

    (D) Stop insulin infusion, recheck glucose in 30 minutes, and, if > 100 mg/dL, give him his usual insulin dose (NPH/regular).

    (E) Give him his usual insulin dose (NPH/regular), and stop insulin infusion 30 minutes later.

43. A 30-year-old man presents with a fracture of the tibia following a fall from a 12-foot ladder in his yard. He has an obvious fracture of the middle third of the tibia with a 5-cm wound and dirt on the end of the protruding fracture fragment. His distal pulses are 2+. Which of the following best describes his injury?

    (A) Type I open fracture

    (B) Type II open fracture

    (C) Type III A open fracture

    (D) Type III B open fracture

    (E) Type III C open fracture

44. Patients at high risk for sudden death should be evaluated and considered for implantation of an implantable cardioverter defibrillator (ICD). Which of the following patients should be evaluated for an ICD implant?

    (A) A 47-year-old man has had an anterior wall myocardial infarction. His ejection fraction is 30%. On 24-hour ambulatory monitor, he has two runs of ventricular tachycardia, each 7 beats long.

    (B) A 27-year-old graduate student has recurrent syncope during oral presentations.

    (C) A 30-year-old woman has palpitations. Her ejection fraction is 60%. Her ECG is normal, and there is no structural heart disease. Her family history is negative for sudden death. A 24-hour ambulatory monitor shows three runs of ventricular tachycardia, each 10 beats long.

    (D) A 33-year-old woman has hypertrophic cardiomyopathy. She has no obstruction and has minimal symptoms. There is no family history of sudden death. A 24-hour ambulatory monitor shows 3,000 premature atrial contractions.

45. A patient with a history of a splenectomy is at increased risk for the development of overwhelming bacteremia with all of the following organisms EXCEPT

    (A) *Streptococcus pneumoniae*
    (B) *Capnocytophaga*
    (C) *Pseudomonas aeruginosa*
    (D) *Neisseria meningitidis*

46. The most successful treatment for a man with chronic nonbacterial prostatitis includes all of the following EXCEPT

    (A) empiric trial of antibiotics directed at *Chlamydia* and *Ureaplasma*
    (B) nonsteroidal agents and sitz baths
    (C) transurethral resection of the prostate
    (D) alpha blockers such as doxazosin
    (E) video urodynamics

47. The prognosis in Perthes disease is better for a child age

    (A) 0 to 5 years
    (B) 5 to 8 years
    (C) 8 to 11 years
    (D) Age is not a factor, only the amount of femoral head involvement

48. Of the following diagnoses, which is associated with a clear secondary gain?

    (A) factitious disorder
    (B) conversion disorder
    (C) somatoform disorder
    (D) malingering
    (E) all of the above

49. A 30-year-old woman is seen in the ED with oliguria. She was given chemotherapy several days ago for the first time for a high-grade lymphoma. She has mild nausea and vomiting. Multiple nodes are evident on examination, but the patient feels there has already been substantial shrinkage. The cause of oliguria is

    (A) tumor lysis syndrome
    (B) acute nephrotoxicity from chemotherapy
    (C) antidiuretic hormone secretion by the lymphoma
    (D) volume depletion due to nausea and vomiting
    (E) bilateral ureteral obstruction by the lymphoma

50. Concerning thyrotoxic crisis, all of the following statements are correct EXCEPT

    (A) the cardinal manifestation is fever
    (B) on the basis of routine thyroid tests, patients in thyroid storm are indistinguishable from those with uncomplicated thyrotoxicosis
    (C) laboratory findings may include hyperglycemia, leukocytosis, and hyponatremia
    (D) therapy includes PTU (propylthiouracil), iodine, beta blockers, and glucocorticoids
    (E) lithium can be used in the treatment

Practice Test 11
Answers and Explanations

1. **(C)** The woman most likely suffers from panic disorder, which is characterized by at least a 1-month history of recurrent panic attacks that develop abruptly and peak within 10 minutes, persistent concern about having additional attacks, or worry about going crazy/losing control/having a heart attack or a significant change in behavior as a result of the attacks. The disorder may or may not be associated with agoraphobia.

2. **(B)** Many cases of so-called degenerative aortic stenosis are associated with inflammatory lesions that resemble the plaque of coronary artery disease. There is a modest relationship between the risk factors associated with the development of coronary artery disease and the development of aortic stenosis. Many valves that are stenotic are congenitally bicuspid. About 1 to 2% of the population has congenitally bicuspid valves and about half of these become stenotic. Rheumatic fever is not common in North America. Angina is a frequent symptom of severe aortic stenosis.

3. **(B)** This is a characteristic presentation of acquired angioedema secondary to ACE inhibitor medications. With no stridor or airway distress, emergency airway establishment (cricothyroidotomy) is not needed, but fiberoptic endoscopic evaluation is.

4. **(B)** The presence of macrophages containing fat (oval bodies) is highly suggestive of prostatic inflammation. These are not seen in healthy men or those with urethritis. The other findings can be seen with many infectious and benign conditions of the urinary tract.

5. **(B)** The third cranial nerve is responsible for extraocular movements except the superior oblique (IV) and the lateral rectus (VI) muscles. Ptosis is a common finding in patients with complete third nerve palsies since the superior branch of the third nerve innervates the levator muscle.

6. **(D)** Lesions of the lung apex can cause Horner's syndrome but are not associated with third nerve palsy. Trauma can cause third nerve palsy, but generally it is very severe trauma with skull base fractures. Aneurysms usually cause third nerve palsy with pupillary involvement (dilatation). Diabetes mellitus and vasculopathic processes commonly cause isolated, pupil-sparing third nerve palsies.

7. **(B)** MRI should be done to rule out tumor or stroke, both of which are unlikely with a normal pupil but are still possible. Blood pressure should be tested as an additional possible vasculopathic risk factor. Sedimentation rate should be tested to help exclude temporal arteritis as a cause for third nerve palsy. Glucose elevation would indicate poor control of diabetes mellitus as a risk factor for third nerve palsy. The chest x-ray would be of low yield in this setting.

8. **(E)** This is a classic case presentation of uterine fibroids. There is a history of increasing menorrhagia, pelvic pressure, and urinary

symptoms. The uterus is enlarged and irregular in size. Since she is not sexually active and her LMP was 3 weeks ago, it is highly unlikely that a pregnancy test would be positive. A CBC may not be abnormal in women with fibroids, except that she may be anemic secondary to the menorrhagia. An elevated CA 125 may be found in cases of epithelial ovarian cancer but is very nonspecific for intra-abdominal pathology in general. Finally, although MRI and pelvic ultrasonography are good for imaging the pelvis, pelvic ultrasound is cheaper, faster, and more readily available, and thus would be the next test obtained at this time. (Beckmann, 531–534)

9. **(C)** Fibroids may be managed medically, surgically, or by observation. Myomectomy refers to removal of the fibroids themselves, whereas hysterectomy is curative in that there is no chance of recurrence. Fibroids are benign, smooth muscle tumors of the uterus and very rarely malignant; thus, there is no need to do a node sampling at the time of surgery. GnRH agonist therapy may be used to shrink fibroids medically by inducing a hypoestrogenic state. Finally, uterine artery embolization is a new experimental procedure in the treatment of fibroids. (Beckmann, 534–537)

10. **(A)** The incidence of malignancy in uterine fibroids is less than 1%. (DeCherney, 733)

11. **(D)** The growth of uterine fibroids is most closely associated with estrogen production. They are most common in African-American women in their 20s and 30s, and regress after menopause as a result of the abrupt decline in endogenous estrogen levels. Progesterone may antagonize the effects of estrogen at the level of the estrogen receptors, and therefore progesterone does not usually result in fibroid growth. The growth of fibroids is not directly related to any of the other hormones listed either. (Beckmann, 535)

12. **(E)** Submucosal fibroids are the type of fibroids most likely associated with menorrhagia as well as recurrent pregnancy losses. In-

tramural and subserosal fibroids may be associated with increased dysmenorrhea or pelvic pain and fullness. Pedunculated fibroids and intraligamentary fibroids may often be asymptomatic and not discovered until routine pelvic exam. (Beckmann, 532)

13. **(B)** MCT can be associated with pheochromocytomas and hyperparathyroidism in multiple endocrine neoplasia type IIa (MEN IIa), pheochromocytomas, and mucosal neuromas in MEN IIb. It is not part of MEN I, which includes pituitary tumors, pancreatic tumors, and hyperparathyroidism. Because it has an autosomal dominant inheritance, family members of a patient with MCT should be screened by doing a Ret oncogene analysis mutation (on chromosome 10).

14. **(D)** The findings of elevated WBC, mostly neutrophils with absolute eosinophilia, basophilia, and monocytosis, as well as elevated platelets are classic for chronic myelogenous leukemia (CML). The enlarged spleen is also very characteristic for this disease entity. The 9,22 translocation of bcr on 22 and c-abl on 9 is also well characterized. Leukemoid reactions seldom produce WBCs higher than 50,000/µL, and there is no associated eosinophilia and basophilia. High-dose chemotherapy with stem cell rescue from a matched sibling donor can be curative in 60 to 90% of cases. Interferon can prolong the chronic phase of this disease.

15. **(B)** Sulfonylureas will enhance beta-cell function and lead to high insulin, C-peptide, and proinsulin levels—a very similar profile to patients with insulinomas. The only way to differentiate both conditions is to send a serum sulfonylurea screen in which the laboratory can detect the sulfonylurea drug.

16. **(E)** Each disorder can manifest with the patient's symptoms.

17. **(A)** The radial nerve passes through the lateral intermuscular septum at the junction of the middle and distal thirds of the humerus. The nerve is prone to injury at that level, as it

is tethered by the intermuscular septum. Wrist and MCP joint extension is affected. IP joint extension is a function of the lumbrical muscles innervated by the median and ulnar nerves.

18–19. (18-E, 19-D) Visual symptoms without headache are not uncommon in patients with migraine. This is especially true when onset occurs later in life. Temporal arteritis should always be a consideration in older patients with visual loss. Headache is not an invariable symptom.

The North American Symptomatic Carotid Endarterectomy Trial was unequivocal in suggesting that patients who were symptomatic from a more than 70% occluded carotid artery had fewer subsequent transient ischemic attacks (TIAs) and strokes when treated surgically as opposed to medically with antiplatelet agents or warfarin. With a less than 70% stenosis, increasing the dose of aspirin or switching to a different antiplatelet agent (such as clopidogrel, ticlopidine, or dipyridamole) may be the proper course of action. Recent literature has suggested that warfarin may not be as effective as aspirin in noncardiac causes of stroke or TIA.

20. (B) The mitral valve is affected in 50 to 60% of cases of rheumatic heart disease. The aortic valve is affected commonly but is generally seen in combination with mitral disease. The tricuspid valve is affected < 10% of the time and is always associated with mitral and aortic disease. The pulmonic valve is almost never affected.

21. (C) Developmental dislocation of the hip is rarely seen in male children. The correct term for this type of dislocation is developmental instead of congenital, as newborns have been observed with concentrically reduced hips at birth that later sublux or dislocate secondary to joint laxity.

22. (B) Although both mitral stenosis and aortic regurgitation cause diastolic murmurs, the symptoms, the rumbling quality of the murmur, and the opening snap all suggest mitral

stenosis. Mitral stenosis is the most common lesion seen with rheumatic heart disease. Aortic stenosis and mitral regurgitation cause systolic murmurs.

23. (C) The BCG vaccine is used in many countries around the world to prevent disseminated tuberculosis (especially meningitis) in children. The effect that it has on giving a false-positive TB skin test usually happens for only a few years after receiving the vaccine. This effect wanes after several years. For that reason, anyone with a positive PPD who has received BCG in the past should be treated as if they have latent TB infection and receive the appropriate therapy.

24. (D) Preeclampsia is cured by delivery. While all of the other aspects mentioned are important in the management of a mother with preeclampsia, especially when the fetus is at or near term, delivery is crucial in the management of this disease.

25. (C) This is a characteristic demographic group and a characteristic presentation of Wegener's granulomatosis. ANCA level is the most specific serologic test for Wegener's granulomatosis.

26. (C) The diagnosis of chronic bacterial prostatitis requires that bacteria be localized to the prostate with repeat urinary cultures and examination of the prostatic secretions. The persistence of pelvic pain may be associated with chronic nonbacterial prostatitis or other conditions.

27. (C) Elderly patients typically undergo atrophy of the brain as a result of the aging process, with resultant stretching of the bridging veins, which increases susceptibility to intracranial hemorrhage with a blow to the head. The threshold for ordering a CT scan of the brain thus should be lower for the elderly than for younger patients. It is often stated that any laceration above the eyebrows that results from blunt trauma in an elderly patient warrants a head CT scan, which allows not only evaluation of the intracranial contents, but also the bones of the skull, and has clear advantage over a skull series. Other studies such as an ECG may be indicated for evaluation of falls in the elderly if there is suspicion of a syncopal episode as the cause of the fall but are not necessary when there is a well-documented mechanical cause for the fall.

28. **(D)** When a patient presents with a food bolus impacted in the esophagus, it generally needs to be removed endoscopically. Equally important, endoscopic exam can identify pathology of the esophagus responsible for the impaction. While a wide variety of "noninvasive" treatments for this condition have been advocated in the past, most are rather ineffective, and some, such as the use of papain, are potentially dangerous. The larger the food bolus and the longer it has been impacted, the greater the risk of pressure necrosis of the esophageal mucus. Papain may increase the risk of esophageal perforation. Ordering a barium swallow may result in aspiration of barium by the patient and may also remain impacted in the esophagus, thus interfering with subsequent endoscopy. Administration of an IV benzodiazepine may temporarily make the patient more comfortable, but at the cost of blunting airway protection reflexes, thus increasing the risk of pulmonary aspiration. The most appropriate action for the patient presented would be to establish an IV line, start fluids, order a chest x-ray, and consult a gastroenterologist for endoscopy. A CT scan of the chest is not appropriate.

29. **(E)** Scabies infestation is treated with permethrin cream. Consideration should be given to also treating all close contacts.

30. **(A)** Testicular torsion must be included in the differential diagnosis of any male presenting with abdominal pain, groin pain, or scrotal pain. Testicular torsion is a true urological emergency. The peak incidence of testicular torsion occurs during puberty, but it may occur at any age. Usually, the testis that

is at risk for torsion is aligned along a horizontal axis rather than along the normal vertical axis. There is often a history of vigorous physical activity or trauma prior to development of a torsion, although the condition may develop during sleep. Typical findings of epididymitis include fever, chills, dysuria, pyuria, and localization of the pain area to a swollen tender epididymis. The epididymis is posterior to and palpably separate from the testicle.

31. **(D)** Sezary syndrome is a subtype of cutaneous T-cell lymphoma (CTCL) characterized by lymphadenopathy and cutaneous erythema. The diagnosis is established by a skin biopsy showing CTCL and the presence of atypical mononuclear cells in the peripheral blood.

32. **(A)** Genetic hemochromatosis, if not detected early in life and treated, most often manifests in later years with *mildly* elevated serum transaminase levels, elevated transferrin saturation, very high serum ferritin levels, and hepatic iron indices over 1.9 μmol/g/year of age. The most common gene defect is C282Y homozygosity.

33. **(E)** Diabetes is not an indication for hepatitis B vaccination, nor is it routine to vaccinate adults without risk factors. Persons at future risk of HBV infection, such as medical, nursing, and dental students, who have no previous history of risk factors for HBV, all should be vaccinated and do not need prevaccination serologies (most cost-effective strategy). Babies born to women who are HBsAg positive all require hepatitis B virus vaccination and hepatitis B hyperimmune globulin as soon as possible after birth, whether premature or mature. An alcoholic with cirrhosis, with negative serology, should be vaccinated, as should any person with chronic non-HBV liver disease. The IV drug abuser is at risk for HBV infection, and the serology profile suggests previous HCV exposure, as well as isolated anti-HBc positivity, which is not always due to HBV infection. In fact, it is not unusual for persons infected with HCV to be

positive for anti-HBc. Thus, HBV vaccination is indicated.

34. **(D)** The patient exhibits features of the anticholinergic toxidrome. The ECG shows a wide QRS complex and a rightward axis shift of the terminal portion of the QRS complex, resulting in a prominent R-wave in lead aVR. This combination of findings is strongly suggestive of a toxic ingestion of a tricyclic antidepressant such as amitriptyline.

35. **(B)** Untreated progressive scoliosis causes severe shortening and rotation of the thoracic spine. Rib cage deformity can be severe, with a significant decrease in pulmonary reserve.

36. **(B)** Given the amount of bleeding and the lack of placenta previa on ultrasound, as well as visualization of uterine source of bleeding on exam, especially with maternal hypertension, placental abruption is the most likely diagnosis.

37. **(A)** Cesarean section is not indicated unless maternal or fetal condition becomes unstable. The current monitor strip shows a reactive fetus with a negative stress test. Maternal vital signs are reassuring.

38. **(E)** While many pregnancy complications are more common with multifetal pregnancy, placental abruption is not one of them. Personal history of prior abruption greatly increases the risk of subsequent abruption while chronic hypertension and preeclampsia are commonly associated conditions. While age and increasing parity have been shown to be risk factors, the association is modest.

39. **(D)** The increase in the patient's blood pressure along with the development of proteinuria make the diagnosis of preeclampsia, and magnesium sulfate therapy is indicated for seizure prophylaxis. Diazepam is not well tolerated by the fetus. With current maternal and fetal stability and labor progress, expectant management of labor is indicated. The fetal monitor strip shows a normal fetal heart rate with good long- and short-term variabil-

ity as well as no decelerations with contractions. With suspected abruption, any attempt to stop labor, especially at this close to term, is ill advised.

40. **(B)** The patient is exhibiting signs and symptoms of magnesium toxicity. Calcium gluconate is the antidote and should be administered promptly in a 1-g dose intravenously. The other medications listed will not reverse the effects of magnesium on respiration and would be potentially dangerous under these circumstances.

41. **(B)** Of the substances listed, heroin is the only intoxication syndrome associated with miosis.

42. **(E)** After recovery from diabetic ketoacidosis (DKA), there should be an overlap of 30 to 60 minutes between starting subcutaneous insulin injection (regular insulin) and stopping the insulin infusion, because the half-life of intravenous insulin is only 8 minutes, and subcutaneous insulin does not start working before 30 minutes.

43. **(D)** Open fractures are graded by the severity of the wound. Treatment is guided by this classification. A small puncture wound less than 1 cm in length, usually caused by a fracture spike, is considered a Type I wound. A Type II wound is greater the 1 cm in length, clean, and the fracture does not have extensive periosteal stripping. Type III wounds have extensive periosteal stripping. A Type III A wound is clean. A Type III B wound is grossly contaminated. A Type III C wound is associated with a vascular injury to the extremity requiring repair. Amputation of an extremity, especially the lower leg, is common with a Type III C open fracture.

44. **(A)** Factors associated with high risk for sudden death include: post–myocardial infarction patients with reduced ejection fractions and nonsustained ventricular tachycardia (VT); patients with structural heart disease and recurrent unexplained syncope; idiopathic cardiomyopathy with syncope or VT;

hypertrophic cardiomyopathy with syncope or VT; right ventricular dysplasia; or long QT syndrome.

45. **(C)** An important function of the spleen is its ability to filter out and opsonize certain organisms, especially encapsulated organisms. Patients with a history of splenectomy, either surgical or autosplenectomy (e.g., sickle cell disease), are at risk for overwhelming bacteremia due to *S. pneumoniae, N. meningitidis, Haemophilus influenzae, Capnocytophaga,* and *Babesia.*

46. **(C)** Although video urodynamics may demonstrate outlet obstruction in some men with symptoms of chronic prostatitis, this disorder is rarely successfully treated with a resection of the prostate. Additionally, repeat courses of antibiotics usually fail to alter the symptoms since a bacterial infection is not the etiology.

47. **(A)** The younger the child, the more likely the better outcome as there is more time for femoral head and acetabular remodeling before growth ceases. Children over the age of 9 have the poorest outcome. The amount of femoral head epiphysis that becomes avascular is also a factor in prognosis.

48. **(D)** By definition, to make a diagnosis of malingering, you must identify a secondary gain.

49. **(A)** This is a typical presentation for tumor lysis syndrome, and thus many patients with

high-grade, bulky lymphomas are generally hospitalized for their first chemotherapy to ensure adequate hydration and urination in the event of tumor lysis. The amount of nausea/vomiting from chemotherapy appears minimal in this patient and would not cause this oliguria. It is unlikely that the ureter is obstructed by lymphoma given the fact that the patient has noted decreases in the palpable nodes. Although acute nephrotoxicity can occur with chemotherapy, the setting of a rapid response to chemotherapy with nausea and vomiting is more consistent with tumor lysis. Lymphomas are not known to secrete antidiuretic hormone, nor is this a likely cause of oliguria.

50. **(C)** Thyroid storm accounts for 1 to 2% of hospital admissions for thyrotoxicosis. Cardinal manifestations include fever > 38.6 to 38.8° C (101.5 to 102° F), tachycardia (out of proportion to the fever), gastrointestinal dysfunction (nausea, vomiting, diarrhea), and change in mental status. Triiodothyronine (T_4) and thyroxine (T_3) values are not particularly different from the values in uncomplicated thyrotoxicosis. Hyperglycemia may result from increased glycogenolysis. Serum electrolytes are usually normal. Leukocytosis, mild hypercalcemia, and abnormal liver function tests can be seen. Lithium may be used in patients who are allergic to iodine, and works by inhibiting thyroid hormone release from the thyroid gland.

Practice Test 12
Questions

1. A 25-year-old woman is found to have a 2-cm thyroid nodule on physical examination. Fine-needle aspiration biopsy (FNAB) is done. All of the following statements are correct EXCEPT

    (A) the risk of cancer in that nodule is about 5%

    (B) papillary carcinoma is the most common thyroid carcinoma

    (C) papillary carcinoma can usually be diagnosed confidently by FNAB

    (D) follicular carcinoma cannot be diagnosed by FNAB

    (E) 80% of follicular neoplasms will be malignant

Items 2–3

A 22-year-old woman complains of palpitations that are of abrupt onset. In general, episodes last minutes and are regular but fast. She recalls at least one episode in which the palpitations were grossly irregular and she was presyncopal. She has a family history of sudden death. Her baseline electrocardiogram (ECG) is shown in Figure 12.1.

2. The cause of the *irregular* palpitations most likely was

    (A) preexcited atrial fibrillation

    (B) atrioventricular (AV) node reentry

    (C) ventricular fibrillation

    (D) complete heart block

3. The correct treatment for this patient would be

    (A) electrophysiologic testing and catheter ablation

    (B) diltiazem

    (C) vagal maneuvers

    (D) digoxin

END OF SET

4. Which of the following statements is true regarding acute bacterial endocarditis?

    (A) Enterococcal endocarditis may be treated with a first-generation cephalosporin.

    (B) Vegetation size is an important determinant for the need of a valve replacement.

    (C) Right-sided endocarditis with methicillin-susceptible *Staphylococcus aureus* in an intravenous drug user may be treated for 2 weeks with nafcillin and gentamicin.

    (D) Development of congestive heart failure (CHF) is not an indication for valve replacement.

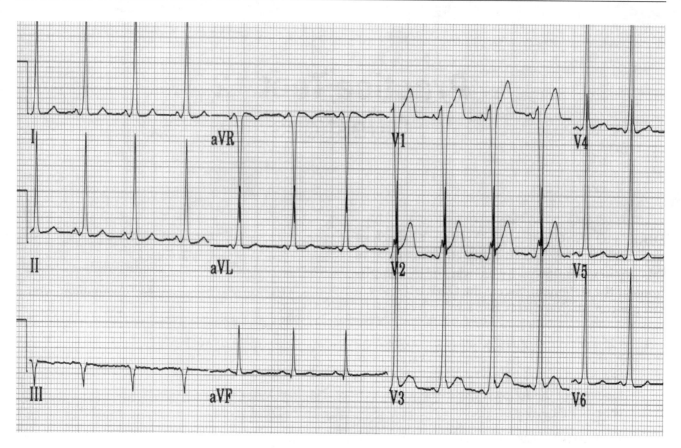

Figure 12.1

5. A 20-year-old patient presents with fever, throat pain, odynophagia, and muffled voice. Examination reveals enlarged tonsils nearly covered with a gray-white exudate. Which of the following is the most likely diagnosis?

   (A) peritonsillar abscess
   (B) deep neck abscess
   (C) herpangina
   (D) *Candida* pharyngitis
   (E) infectious mononucleosis

6. What percentage of men will experience symptoms of prostatitis in their lifetime?

   (A) 10%
   (B) 25%
   (C) 50%
   (D) 100%

Items 7–9

A 50-year-old woman presents with a history of blurred vision in the right eye. Her onset is acute. She has no pain. On physical examination, the patient appears to be well. Funduscopic examination reveals a creamy-white lesion and subretinal fluid in the superotemporal portion of the macula. The lesion is approximately 3 disc diameters in size. A second creamy-white lesion is seen in the superonasal quadrant. The left eye is normal.

7. The most important step in the patient's management is to

   (A) begin chemotherapy
   (B) begin radiation therapy
   (C) determine the primary
   (D) begin with antibiotic therapy
   (E) perform an eye tissue biopsy

8. This patient's workup will focus on

    (A) hematologic studies for a clotting disorder
    (B) evaluation for hypertension
    (C) breast examination
    (D) family history of visual loss that is autosomal dominant
    (E) family history of recent raw meat ingestion

9. The most important step in the patient's management is to

    (A) begin chemotherapy
    (B) begin radiation therapy
    (C) determine the primary
    (D) begin with antibiotic therapy
    (E) perform an eye tissue biopsy

END OF SET

10. Each of the following findings is typical of acute appendicitis EXCEPT

    (A) emesis preceding development of abdominal pain
    (B) low-grade fever
    (C) change in the character and location of pain over a number of hours
    (D) anorexia
    (E) leukocytosis

11. A 24-year-old woman being evaluated for lower abdominal pain is found to have significant cervical motion tenderness (CMT). Which of the following statements is most accurate regarding this physical finding?

    (A) Presence of CMT is diagnostic of pelvic inflammatory disease (PID).
    (B) Presence of CMT essentially excludes the presence of acute appendicitis.
    (C) Presence of CMT excludes ectopic pregnancy as the cause of the patient's pain.
    (D) CMT is a nonspecific finding requiring correlation with other clinical data.

12. The symptoms of acute bacterial prostatitis include all of the following EXCEPT

    (A) fever
    (B) urinary frequency and urgency
    (C) myalgia
    (D) gross hematuria
    (E) low back pain

13. All of the following are risk factors for preeclampsia EXCEPT

    (A) obesity
    (B) nulliparity
    (C) renal disease
    (D) diabetes
    (E) family history of preeclampsia/eclampsia

14. Regarding the use of implantable cardioverter defibrillators (ICDs), all of the following statements are true EXCEPT

    (A) ICDs are more effective than antiarrhythmic drugs in reducing arrhythmic cardiac death
    (B) in patients with ICDs, sudden cardiac death is virtually eliminated
    (C) ICDs are superior to antiarrhythmic drugs in prolonging survival in patients who have survived life-threatening arrhythmias
    (D) ICDs are indicated in patients with cardiac arrests that occur without myocardial infarction

15. The presence of which of the following devices in a patient prevents the use of a magnetic resonance imaging (MRI) scan in the workup of a patient suspected of having a lumbar spine tumor?

    (A) total hip arthroplasty
    (B) implanted bone growth stimulator in the lower leg for nonunion of the tibia
    (C) plates and screws in the foramen used for fracture fixation
    (D) pacemaker
    (E) all of the above

16. Bile acid sequestrants are indicated in the treatment of

   (A) increased low-density lipoprotein (LDL)-C
   (B) decreased high-density lipoprotein (HDL)-C
   (C) increased triglycerides
   (D) A and B
   (E) all of the above

17. A 78-year-old woman is brought by her son to the ED with change in mental status for the past few weeks. She is lethargic and very pale with periorbital edema and swelling of her extremities. She has a blood pressure of 100/60 mm Hg, pulse 50/min, temperature 31/3° C (88° F), oxygen saturation 84%, a serum sodium 125 mEq/L, and blood glucose 52 mg/dL. Your immediate management includes

   (A) normal saline infusion
   (B) electric warming blankets
   (C) hydrocortisone 100 mg intravenously (IV), then 300 μg of levothyroxine IV
   (D) hydrocortisone 100 mg IV, then 100 μg of levothyroxine IV
   (E) levothyroxine 100 μg IV

18. A 22-year-old man presents with a 4-week history of intermittent fevers, sore throat, lymphadenopathy, and tender splenomegaly. He is noted to have a hemoglobin of 14.7 g/dL; white blood count (WBC) 17,000/μL with 70% lymphocytosis, some of which have atypical feature; and platelet count 310,000/μL. Mild transaminitis is evident as well. Which test would most likely explain this patient's illness?

   (A) human immunodeficiency virus (HIV) serology
   (B) bone marrow analysis
   (C) lymph node biopsy
   (D) flow cytometry of the lymphocytes
   (E) Epstein–Barr virus (EBV) titers

19. A consult is called on a 63-year-old man who has just undergone cardiac surgery. The surgery team states that the patient is very psychotic and having auditory hallucinations, but that he has no prior psychiatric history. Which of the following would be the LEAST likely diagnosis?

   (A) alcohol withdrawal
   (B) schizophrenia
   (C) adverse reaction to general anesthesia
   (D) delirium

20. A 22-year-old white man, status post motor vehicle accident in which he totaled his car, was brought to the ED. He reports feeling increased energy, with little to no sleep that night. Earlier that day, he was seen running naked in his dorm. He also noted that he was hearing voices telling him that his parents were evil demons. The most likely diagnosis is

   (A) Bipolar Disorder, Manic with mood-incongruent psychotic features
   (B) Bipolar Disorder, Manic with mood-congruent psychotic features
   (C) Bipolar Disorder, Mixed with mood-congruent psychotic features
   (D) Bipolar Disorder, Depressed with mood-congruent psychotic features

21. A 63-year-old man noted blood in his stool on several occasions during the past several months. He has also noted some intermittent fatigue and dyspnea on exertion. He has been using aspirin frequently for headaches. He denies an alcohol or tobacco history and has not lost weight. His exam is benign except for external hemorrhoids. Laboratory studies were done as follows:

Hemoglobin	10.5 g/dL
MCHC	33.5 g/dL
MCV	72 fL
WBC	9,200/μL
Neutrophils	75%
Lymphocytes	16%
Platelet count	1,000,000/μL
Ferritin	5 μg/mL
BUN	9 mg/dL

Cr	1.0 mg/dL
Total bilirubin	0.8 mg/dL
Alk Phos	75 U/L
LDH	Normal
ALT/AST	25/24
Hemoccult	Positive

Chest x-ray was normal, as were an upper endoscopy and colonoscopy. Which of the following is the most appropriate therapy for the elevated platelet count?

(A) hydrea

(B) splenectomy

(C) interferon therapy

(D) erythropoietin

(E) iron

22. Appropriate therapy for an infected dog bite would include

(A) ciprofloxacin

(B) cephalexin

(C) amoxicillin–clavulanate

(D) clindamycin

23. Which of the following is the pathophysiology of cholesteatoma?

(A) cholesterol-based neoplasm from retained blood in the middle ear

(B) neoplasm of the middle ear mucosa

(C) squamous cells coalescing on the medial surface of the tympanic membrane

(D) plaque formation in the fibrous layer of the tympanic membrane

(E) neoplasm from the endolymphatic sac

24. Benign prostatic hyperplasia (BPH) develops in which region of the prostate?

(A) peripheral zone

(B) transition zone

(C) anterior fibromuscular stroma

(D) bladder neck region

25. Which of the following tests is NOT required in the initial evaluation of a man with BPH?

(A) serum creatinine

(B) urinalysis

(C) serum prostate-specific antigen (PSA)

(D) bladder ultrasound for calculation postvoid residual

(E) digital rectal examination

26. A 42-year-old woman with a previously diagnosed autoimmune condition presents with the rash shown in Figure 12.2. What is it called?

(A) Janeway lesions

(B) Gottron's papules

(C) Lisch nodules

(D) Koenen's tumors

(E) Angioid streaks

27. A 34-year-old man with a history of heavy alcohol use is seen in the ED with a 48-hour history of constant bandlike upper abdominal pain, nausea, and some vomiting. All of the following would support admission to the intensive care unit (ICU) EXCEPT

(A) serum hemoglobin 17.1 g/dL

(B) serum creatinine 3.7 mg/dL

(C) serum amylase 3,627 U/L

(D) Pa 02 53 mm Hg

(E) arterial pH 7.17

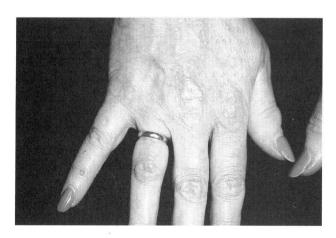

Figure 12.2

28. All of the following should be repaired surgically in a middle-aged, fit patient EXCEPT

   (A) right inguinal hernia, moderate in size, uncomfortable climbing stairs

   (B) incisional hernia, small, uncomfortable upon lifting boxes

   (C) sliding hiatal hernia, moderate, occasional heartburn

   (D) paraesophageal hernia, moderate in size, asymptomatic

   (E) complete malrotation on upper gastrointestinal (GI) barium study, occasional postprandial bloating

29. A 25-year-old G2P1 woman who is currently 28 weeks pregnant stumbles as she is getting out of her car and falls to the ground, striking her abdomen and abrading both hands and knees. There is no loss of consciousness and her only significant complaint is soreness of the lower abdomen. Vital signs are normal. The abdomen is soft and minimally tender, with the uterine fundus palpable midway between the umbilicus and the xiphoid. Fetal heart tones are present at 140 bpm by Doppler. There are no uterine contractions noted, and bowel sounds are normal. The patient has no vaginal bleeding or fluid leakage. Which of the following represents the most appropriate course of action at this time?

   (A) Order an obstetrical ultrasound and discharge the patient if this is normal.

   (B) Order a computed tomography (CT) scan of the abdomen.

   (C) Request plain films of the abdomen.

   (D) Initially, evaluate the patient with an obstetrical ultrasound and, if normal, send her to the labor and delivery suite for at least 4 hours of fetal monitoring.

   (E) Reassure the patient and discharge her home with instructions to follow up with her gynecologist tomorrow.

30. A 25-year-old man returns from a camping trip in North Carolina in mid-May complaining of 3 days of mild flulike symptoms associated with dull headache and a fever to 39.7° C (103.6° F). Exam shows no nuchal rigidity and a nonfocal neurological exam. A very faint erythematous rash is noted around the wrists and ankles. His WBC is 8.5, platelets are low at 105,000, and serum sodium is low at 129. Each of the following statements is true EXCEPT

   (A) doxycycline is the usual drug of choice for treatment

   (B) serologic testing is now widely available, and antibiotic therapy should not be used unless positive

   (C) up to 17% of affected patients never develop a rash with this illness

   (D) this is a rickettsial disease

   (E) this is a tick-borne illness, but only about 50% of affected patients recall tick exposure

31. The 72-year-old woman shown in Figure 12.3 presented with a pruritic generalized rash characterized by urticarial plaques and bullae. Direct immunofluorescence reveals which of the following patterns?

   (A) linear immunoglobulin G (IgG) and C3 along the basement membrane

   (B) linear IgA along the basement membrane

   (C) granular deposits of IgA at tips of the dermal papillae

   (D) IgG and C3 between keratinocytes

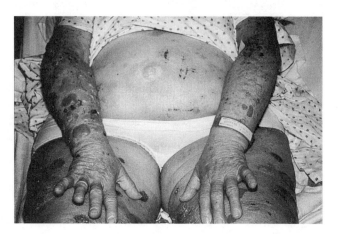

Figure 12.3

32. A 34-year-old G5P5 woman is admitted to the hospital with severe, acute upper abdominal pain, with nausea. She is afebrile. Her exam and laboratory tests are consistent with a moderately severe case of acute pancreatitis. An abdominal ultrasound exam reveals multiple small gallstones within an otherwise normal gallbladder, and a swollen pancreas with some peripancreatic fluid collections. The biliary tree is normal. Which of the following best explains why enteral feeding via a nasojejunal (NJ) feeding tube is preferable to total parenteral nutrition (TPN) and bowel rest?

   (A) NJ tube feedings probably decrease bacterial translocation from the gut in contrast to feeding by TPN.

   (B) NJ tube feedings include glutamine, which is difficult to give via TPN, and this improves patient mortality.

   (C) NJ tube feedings cost less than feeding by TPN.

   (D) NJ tube feedings enhance GI motility, especially if there is an ileus.

33. The acute treatment of a man with acute bacterial prostatitis can include all of the following EXCEPT

   (A) placement of a urethral catheter

   (B) oral antibiotic therapy for 2 to 4 weeks

   (C) IV antibiotic therapy

   (D) transrectal ultrasound

34. Which of the following is a potential acute airway emergency?

   (A) epiglottitis

   (B) vocal cord paralysis

   (C) deep neck abscess

   (D) peritonsillar abscess

   (E) lingual tonsillitis

35. A 57-year-old man has a history of lung cancer. He presents to the ED complaining of severe fatigue, dizziness, and shortness of breath. His chest x-ray shows cardiomegaly and a pleural effusion. His blood pressure was 80/60, pulse 110 bpm, and respiratory rate 20. His echocardiogram is shown in Figure 12.4. The most likely diagnosis is

   (A) incipient cardiac tamponade

   (B) acute myocardial infarction

   (C) pneumothorax

   (D) aortic dissection

Items 36–38

A 72-year-old left-handed man with hypertension and a long history of smoking presents to the ED with the acute onset 2 hours prior of an inability to speak, right homonymous hemianopsia, and weakness of his right face and arm more than leg. His initial blood pressure is 190/110, and his heart rate is 76 and regular. A CT scan of his brain obtained in the ED is normal.

36. Your initial diagnosis is

   (A) left basal ganglia hemorrhage

   (B) left anterior cerebral artery infarct

   (C) left middle cerebral artery infarct

   (D) left frontal lobe tumor

   (E) right middle cerebral artery infarct

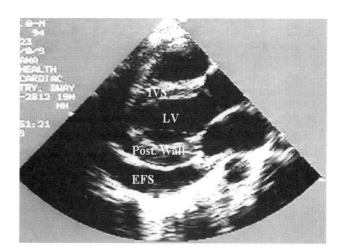

Figure 12.4

37. Initial therapeutic management should include

    (A) aggressive control of blood pressure
    (B) IV heparin
    (C) IV tissue plasminogen activator (TPA)
    (D) IV mannitol
    (E) observation only

38. This patient has a repeat CT scan of the brain 48 hours after onset of symptoms (see Figure 12.5). Seventy-two hours after onset of symptoms, the patient becomes acutely somnolent, with new onset of left pupil dilatation. Your next course of action should be

    (A) hyperventilation
    (B) mannitol
    (C) dexamethasone
    (D) neurosurgical consultation
    (E) immediate CT scan of the brain

END OF SET

39. A 50-year-old woman is seen with the MRI scan you ordered for workup of a 4-cm thigh mass. The MRI image is consistent with what may be a sarcoma. The radiologist has recom-

mended a needle biopsy. The next most appropriate step is

    (A) open excisional biopsy
    (B) CT-directed needle biopsy as suggested by the radiologist
    (C) CT scan of the chest
    (D) referral to a musculoskeletal tumor surgeon

40. A 42-year-old woman presents for a routine physical with no complaints. During the exam, a 1.4-cm mass in the upper outer quadrant of the left breast is detected. It has not been previously documented and feels firm. The patient is sent for a mammogram, which by report is negative. The next step is to

    (A) observe the patient through several menstrual cycles
    (B) reassure the patient that she does not have breast cancer with a negative mammogram
    (C) repeat the mammogram in 6 months
    (D) refer the patient to a surgeon for biopsy
    (E) attempt to shrink the mass with estrogen and progesterone

41. Depressive symptoms may be associated with

    (A) schizophrenia
    (B) substance abuse
    (C) cyclothymia
    (D) anxiety disorders
    (E) all of the above

42. Which of the following is not a vegetative sign in depression?

    (A) decreased libido
    (B) weight loss
    (C) abnormal menses
    (D) fatigability
    (E) obsessive rumination

43. Niacin is indicated for the treatment of

    (A) increased LDL-C
    (B) decreased HDL-C

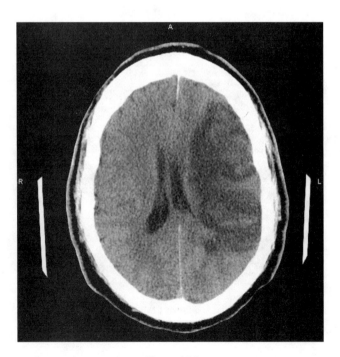

Figure 12.5

(C) increased triglycerides

(D) A and B

(E) all of the above

44. The fibrate gemfibrozil is useful in the treatment of

(A) increased triglycerides

(B) increased LDL-C

(C) decreased HDL-C

(D) A and B

(E) A and C

45. Which of the following best describes a comminuted fracture?

(A) a fracture communicating with a joint

(B) a fracture consisting of many fragments

(C) a fracture caused by a twisting movement

(D) a fracture in which the bone penetrates the skin

46. A patient involved in a motor vehicle accident is admitted to the ED. The abdomen, chest, and head have been evaluated and cleared. Orthopedic injuries are listed below. Which injury should be treated most urgently?

(A) closed left femur fracture

(B) L3 compression fracture

(C) closed right radius and ulna fracture

(D) closed left humerus fracture with nerve deficit

(E) posterior dislocation right hip

47. A 45-year-old man falls from a roof and lands on his feet. He sustains a fracture of the right os calcis. What other injury is he at high risk for?

(A) dislocation of the hip

(B) fracture of the ankle

(C) compression fracture of the lumbar spine

(D) fracture of the pelvis

(E) fracture of the femur

DIRECTIONS (Questions 48 through 50): Each group of items in this section consists of lettered headings followed by a set of numbered words or phrases. For each numbered word or phrase, select the ONE lettered heading that is most closely associated with it. Each lettered heading may be selected once, more than once, or not at all.

<u>Items 48–50</u>

Match the most appropriate choice of birth control to the clinical scenario.

(A) rhythm

(B) oral contraceptives

(C) oral contraceptives plus condoms

(D) bilateral tubal ligation

(E) abstinence

48. A 15-year-old nulligravid teenager who presents to the gynecologist for the first time and requests birth control. She has been sexually active for 6 months now with two different partners.

49. A 43-year-old G3P2012 woman who has completed her childbearing.

50. A 26-year-old G1P1001 woman who is in a 4-year monogamous relationship.

END OF SET

Practice Test 12
Answers and Explanations

1. **(E)** Cytologic findings are diagnostic in almost 85% of specimens. The remaining 15% are nondiagnostic; in this case, the nodule needs to be rebiopsied. When diagnostic, cancer is found in about 5% of cases, and it is usually of the papillary type. Follicular carcinoma cannot be diagnosed by FNAB, because the criterion for malignancy is capsular/vascular invasion, which can be seen only when the entire specimen is excised surgically. When the biopsy shows a follicular neoplasm, it means that the lesion is indeterminate and suspicious, and surgery needs to be done so that the entire specimen can be examined for capsular/vascular invasion. Almost 15 to 20% of follicular neoplasms will end up being follicular carcinomas on final surgical pathology; the remainder will be benign follicular adenomas.

2. **(A)** The baseline ECG demonstrates pre-excitation consistent with Wolff–Parkinson–White (WPW) syndrome. Atrial fibrillation is often poorly tolerated in people with WPW syndrome, particularly in those with rapidly conducting pathways. Most of this patient's symptoms are likely AV reentrant tachycardia. This involves a reentrant loop using both the AV node and the accessory pathway. Although AV node reentry is possible in patients with WPW syndrome, this patient's symptoms suggest an irregular rhythm. Although ventricular fibrillation is a potential consequence of preexcited atrial fibrillation in patients with very rapidly conducting pathways, this rhythm is generally catastrophic. There is no reason to suspect heart block.

3. **(A)** Symptomatic patients with WPW, particularly those with atrial fibrillation, are at potential risk of sudden death. Therefore, ablation is indicated. While vagal maneuvers may terminate reentrant arrhythmias, the risk of sudden death precludes using this alone. Also, atrial fibrillation does not terminate with vagal maneuvers. Drugs that affect the AV node can theoretically make atrial fibrillation more dangerous in patients with WPW syndrome by leaving the accessory pathway unopposed.

4. **(C)** The main criteria for valve replacement in endocarditis include the development of CHF, multiple embolic events, a valvular abscess, and fungal endocarditis. Vegetation size alone is not an indication for an operation. Enterococcal endocarditis should be treated with ampicillin or vancomycin plus an aminoglycoside because ampicillin or vancomycin alone would not be bactericidal and endocarditis must be treated with a bactericidal regimen or failure may result. There are studies that show that intravenous drug users with uncomplicated right-sided endocarditis may be treated with 2 weeks of intravenous therapy.

5. **(E)** Infectious mononucleosis typically causes tonsil hypertrophy, muffled voice, and odynophagia. The gray-white exudate can mimic streptococcal tonsillitis. The other key distinguishing features of mononucleosis are the abnormal complete blood count, systemic malaise, and splenomegaly.

6. **(C)** Approximately 50% of men will experience symptoms of prostatitis in their lifetime. Approximately 25% of men with voiding symptoms have prostatitis.

7. **(C)** Metastatic carcinoma to the choroid is associated with creamy-white lesions. In women of this age, metastatic lesions are the most common cause for creamy-white subretinal lesions. Best's disease can cause an "egg yolk" lesion of the macula that may appear whitish but is usually bilateral and is usually associated with normal to slightly decreased vision in most patients. When "scrambled," the lesion can be associated with decreased vision. Age-related macular degeneration usually occurs at a slightly older age and is often associated with hemorrhage and fluid in the macula but not creamy-white lesions. Creamy-white lesions are not characteristic of age-related macular degeneration. The presence of *Toxoplasma* is often associated with cells within the vitreous and an inflammatory lesion rather than a subretinal creamy-white lesion.

8. **(C)** The primary site of the metastatic lesion must be determined. The form of therapy will depend on the sensitivity of the metastatic lesion to different treatment modalities such as chemotherapy or radiation therapy. Surgeon preference must also be considered.

9. **(C)** Determining the primary site of cancer is the most important step in designing a treatment regimen. Chemotherapy is the most frequently used modality for the treatment of metastatic carcinoma to the eye. Many lesions may be chemosensitive. Radiosensitivity is also noted and is the treatment of second choice since radiation therapy can be a long-standing complication.

10. **(A)** Acute appendicitis is a common entity seen in the ED that all too often presents atypically. Taking a good history and doing a careful exam is essential. Excessive reliance on labs and imaging risks serious misdiagnosis. When patients present with the association of abdominal pain and emesis, it is very helpful to know that pain preceding emesis is commonly associated with surgical problems while the opposite pattern is more often seen with nonsurgical disorders. Low-grade temperature is common in appendicitis, but many patients are afebrile. Dull, poorly localized pain that intensifies and localizes to the right lower quadrant over a number of hours is very suggestive of appendicitis. Anorexia occurs in most patients with appendicitis but not all. Leukocytosis is commonly seen in acute appendicitis, but a normal white cell count does not exclude appendicitis.

11. **(D)** CMT is a nonspecific finding and implies localized peritoneal irritation in the pelvis. CMT alone does not establish a diagnosis of PID. PID can cause CMT, but so can other conditions including ectopic pregnancy and appendicitis. When we contemplate a diagnosis of PID, we need to review appropriate history and exam and get labs including beta human chorionic gonadotropin (hCG), urinalysis, and white count. Absence of cervical discharge should make us rethink a tentative diagnosis of PID.

12. **(D)** The symptoms of acute bacterial prostatitis include all of the above except for gross hematuria. Additionally, a digital rectal examination would reveal an enlarged and very tender prostate gland.

13. **(A)** While rapid weight gain during later pregnancy can be a warning sign of developing preeclampsia, baseline obesity is not one of the risk factors cited for preeclampsia.

14. **(B)** All of the other statements regarding the use of ICDs are correct. Because of the nature of the underlying heart disease in these patients, despite ICD treatment, 38% of all cardiac deaths are arrhythmic.

15. **(D)** An MRI scan will interfere with the function of a pacemaker. The presence of surgical-grade metal in the body is generally not a problem as long as it is not in the area to be imaged. Surgical-grade metals will not attract

a magnet but will obscure an MRI image if in the area of the field.

16. **(A)** Bile acid sequestrants are indicated only in the therapy of an elevated LDL-C. At maximal dose, they can lower LDL-C by at least 20%. They have little effect on HDL-C and increase triglycerides.

17. **(C)** This case is a classic example of myxedema coma. The hypoglycemia should make you suspect a coexistent adrenal insufficiency. It is extremely important to administer hydrocortisone before levothyroxine; otherwise, an adrenal crisis can be precipitated because thyroid hormones increase the catabolism of cortisol. An initial bolus of 300 μg of levothyroxine is necessary to replete the extrathyroidal thyroxine (T_4) pool. Hyponatremia is caused by impaired water excretion; therefore, fluid restriction can correct hyponatremia. If there is a severe hyponatremia (serum sodium < 120 mEq/L), a small amount of hypertonic saline can be given. Electric warming blankets should not be used because they can cause vasodilation and precipitate a hypotensive shock.

18. **(E)** The patient has a lymphocytosis, tender splenomegaly, and lymphadenopathy consistent with EBV or mononucleosis (Monospot test would be more cost-effective and would make the diagnosis). Flow cytometry would most likely show that these are activated T lymphocytes and thus not likely to be chronic lymphocytic leukemia (CLL). This patient is also too young to have CLL. Although acute HIV infection can present with fever, lymphocytosis, and lymphadenopathy, usually tender splenomegaly is not in the differential. Neither a lymph node biopsy nor bone marrow evaluation would be useful in making this diagnosis.

19. **(B)** Due to the age of the patient, this is unlikely to be a first episode of schizophrenia.

20. **(A)** The patient's diagnosis is Bipolar Disorder, Manic with psychotic features that are not consistent or congruent with his elated mood.

21. **(E)** The issue is whether this is a primary thrombocytosis or a reactive thrombocytosis. Primary thrombocytosis usually represents a myeloproliferative disorder, whereas reactive thrombocytosis can be from many causes. The patient is clearly iron deficient with a microcytic anemia and low ferritin. Most likely with the history of chronic aspirin use, the patient has had intermittent chronic blood loss. In addition, he also has external hemorrhoids that could contribute. He could have an occult cancer, but a workup revealed no evidence of cancer. Iron deficiency often causes thrombocytosis, as does active bleeding. Often, platelet counts can exceed 1 million and fall to normal with the correction of the iron deficiency. Therefore, iron therapy is indicated. Hydrea is generally given in myeloproliferative disorders but there is no evidence of chronic myelogenous leukemia (CML) or polycythemia vera (PV), in which an erythrocytosis can be masked with chronic blood loss. Iron therapy can be instituted if the platelet count is not corrected, and a workup for essential thrombocytosis or PV could be pursued. Interferon again is given in a myeloproliferative state. Splenectomy is not appropriate and could further raise the platelet count.

22. **(C)** Dog bites are usually polymicrobial and must be treated with an agent that can target gram-positive organisms, gram-negative organisms, and anaerobes. *Pasteurella multocida* is susceptible to amoxicillin–clavulanate. Cephalexin does not have broad enough activity (no anaerobic activity and no activity against *Pasteurella*). A quinolone or clindamycin might be reasonable when combined with other agents, but they should not be used alone.

23. **(C)** The term *cholesteatoma* is unfortunate because it is neither a neoplasm nor cholesterol based, but rather is the result of proliferating squamous cells from the lateral surface of the tympanic membrane becoming trapped in the middle ear space medial to the tympanic membrane, where they form an expanding and destructive tissue mass.

24. **(B)** BPH develops in the transition zone of the prostate and is not palpable on digital rectal examination.

25. **(D)** Each of these tests may be performed during the initial evaluation of a man with BPH. However, the bladder ultrasound is to be considered but is not required in the initial testing.

26. **(B)** Gottron's papules, erythematous papules overlying the knuckles, are a pathognomonic lesion of dermatomyositis.

27. **(C)** The degree of elevation of the serum amylase or lipase level does not correlate with severity of disease or risk of complications. In contrast, significant end-organ failure as well as acidosis and severe volume depletion (very high serum hemoglobin at presentation) mandate care in an ICU, as they predict severe pancreatitis and, more likely, a complicated course.

28. **(C)** A sliding hiatal (diaphragmatic) hernia in and of itself does not require surgery. The other situations all require surgery because they are true hernias that are symptomatic, or are situations in which torsion or twisting of the hernia or a loop of bowel entrapped at the root of the mesentery by adhesive bands can quickly result in necrotic, gangrenous bowel with considerable morbidity and mortality. An elderly patient or a patient with serious comorbidities (e.g., cardiovascular disease) with an asymptomatic paraesophageal hernia or malrotation would not routinely require surgical repair.

29. **(D)** The placenta, though surrounded by the muscular uterus, is moderately vulnerable to blunt trauma and has been compared to a potato chip sitting inside a tennis ball. Traumatic abruption can occur with relatively minor trauma, and suggestive findings such as uterine irritability and/or vaginal bleeding may not be present on initial exam. Even obstetrical ultrasound may fail to identify a small abruption of the placenta. Fetal monitoring is far more sensitive. After general evaluation for maternal injuries in the ED, gravidas at or beyond 20 weeks' gestation should be sent to a labor and delivery suite for fetal monitoring to look for contractions or evidence of fetal distress for at least 4 hours prior to discharge. Plain films of the abdomen are of no value in this case and would unnecessarily expose the fetus to a small amount of ionizing radiation. The uterus, fetus, and amniotic fluid actually protect the bowel and intra-abdominal viscera from blunt trauma in pregnancy. A CT scan does not appear to be indicated on the basis of history or exam and would inappropriately expose the fetus to a relatively large dose of ionizing radiation.

30. **(B)** Rocky Mountain spotted fever (RMSF) is a tick-borne illness caused by *Rickettsia rickettsii*. Most cases occur in the eastern United States, especially the mid-Atlantic states. It is seen in endemic areas from early spring through late fall. Only about half of the patients who develop RMSF recall tick exposure. The characteristic rash typically begins around the third day of illness as a faint eruption around the wrists and ankles and becomes purpuric as it spreads centrally. Rash never develops in a small but significant number of patients. Headache, malaise, and high fever are common. Typical lab findings include hyponatremia, thrombocytopenia, and a relatively normal white blood cell count. Do not delay treatment for serologic confirmation of the illness as complications may include shock, seizures, and death and the treatment is relatively benign. Currently, the preferred treatment for adults and children older than 9 years is a tetracycline such as doxycycline.

31. **(A)** Bullous pemphigoid is characterized by a linear distribution of IgG and C3 along the basement membrane with direct immunofluorescence.

32. **(A)** Glutamine is difficult, but not impossible, to incorporate into TPN. However, there is not clear evidence that NJ tube feedings with glutamine improve patient mortality.

While NJ tube feedings are not contraindicated with an ileus, there is no evidence that they enhance GI motility. Although TPN *is* more expensive, that in itself is not a compelling reason to use NJ tube feedings. The risk of sepsis and end-organ failure is felt to be more likely with bowel rest and TPN than with NJ tube feedings and has, in recent years, become a major reason for enteral versus parenteral feeding in persons with moderate to severe acute pancreatitis who cannot eat by mouth for many days.

33. **(A)** Men with an acute bacterial infection of the prostate suggested by symptoms and digital rectal exam should not be instrumented with a urethral catheter. If the patient has urinary retention, a percutaneous cystostomy should be placed.

34. **(A)** Epiglottitis, although more rarely seen since immunization for *Haemophilus influenzae*, is a true airway emergency, and a specialist able to secure an airway should be called immediately.

35. **(A)** Malignant pericardial effusions commonly result from lung and breast cancers. Although the effusion can take time to accumulate, some patients will present with acute hemodynamic compromise and require urgent pericardiocentesis. The echo pictured is consistent with this diagnosis and shows a large pericardial effusion.

36–38. **(36-C, 37-C, 38-A)** This patient did indeed suffer an acute left middle cerebral infarction. The extent of the deficits suggests internal artery occlusion. Despite being left-handed, his language centers are in the left hemisphere as they are in 85 to 90% of left-handed people.

Intravenous TPA has been shown to reduce long-term disability when initiated within 3 hours of onset of symptoms attributable to cortical infarct. The benefits of IV heparin in this clinical setting are unclear, and there may be risk of hemorrhage . Aggressive lowering of blood pressure may actually worsen the clinical deficits due to reduction of blood flow to the injured (but not dead) areas of infarcted brain.

CT scan of the brain will not demonstrate cerebral infarction within the first 24 to 48 hours after onset. Its main utility in the emergency setting is to document prior infarction and to exclude hemorrhage. While signs of increased intracranial pressure will be seen on CT scan, it should not be obtained in lieu of urgent treatment. Hyperventilation causes a decrease in PCO_2 with immediate cerebral vasoconstriction and decrease in intracranial pressure. Mannitol may not become effective for more than 20 to 30 minutes, and dexamethasone will be ineffective on the cytotoxic edema seen in postinfarct swelling.

39. **(C)** If the lesion is metastatic to lung, then a needle or open biopsy is needed for diagnosis. An open biopsy will provide more tissue, which may be needed for an accurate diagnosis. If a metastatic workup is negative, then referral to a musculoskeletal tumor surgeon should be done before biopsy. The surgeon will plan the best way to do the biopsy, keeping tissue planes and muscle compartments in mind to avoid unnecessary tissue contamination with tumor cells. If resection of the tumor is necessary, the biopsy tract (open or needle) should be excised.

40. **(D)** Ten to fifteen percent of biopsy-proven breast cancers are negative on mammograms, especially if the mammogram was a screening rather than diagnostic mammogram. A negative mammogram, especially in a young woman, is not a reason not to evaluate a suspicious mass. A nonsuspect mass might be observed through a menstrual cycle. Waiting 6 months to repeat a mammogram is not appropriate. Estrogen and progesterone are unlikely to have any effect on any masses in a premenopausal female.

41. **(E)** All of the above diagnoses have been associated with depressive symptoms.

42. **(E)** Obsessive rumination, although associated with diagnosis of depression, is not a vegetative symptom.

43. **(E)** Niacin (nicotinic acid) is known to favorably influence the level of all three lipid fractions. At therapeutic doses, triglycerides may be lowered by at least 30 to 40%, LDL-C by 15 to 30%, and HDL-C may be increased by more than 15 to 25%.

44. **(E)** Gemfibrozil lowers triglycerides by about 40%, and increases HDL-C by about 10%. It has minor effects on LDL-C. The newer agent fenofibrate has a greater and more consistent LDL-C lowering effect.

45. **(B)** The ability to accurately describe a fracture is an essential skill of ED physicians. Treatment of injuries and the speed necessary for this treatment is dictated by the circumstances of the injury, the condition of the patient, and the actual injuries. Plans for emergency treatment often must be formulated prior to the patient actually being seen by a specialist. Unnecessary delay increases both morbidity and mortality.

46. **(E)** Trauma is one of the main causes of avascular necrosis of the hip. A dislocation interrupts the vascular supply to the head of the femur from the joint capsule. The longer the delay in reduction, the greater the risk of avascular necrosis. Emergent reduction is essential and should be performed even before workup of a multiple trauma patient is complete.

47. **(C)** A person falling from height is at risk for all of the injuries listed. When landing on the feet or in a sitting position, the spine is axially loaded, putting the lumbar and lower thoracic spine at high risk for a compression fracture. Careful evaluation of the spine in this situation is necessary.

48. **(C)** Although in an ideal world, a 15-year-old girl should be abstaining from sexual relations, if she is already sexually active, "just saying no" is probably not going to work. She needs to be protected from sexually transmitted infections (STIs) as well as unplanned pregnancy. In her case, condoms are not enough because of patient compliance. Thus, a hormonal back-up method such as the oral contraceptive or depo-medroxyprogesterone acetate is recommended. *(Beckmann, 297–312)*

49. **(D)** Since she has completed her childbearing, the most effective form of birth control for her is tubal sterilization, which carries a 0.3% failure rate. *(Beckmann, 317–322)*

50. **(B)** Since she is in a monogamous relationship, STI protection is probably not a priority. However, since she has not yet attained desired family size, sterilization would not be an option either. Hormonal contraception such as the oral contraceptive would be the ideal choice here. Rhythm is not very effective, and completely unrealistic in women who have the slightest variation in cycle length. *(Beckmann, 297–312)*

Practice Test 13
Questions

DIRECTIONS (Questions 1 through 50): Each of the numbered items or incomplete statements in this section is followed by answers or by completions of the statement. Select the ONE lettered answer or completion that is BEST in each case.

Items 1–5

A 24-year-old G2P0020 woman, last menstrual period (LMP) 1 week ago, presents to the emergency department (ED) of an inner-city hospital with bilateral lower abdominal pain. She is sexually active with two partners, and not using any birth control. On admission, her temperature is 37.5° C (99.6° F), pulse 84/reg. Abdominal exam reveals diffuse tenderness with mild guarding and rebound. Speculum exam reveals a mucopurulent cervical discharge.

1. The most important laboratory study in the workup at this point would be

   (A) cervical cultures for gonorrhea and chlamydia
   (B) a wet prep
   (C) a Pap smear
   (D) vaginal cytology for determination of a maturation index
   (E) cervical mucus for spinnbarkeit

2. On this patient's bimanual exam, one is likely to find all of the following EXCEPT

   (A) cervical motion tenderness
   (B) mild adnexal enlargement
   (C) nulliparous cervical os
   (D) uterine prolapse
   (E) adnexal tenderness

3. All of the following studies should be obtained immediately EXCEPT

   (A) complete blood count (CBC) with differential
   (B) pelvic ultrasound
   (C) serum beta human chorionic gonadotropin (hCG)
   (D) Gram stain of cervical discharge
   (E) hysterosalpingogram (HSG)

4. The most likely primary causative organism is

   (A) herpes simplex type 2
   (B) *Chlamydia trachomatis*
   (C) *Treponema pallidum*
   (D) *Mycobacterium tuberculosis*
   (E) *Gardnerella vaginalis*

5. The treatment of choice would be to institute antibiotic therapy with

   (A) acyclovir
   (B) doxycycline only
   (C) ceftriaxone and doxycycline
   (D) rifampin
   (E) metronidazole

END OF SET

6. The most serious complication following supracondylar fracture of the humerus in a child is

   (A) tardy ulnar nerve palsy
   (B) Volkmann's ischemic contracture
   (C) nonunion of the fracture
   (D) loss of the carrying angle of the elbow (gunstock deformity)
   (E) articular disruption

7. Amphotericin may account for all the following side effects EXCEPT

   (A) hypokalemia
   (B) hypomagnesemia
   (C) renal insufficiency
   (D) diffuse erythroderma that responds to slowing the infusion
   (E) rigors during administration of the drug

8. Maternal pre- and periconceptual consumption of at least 0.4 mg of folic acid/day is recommended to help prevent

   (A) congenital heart anomalies
   (B) neural tube defects (NTDs)
   (C) mental retardation
   (D) cerebral palsy
   (E) gestational diabetes

9. When present 1 day after injury, which of the following is an indication for surgical repair of an inferior wall blowout fracture?

   (A) any displaced fracture on coronal computed tomography (CT) scan
   (B) herniation of orbital fat into maxillary sinus
   (C) proptosis
   (D) periorbital ecchymosis
   (E) entropion at least 5 mm

10. A 62-year-old man with a 2-year history of hypertension treated with atenolol presents with complaints of the inability to achieve a rigid erotic erection for 6 months. The initial evaluation fails to reveal a specific abnormality, and the serum hormone levels are normal. What is the best initial therapy?

    (A) Refer patient for psychological therapy for sexual dysfunction.
    (B) Prescribe sildenafil at a dose of 100 mg.
    (C) Perform further diagnostic testing such as duplex ultrasound of the penis.
    (D) Change antihypertensive medications and have patient return for follow-up evaluation.

11. A 70-year-old man presents with a 1-week history of persistent throbbing headache. He denies trauma. He has exquisite tenderness and swelling over the right temple. His neurological exam is normal. His erythrocyte sedimentation rate (ESR) is 90 mm/hr. The most appropriate next step is to

    (A) order a carboxyhemoglobin level
    (B) start oral prednisone
    (C) schedule a magnetic resonance imaging (MRI) scan of the brain
    (D) start indomethacin
    (E) order a duplex scan of the carotid arteries

12. Potential complications of atrial fibrillation include all the following EXCEPT

    (A) embolism and stroke
    (B) bleeding secondary to anticoagulation
    (C) congestive heart failure
    (D) ischemic cardiomyopathy
    (E) rate-related atrial myopathy

13. A patient involved in a motor vehicle accident is admitted to the hospital with multiple injuries. The abdomen and head have been evaluated. Other injuries are listed below. Which injury should be treated most urgently?

    (A) closed right femur fracture
    (B) open left tibia fracture
    (C) left central acetabular fracture
    (D) closed left humerus fracture with nerve deficit
    (E) T8 compression fracture

14. A 40-year-old man is seen in your office for regular checkup. On physical examination, a

right carotid bruit is heard. A Doppler ultrasound of the carotids reveals a 1.6-cm thyroid nodule in the left lobe. Serum thyroid-stimulating hormone (TSH) level is < 0.01 μU/mL (N: 0.4–4.8). What would you do next?

(A) fine-needle aspiration biopsy (FNAB) of the nodule

(B) check free thyroxine (T_4) and total triiodothyronine (T_3)

(C) 24-hour radioactive iodine uptake and scan

(D) A and B

(E) B and C

(F) A and C

15. A young, unidentified man was brought to the ED after he was found wandering the streets. He was alert but unable to identify himself. He was unable to give any information about where he lived. Upon investigation, his family was found, and it was learned that the patient was from a city 3 hours away. This is most likely

(A) dissociated amnesia

(B) depersonalization disorder

(C) dissociative disorder not otherwise specified (NOS)

(D) dissociative fugue

16. Osgood–Schlatter disease is a condition affecting the

(A) second metatarsal

(B) femur

(C) tarsal navicular

(D) tibia

(E) calcaneus

17. A 43-year-old woman is admitted with syncope and severe episodes of dizziness over the last week. Her past history is benign other than for mild hypertension. She was placed on erythromycin for a respiratory tract infection about 10 days prior to presentation. In the ED, she complains of dizziness, and on monitor, torsades de pointes is seen. The most likely reason for this is

(A) the patient's triamterine/hydrochlorothiazide

(B) over-the-counter diphenhydramine

(C) erythromycin

(D) congenital long QT syndrome

18. A 46-year-old man is admitted to the hospital with pneumococcal pneumonia. He has a right lower lobe infiltrate. Ceftriaxone therapy is initiated; however, 48 hours later he begins to have increased fevers to 39 to 40° C (102.2–104° F) and appears more tachypneic. What scenario would best explain his failure to improve?

(A) He has developed a parapneumonic effusion, and a chest CT scan should be obtained.

(B) He has developed a parapneumonic effusion, but it should be taken care of with antibiotic therapy.

(C) He has developed a beta-lactam allergy to the ceftriaxone.

(D) This is the expected course for someone with pneumococcal pneumonia.

19. Nägele's rule describes how to derive an estimated date of delivery based on the first day of the last normal period. The rule is

(A) count ahead 9 months and add 2 weeks

(B) count back 2 months and add 1 week

(C) count back 3 months and add 1 week

(D) count back 3 months and add 10 days

20. Which of the following is the most likely cause of significant epistaxis in a 14-year-old boy?

(A) hemangiopericytoma

(B) nasal polyp

(C) ossifying fibroma

(D) pyogenic granuloma

(E) nasopharyngeal angiofibroma

21. The initial evaluation of a man presenting with the chief complaint of the inability to achieve an erotic erection includes all of the following EXCEPT

    (A) examination of peripheral pulses
    (B) palpation of testicular size and consistency
    (C) serum prostate-specific antigen (PSA)
    (D) neurologic examination of pelvis and lower extremities
    (E) serum testosterone and prolactin

22. A 50-year-old woman with hemoccult-positive stools found on routine physical exam is subsequently diagnosed with colon cancer after colonoscopy. She undergoes surgery with excision of the tumor and an end-to-end anastomosis of her remaining bowel. The pathology demonstrated a 5-cm adenocarcinoma of the bowel wall not beyond the muscularis. Twenty lymph nodes were removed and were found to be negative. A staging workup with carcinoembryonic antigen (CEA), liver ultrasound, and chest x-ray were negative. What is the next best therapeutic option for this patient?

    (A) adjuvant chemotherapy with 5-fluorouracil (FU) and leucovorin
    (B) radiation therapy to the colon in the region of the hemicolectomy/lymph node dissection
    (C) adjuvant chemotherapy with 5-FU and levamisole
    (D) annual evaluation and colonoscopy
    (E) COX-1 or -2 inhibitors

23. A 56-year-old man with history of hypertension, coronary artery disease (CAD), asthma, and renal insufficiency is admitted to the hospital with pneumonia and asthma exacerbation. One day later, the patient is transferred to the intensive care unit (ICU) in respiratory failure. His hospital course is complicated by sepsis and hypotension, necessitating dopamine infusion. One week after his transfer to the unit, thyroid function tests show a total T_4 of 3.8 μg/dL (N: 4.2–12), a total T_3 of 35 ng/dL (N: 90–200), a T_3-resin uptake of 45%

(N: 25–35%), and a TSH of < 0.01 μU/mL (N: 0.4–4.8). A diagnosis of central hypothyroidism is made by the resident. MRI of the pituitary gland shows a 5-mm adenoma. The resident calls for advice. What would you tell him?

    (A) Start levothyroxine 25 μg/day and consult neurosurgery.
    (B) Consult neurosurgery.
    (C) Send prolactin, luteinizing hormone (LH), follicle-stimulating hormone (FSH), testosterone, insulin-like growth factor-1 (IGF-1), and cortisol, then start levothyroxine 25 μg/day.
    (D) Perform a 24-hour radioactive iodine uptake and scan.
    (E) none of the above

24. A 60-year-old woman is seen in the office complaining of fatigue and swollen legs. Her lung fields are clear to auscultation, but her neck veins are elevated and her liver is somewhat enlarged. A systolic murmur is heard, which increases during inspiration. The most likely diagnosis is

    (A) mitral regurgitation
    (B) mitral stenosis and biventricular failure
    (C) systolic failure
    (D) left heart failure
    (E) right heart failure

25. A 63-year-old diabetic is brought to the ED by family members because the patient has altered mental status. The patient is known to be poorly compliant with insulin therapy. On exam the left eye appears to be swollen, and a black eschar is seen inside the left nares. The initial laboratory studies reveal a serum glucose of 930 mg/dL and the pH is 7.1. What organism is responsible for the patient's presentation?

    (A) *Pseudomonas aeruginosa*
    (B) *Mucor*
    (C) *Aspergillus fumigatus*
    (D) *Histoplasma capsulatum*

26. A 34-year-old nonsmoking monument engraver presents with cough and chest pain. What do you expect to find on his chest radiograph?

   (A) pleural plaques
   (B) eggshell calcification of the hilar lymph nodes
   (C) alveolar infiltrates
   (D) cardiomegaly
   (E) none of the above

27. A 5-year-old child presents with a midline neck mass at the level of the hyoid bone, with erythema, tenderness, and fluctuance. Which of the following is the most likely diagnosis?

   (A) infected dermoid cyst
   (B) infected branchial cleft cyst
   (C) infected thyroglossal duct cyst
   (D) simple neck abscess
   (E) suppurative lymphadenitis

28. Which of the following would cause you to make the diagnosis of severe preecclampsia, when associated with other signs and symptoms of preeclampsia, for a pregnant woman in the late second or third trimester?

   (A) paresthesias in the hands or feet
   (B) 1+ proteinuria
   (C) platelet count of 300,000
   (D) intrauterine fetal growth retardation
   (E) nonreactive nonstress testing

29. A 30-year-old woman was in good health until 1 week before coming to the ED. She has had a low-grade fever for a week and progressively worsening chest pains. Pain is relieved when she leans forward and worse when she takes a deep breath. On physical exam, a three-component, high-pitched, scratchy sound is heard at the left sternal border. The most likely diagnosis is

   (A) acute myocardial infarction (MI)
   (B) viral pleurisy
   (C) viral pericarditis
   (D) bacterial pneumonia

30. Common causes of dilated cardiomyopathy include all of the following EXCEPT

   (A) alcohol abuse
   (B) long-standing hypertension
   (C) idiopathic
   (D) viral infections of the heart
   (E) bacterial infection of the heart

31. Which of the following is a risk factor in the development of a nonunion in a fracture?

   (A) smoking
   (B) obesity
   (C) age
   (D) diabetes
   (E) rheumatoid arthritis

Items 32–35

32. A 32-year-old woman presents to the ED with the sudden onset of the "worst headache of her life." She has no prior history of headache or other medical problems. A CT scan of the brain is normal. Your next course of action should be

   (A) MRI of the brain
   (B) lumbar puncture
   (C) electroencephalogram (EEG)
   (D) treatment with meperidine
   (E) treatment with sumatriptan

33. A lumbar puncture is performed and is described as grossly bloody but "traumatic." In order to confirm subarachnoid hemorrhage, you should

   (A) measure red blood cell count in tubes 1 and 4
   (B) obtain cerebral arteriogram
   (C) centrifuge the cerebrospinal fluid (CSF) to look for xanthochromia
   (D) A and C
   (E) A, B, and C

34. Subarachnoid hemorrhage is diagnosed. The patient's examination reveals her to be awake and alert, with a right pupillary mydriasis, right ptosis, and fixed abduction of the right eye. The likely etiology of the hemorrhage is

   (A) anterior communicating artery aneurysm
   (B) middle cerebral artery aneurysm
   (C) posterior communicating artery aneurysm
   (D) cerebellar hemorrhage
   (E) herpes simplex encephalitis

35. A cerebral aneurysm is diagnosed. Your next therapeutic course of action should include

   (A) initiating nimodipine
   (B) immediate neurosurgery to clip the aneurysm
   (C) initiating anticonvulsant therapy
   (D) initiating dexamethasone therapy
   (E) A and C
   (F) A, B, and C
   (G) A, B, C, and D

END OF SET

36. An awake, alert, unrestrained driver involved in a motor vehicle accident is admitted to the ED for evaluation. The vertebrae that must be visualized on a lateral C-spine x-ray to provide an adequate assessment of possible injury are from occiput to

   (A) C6
   (B) C6 and superior aspect of C7
   (C) C7
   (D) C7 and the superior aspect of T1
   (E) any of the above if the patient does not have neck pain

37. A 45-year-old woman presents to your office for a health check as a new patient. She has a history of chronic active hepatitis C with persistent abnormalities in liver function tests. There is a strong family history of premature CAD. She has normal periods. On exam, she has thickening of the Achilles tendons. Laboratory studies show a cholesterol of 350 mg/dL, high-density lipoprotein (HDL)-C 54 mg/dL, and triglycerides 154 mg/dL. Her fasting glucose is 114 mg/dL. What is the best therapy for her dyslipidemia?

   (A) diet
   (B) cholestyramine
   (C) atorvastatin
   (D) niacin
   (E) fenofibrate

38. High-dose chemotherapy and radiation followed by stem cell rescue in the autologous setting has been shown in randomized trials to prolong survival compared with more conventional treatment in

   (A) acute lymphocytic leukemia (ALL)
   (B) multiple myeloma (MM)
   (C) chronic myelogenous leukemia (CML)
   (D) chronic lymphocytic leukemia (CLL)

39. A 56-year-old woman presents with a chief complaint of heart palpitations, sweating, fear of dying, and paresthesias. She is able to go to work every day at an accounting firm that is on the sixth floor, but is unable to take the elevator. She has had persistent concern about these discrete episodes for 2 months. The most accurate diagnosis is

   (A) generalized anxiety disorder
   (B) panic disorder with agoraphobia
   (C) dysthymia
   (D) panic disorder without agoraphobia

40. A young woman presents to the ED after being raped at gunpoint approximately 1 week ago. During the interview, the patient is extremely tearful and has difficulty recalling the events. She described feelings of being in a daze and that the event was not real. She is withdrawn, has nightmares, and is unable to leave her home without anxiety. The most likely diagnosis is

   (A) post-traumatic stress disorder
   (B) depression
   (C) generalized anxiety disorder
   (D) acute stress disorder

41. A 35-year-old woman was recently diagnosed with antithrombin III deficiency. Although she has had no thrombotic episodes, her affected brother has had recurrent pulmonary embolisms. She is now pregnant for the first time. What should be done during pregnancy to prevent a thrombotic event?

   (A) Insert an intraventricular catheter (IVC) filter.
   (B) Do not initiate prophylaxis, but monitor the patient carefully for an event.
   (C) Begin warfarin immediately and continue through the pregnancy.
   (D) Begin subcutaneous heparin or low-molecular-weight heparin immediately and continue through pregnancy.
   (E) Begin aspirin in the third trimester and continue through the delivery.

42. Which medications should be avoided by a man with a history of an enlarged prostate and voiding symptoms?

   (A) over-the-counter cold medications containing anticholinergic agents
   (B) diuretics such as furosemide
   (C) sildenafil
   (D) beta blockers for hypertension therapy

43. Each of the following interventions in the ED has been shown to reduce mortality among patients who sustain major burns EXCEPT

   (A) endotracheal intubation for patients with evidence of injury to the respiratory tract
   (B) administration of broad-spectrum antibiotics
   (C) aggressive fluid resuscitation
   (D) prompt transfer to a regional burn center following initial stabilization

44. A toddler with a 20-cm in diameter congenital nevus overlying the buttock is at increased risk for

   (A) basal cell carcinoma
   (B) melanoma

   (C) alopecia mucinosa
   (D) ankylosing spondylitis

45. The "blueberry muffin" lesions of congenital rubella represent which of the following processes?

   (A) leukocytoclastic vasculits
   (B) erythropoiesis
   (C) angiogenesis
   (D) hemorrhage
   (E) abscess formation

46. Which of the following conditions may benefit from a gluten-free diet?

   (A) bullous pemphigoid
   (B) linear immunoglobulin A (IgA) bullous dermatosis
   (C) dermatitis herpetiformis
   (D) pemphigus vulgaris
   (E) epidermolysis bullosa acquisita

47. All of the following can worsen heartburn in a patient with gastroesophageal reflux disease EXCEPT

   (A) peppermint hard candy
   (B) fruit juice
   (C) verapamil
   (D) chocolate
   (E) lemon hard candy
   (F) fried chicken
   (G) cheese pizza

48. All of the following are true concerning porphyria EXCEPT

   (A) urine aminolevulinic acid (ALA) is always positive during an abdominal crisis
   (B) diabetes insipidus may occur with painful abdominal crises
   (C) acute intermittent porphyria does not include skin manifestations
   (D) elevated total body iron stores may worsen porphyria cutanea tarda

49. A 62-year-old woman complains of intermittent episodes of "coughing small amounts of food across the room." This usually occurs 30 to 60 minutes after eating, especially with dry foods such as tuna or chicken. Rarely, toward the end of a meal, she feels a fullness in the back of her throat. The food that comes out appears undigested. She denies weight loss or dysphagia. At endoscopy, upon trying to enter the upper esophagus, the following is photographed (see Figure 13.1). The most likely diagnosis is

(A) esophageal adenocarcinoma
(B) achalasia
(C) Zenker's diverticulum
(D) gastric outlet obstruction
(E) esophageal cancer, squamous cell type

50. A 19-year-old woman is seen for new odynophagia. She has no medical history, and takes no medications except a few ibuprofen after long-distance running. She denies fever, oral ulcers, or unprotected sexual intercourse. Her physical exam is normal. Fluids or solids by mouth elicit pain in her midchest. The following is the only abnormal finding noted at endoscopy, which is in the midesophagus (see Figure 13.2). Which of the following diagnoses most likely explains her symptoms and this endoscopic finding?

(A) pill esophagitis
(B) herpes simplex esophagitis
(C) squamous cell carcinoma of the esophagus
(D) *Candida* esophagitis
(E) Barrett's esophagus

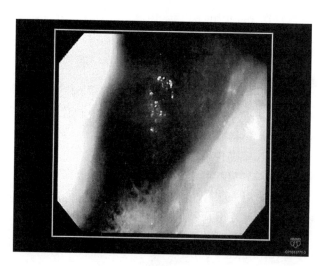

Figure 13.1

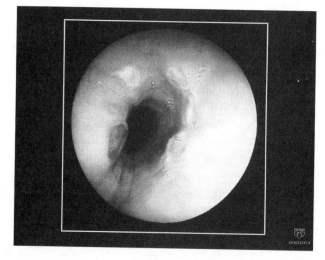

Figure 13.2

Practice Test 13
Answers and Explanations

1. **(A)** This patient is at risk for sexually transmitted infection (STI), and in this case with *Chlamydia trachomatis.* Specifically, she has multiple partners, unprotected sex, and presents 1 week post-menses with a low-grade fever, lower abdominal pain, and a mucopurulent cervical discharge. The most important thing before starting her on antibiotic therapy would be to obtain cervical cultures for gonorrhea and chlamydia. It is also important to get a wet prep, looking for other STIs such as *Trichomonas,* but this patient demonstrates a more acute presentation than that seen with trichomoniasis. A Pap smear is also important, but is not the most crucially related to her current illness. Finally, maturation index and a cervical mucous check for spinnbarkeit (estrogen-related stretchability) are used in the evaluation of ovulation and of no importance here. *(Beckmann, 338–339)*

2. **(D)** Cervical motion tenderness, adnexal tenderness, and possible adnexal enlargement due to tubo-ovarian abscesses are all associated with either acute STI with *Chlamydia* or pelvic inflammatory disease in general. In this case, the woman has only had two prior pregnancies, both of which were abortions (either elective or spontaneous), and thus she would have a nullipous cervical os. Uterine prolapse and pelvic relaxation in general are usually associated with old age and/or multiparity, which is not the case here. *(Beckmann, 353–355)*

3. **(E)** HSG is contraindicated when there is acute pelvic infection. All of the other studies are appropriate and necessary. A CBC with differential is important to evaluate for elevation in the WBC count as an indicator of the severity of infection. Pelvic ultrasound is necessary to rule out adnexal pathology (i.e., tubo-ovarian abscess). A Gram stain of the cervical discharge can lead to rapid diagnosis of gonorrhea infection if there are gram-negative intracellular diplococci. Finally, a pregnancy test is also crucial, because this may affect your choice of antibiotic therapy. *(Beckmann, 337–342)*

4. **(B)** Although pelvic inflammatory disease (PID) is usually polymicrobial, the predominant pathogen is *Chlamydia trachomatis.* Herpes simplex virus (HSV) type 2 or genital herpes presents with painful vesicles, fever, and inguinal lymphadenopathy. *Treponema pallidum* is the causative agent of syphilis, which presents with a painless ulcer known as a chancre. *Mycobacterium tuberculosis* is a cause of genital tuberculosis (TB), relatively uncommon in the United States, and is usually preceded by spread from TB elsewhere, rather than being an STI. Finally, *Gardnerella vaginalis* is the causative organism in bacterial vaginosis and is a minor pathogen, not associated with a fever or abdominal pain. *(Beckmann, 336–349)*

5. **(C)** This patient seems to be presenting with PID, and therefore both chlamydia and gonorrhea must be presumptively treated. Since she is not quite ill enough to be admitted, she may be treated on an outpatient basis with ceftriaxone (125 mg IM) for gonorrhea, and 2 weeks of doxycycline (100 mg bid) for the chlamydia. Doxycycline alone is not suffi-

cient. Acyclovir (400 mg tid × 7 days) is used in the treatment of HSV, and rifampin is used in the treatment of TB. Metronidazole is used in the treatment of bacterial vaginosis and trichomoniasis or may be used in combination with a cephalosporin for treating PID-related gram-negative anaerobes below the diaphragm as an inpatient. *(Beckmann, 343–349)*

6. **(B)** Obstruction to venous outflow from severe swelling produces muscle ischemia commonly known as compartment syndrome. Muscle cell death occurs in roughly 6 hours unless the compartment pressures are relieved by performing fasciotomies on the foramen. The radial pulse is often still present. Muscle death leads to fibrosis, severe contractures, and a useless arm.

7. **(D)** Amphotericin is an antifungal agent that has numerous side effects including renal wasting of potassium, bicarbonate, and magnesium as well causing renal insufficiency. Some patients may complain of rigors during the infusion. Vancomycin is responsible for causing "red man syndrome," a diffuse erythroderma due to histamine release during the infusion. Red man syndrome is treated by giving the patient diphenhydramine and slowing the rate of the infusion.

8. **(B)** Consumption of 0.4 mg of folic acid in the months prior to and during very early pregnancy is felt to have the potential to decrease the incidence of NTDs by as much as 75%.

9. **(E)** Many displaced fractures do not require repair; most orbital blowout fractures have some herniated fat; proptosis and periorbital edema are common in the period immediately after injury and usually resolve; entropion at 1 day after injury indicates a large fracture with significant volume loss, which will require surgical repair.

10. **(D)** Although an initial trial of sildenafil is an acceptable option, this patient has no risk factors for vascular disease other than the hypertension. Medications such as beta blockers are well known to cause erectile dysfunction. It would be best to change medications to agents such as an angiotensin-converting enzyme (ACE) inhibitor or an alpha blocker and reevaluate this patient.

11. **(B)** Temporal arteritis is a relatively common entity in older patients, characterized by headache associated with swelling and tenderness over the temporal artery. The pulse may be diminished or absent over this artery. The ESR is typically elevated, and the patient may have a low-grade fever. Some of these patients will additionally have associated myalgias and generalized weakness with a mild normochromic anemia, a condition called polymyalgia rheumatica. Definitive diagnosis requires biopsy of the temporal artery, but preliminary diagnosis can be made with relative confidence based on clinical findings. Do not delay treatment with prednisone; doing so runs the risk of permanent loss of vision. The biopsy can be done within a week of initiation of steroids. Nonsteroidal anti-inflammatory drugs (NSAIDs), such as indomethacin, are not indicated. Imaging procedures such as CT or MRI of the brain or a carotid duplex scan are not helpful for patients who have clinical findings consistent with temporal arteritis. A carboxyhemoglobin level to rule out CO intoxication as a cause of headache may be very appropriate if history and exam shows no other cause of headache.

12. **(D)** If cardiomyopathy is seen as a complication of atrial fibrillation, it is likely a rate-related cardiomyopathy due to rapid ventricular response. Atrial fibrillation can occur in patients with ischemic cardiomyopathy, but the arrhythmia is secondary to the underlying process.

13. **(B)** The treatment of open fractures takes precedence over all of the above closed injuries. The wound should be sharply debrided, then irrigated with multiple liters of sterile saline. One or more IV antibiotics should be administered, depending on the severity of the wound. Tetanus prophylaxis is

also necessary. Debridement and irrigation of the wound should be done within 12 hours of injury.

14. **(E)** Thyroid nodules can be found incidentally on ultrasonographic studies in approximately 30% of people. The incidence of cancer in an isolated nodule is about 5%. However, a toxic nodule (suppressed TSH with hot nodule on scan) is virtually never malignant. In a patient with a nodule that is palpable or nonpalpable but at least 1 to 1.5 cm and a normal TSH, FNAB is the next step. Some experts recommend FNAB if the nodule is at least 1 cm, others recommend 1.5 cm. In patients who had radiation to their neck at an age < 20, FNAB should be performed regardless of the size. In the case presented, since the TSH is suppressed, FNAB is not indicated; free T_4 and total T_3 are important to obtain, to see if the patient has subclinical (normal free T_4 and T_3) or clinical hyperthyroidism. If he has subclinical hyperthroidism, no therapy is indicated (indications to treat are atrial fibrillation, osteopenia/osteoporosis, symptoms, or > 60 years of age). The scan is also indicated, because a suppressed TSH is not necessarily linked to the nodule, which might be a cold nodule with underlying Graves' disease or multinodular goiter; in that case, FNAB of the nodule will be indicated.

15. **(D)** Fugue may follow emotional stress. A patient may travel away from home and have a loss of identity.

16. **(D)** Osgood–Schlatter disease is an apophysitis affecting the tibial tubercular apophysis. It is commonly seen in teenage males, and is also known as a "growing pain." Treatment is rest or casting if severe. When growth ends and this apophysis closes, symptoms will cease.

17. **(C)** At age 43, it is unlikely that the patient would have her first presentation with the long QT syndrome. Although diuretics may make a patient more susceptible to arrhythmias because of hypokalemia, this is unlikely the cause of this patient's rhythm disturbance. Diphenhydramine is not associated with torsades. Erythromycin, a widely used antibiotic, infrequently causes QT prolongation and torsades de pointes. Significantly more cases of arrhythmias occur in women compared with men. In vitro experiments suggest a gender difference in cardiac repolarization response to erythromycin as a potential contributing factor.

18. **(A)** A fever that develops in a patient already receiving antibiotics is always of great concern and must be investigated. A drug fever secondary to antibiotics would usually not occur this soon; often, it is around a week after starting. The typical patient should improve after starting antibiotics for pneumococcal pneumonia unless there is a complication. One should always exclude the presence of a pleural effusion. If it is significant, it must be aspirated to exclude an empyema as the source of the fever. In addition to antibiotic therapy, an empyema requires drainage.

19. **(C)** The accuracy of the date depends on a 28-day cycle and an accurate LMP.

20. **(E)** All lesions are rare except nasal polyps, which rarely cause significant epistaxis, but nasopharyngeal angiofibroma is invariably seen in peripubescent males and is associated with significant epistaxis.

21. **(C)** The initial physical examination should include a careful review of the neurologic and vascular condition of the patient as well as an evaluation of the genitalia. The gonads should be examined for signs of testicular atrophy. Laboratory testing should include serum testosterone and prolactin levels but without a serum PSA.

22. **(D)** This represents a Stage I or Duke's A colon cancer. Neither chemotherapy nor radiation therapy have been shown to have any benefit in early-stage colon cancer. To date, sulindac and the more selective COX-2 inhibitor celecoxib have been shown in early-

phase trials to reduce polyp size, but this is currently in clinical trials. Thus, most experts recommend annual colonoscopy and physical exams with blood work.

23. **(E)** This patient has euthyroid sick syndrome. A significant systemic illness will alter thyroid function tests, because of the presence of circulating inhibitors (?fatty acids) of hormone binding and the reduction in activity of a deiodinase enzyme involved in conversion of T_4 to the more active thyroid hormone T_3. Also, cytokines such as interleukin-1 and tumor necrosis factor may have inhibitory effects on the pituitary gland. All these changes result in a low T_3 (consistent feature), low T_4 (more seriously ill patients), and low TSH (more lowered by glucocorticoids, dopamine, somatostatin). The T_3-resin uptake is high, due to decrease in the intensity of protein binding (thyroxine-binding globulin [TBG]) from the circulating inhibitors. In chronically ill patients, serum TBG concentration is subnormal due to decreased liver production. In euthyroid sick syndrome, serum concentrations of reverse T_3 (rT_3) are high because of decreased plasma clearance.

In central hypothyroidism, thyroid hormone levels are not so low. There is usually continued low-level synthesis and secretion of both T_4 and T_3 from an intact thyroid gland. The T_3-resin uptake is usually low (as opposed to high in euthyroid sick).

The pituitary adenoma is an incidentaloma, which can be found in 10 to 20% of normal people. Neurosurgery consultation is not necessary unless hormonal hypersecretion is documented (acromegaly, Cushing's), except for prolactinomas for which treatment is medical. Also, a 5-mm adenoma (microadenoma) would not cause hormonal deficiencies or visual field abnormalities.

24. **(E)** The murmur described is consistent with tricuspid regurgitation. In isolated right heart failure, signs and symptoms of left heart failure are not present. In right heart failure, the heart's ability to pump blood to the left side is reduced and the left ventricular end-diastolic pressure (LVEDP) may be low. The most com-

mon cause of right heart failure is left heart failure. However, right heart failure can occur as a result of right ventricular infarction, pulmonary embolism, or cor pulmonale. Signs and symptoms of right heart failure include elevated central venous pressure leading to neck vein elevation and hepatic congestion, edema of the lower extremities, and ascities in severe cases.

25. **(B)** Diabetic patients presenting with diabetic ketoacidosis, sinusitis, and headache or altered mental status should be presumed to have a *Mucor* rhinocerebral infection. The process may be rapidly progressive and can lead to loss of vision, cranial nerve abnormalities, and cavernous sinus and internal carotid artery thrombosis. The patient will require long-term antifungal therapy as well as prompt evaluation by an otolaryngologist for resection and debridement.

26. **(B)** This patient is at risk for silicosis because of his profession. The characteristic finding on chest radiograph is eggshell calcification of the hilar lymph nodes.

27. **(C)** In a young child, a thyroglossal duct cyst is the most common cause of midline neck mass, which can be asymptomatic and unnoticed until it becomes infected. Branchial cleft cysts are lateral, and neck abscesses and suppurative lymphadenitis are almost always lateral.

28. **(D)** Paresthesias of the hands and feet, while common in pregnancy, are not one of the symptoms associated with preeclampsia. In order for preeclampsia to be defined as severe secondary to proteinuria criteria, more than 2+ proteinuria must be persistently present. A platelet count of 350,000 is modestly elevated. Preeclampsia can be associated with thrombocytopenia, not an elevated platelet count. While nonstress testing is an important component of fetal evaluation, a nonreactive test is not one of the criteria for disease severity. However, when associated with other signs and symptoms of pre-

eclampsia, fetal growth retardation is felt to be an indicator of severe disease.

29. **(C)** Viral infections are the most common cause of pericarditis. The low-grade fever and absence of respiratory symptoms makes either a bacterial infection or pleurisy likely.

30. **(E)** Most cases of cardiomyopathy are idiopathic. Other causes are as listed in the question. In addition, cocaine abuse and specific chemotherapeutic agents such as daunorubicin can cause cardiomyopathy.

31. **(A)** The use of tobacco products of any kind interferes with fracture healing secondary to the vasoconstrictive effect of nicotine at the fracture site. Many physicians treating nonunions monitor nicotine levels in noncompliant patients with a history of tobacco use.

32–35. **(32-B, 33-D, 34-C, 35-F)** While CT scan of the head will diagnose the majority of subarachnoid hemorrhages, 10 to 15% will be missed. In the setting of acute and first-time headache, this diagnosis should always be strongly suspected, and lumbar puncture should be performed. A normal CSF exam may then allow for a more leisurely diagnostic workup for the etiology of the headache.

In a traumatic spinal tap, the number of red blood cells will significantly decrease between tube 1 and tube 4, and xanthochromic spinal fluid will not be seen. The risks of arteriogram are not warranted until subarachnoid hemorrhage is confirmed.

In the setting of subarachnoid hemorrhage, an oculomotor cranial nerve palsy (III) in an awake patient suggests an aneurysm at the junction of the internal carotid and posterior communicating artery, which lies just lateral to the third cranial nerve as it exits the midbrain. This is also the most common site for cerebral aneurysm with the anterior cerebral artery–anterior communicating artery junction being next most common.

Nimodipine is a potent vasodilator and may help to prevent cerebral infarct, which may result from arterial spasm induced from the hemorrhage. As the risk of rebleeding is

highest in the first 24 hours, anticonvulsant therapy is often used to prevent seizure and its accompanying risk of hypertension and increased intracranial pressure. Immediate neurosurgery may decrease the risk of rebleeding and allow for more aggressive treatment of the vasospasm (which is highest 3 to 7 days after hemorrhage) without increasing risk of reruption.

36. **(D)** Severe injuries to the C7/T1 area can go unrecognized unless T1 is visualized on a lateral film. If difficult to obtain, a CT scan of the area is necessary.

37. **(B)** This patient has heterozygous familial hypercholesterolemia (cholesterol > 300 mg/dL, premature CAD in the family, Achilles tendon xanthomas). A reasonable first choice of therapy is cholestyramine, especially since hepatic hydroxymethylglutaryl coenzyme A (HMG-CoA) reductase inhibitors and niacin can cause abnormal liver function tests, which is not warranted in this patient who has chronic active hepatitis. Commonly, a combination therapy is necessary to lower cholesterol to normal in these patients. If cholestyramine does not work effectively, then adding a low-dose HMG-CoA reductase inhibitor would be an option, with very careful monitoring of liver function tests.

38. **(B)** A large, randomized trial conducted in Europe has shown that this management strategy prolongs survival in myeloma patients. Allogeneic transplant has curative potential in CML. The lymphocytes in CLL cannot be fully eradicated in patients to undergo autologous transplant, as is the case with ALL.

39. **(B)** Due to the combination of inability to take the elevator and ability to go to work daily

40. **(D)** Because it has been less than 1 month, A would be incorrect.

41. **(D)** Thrombotic complications in those with inherited hypercoagulable states can be pre-

cipitated by a secondary event such as surgery, trauma, pregnancy, or immobilization. Even though she has been asymptomatic in the past, pregnancy is a high-risk state and thus prophylactic therapy is absolutely necessary. The safest regimen is subcutaneous heparin. Antithrombin III concentrate in the peripartum period can also be used. Warfarin is contraindicated during the first trimester since it is a known teratogen. It can cause malformations such as depressed nasal bridge, stippled epiphyses, and nasal hypoplasia. Fetal and maternal hemorrhage risks are also higher. An IVC filter may prevent pulmonary embolism (PE) but will not prevent deep venous thrombosis (DVT) formation. Aspirin therapy is inadequate and, when used in the third trimester, can again increase the risk of maternal or fetal bleed.

42. **(A)** Anticholinergic agents contained in many over-the-counter cold formulations can precipitate acute urinary retention in men with benign prostatic hypertrophy (BPH).

43. **(B)** Empiric administration of antibiotics has not been shown to be of any value in the treatment of patients who sustain major burns. Prompt stabilization with appropriate attention to the patient's airway and aggressive fluid resuscitation followed by transfer to a regional burn center can greatly reduce mortality among these patients.

44. **(B)** A large congenital nevus is associated with an increased risk of melanoma.

45. **(B)** The so-called "blueberry muffin" lesions seen in a variety of congenital infectious diseases including rubella represent extramedullary hematopoiesis.

46. **(C)** Cutaneous IgA immune complexes in dermatitis herpetiformis may clear with strict adherence to a gluten-free diet.

47. **(E)** Fatty foods, chocolate, and mint all can diminish the lower esophageal sphincter pressure and promote acid reflux. Acidic/spicy/hyperosmolar foods can worsen heart-

burn by directly irritating nerve endings in the esophagus. Nonmint, nonchocolate gum and hard candies may help prevent heartburn by stimulating the secretion of bicarbonate-rich saliva. Calcium channel blockers can worsen heartburn by decreasing esophageal smooth muscle contractility.

48. **(B)** Patients with painful abdominal crises often have hyponatremia due to the syndrome of inappropriate antidiuretic hormone secretion (SIADH). The other options are correct.

49. **(C)** Esophageal adenocarcinoma involves the distal esophagus. This and gastric outlet obstruction would more likely present with weight loss, dysphagia, or vomiting of partially digested old food. Achalasia could present with these symptoms, as well as dysphagia and weight loss, but the endoscopic photo shows a blind pouch at the point of trying to enter the upper esophagus, which, given her history, is typical of a Zenker's diverticulum. Squamous cell carcinoma of the esophagus could involve the upper esophagus with high, obstructive symptoms, but weight loss, more dysphagia, and different findings at endoscopy (e.g., a stenosing epithelial tumor) would be expected.

50. **(A)** Pill esophagitis can produce multiple, painful, circumferential ulcerations in the mid- or distal esophagus (i.e., a pill sticks just above the aortic impression or lower esophageal sphincter, causing ulceration and pain). *Candida* esophagitis more often causes dysphagia rather than odynophagia, and this endoscopic picture is not that of *Candida* esophagitis. Barrett's esophagus can be complicated by ulcers at its upper border (its most proximal extent) in the esophagus, but the orange tongues of metaplastic epithelium should be seen just distal to the ulcerations. The clinical and endoscopic findings do not suggest squamous cell carcinoma of the esophagus. Herpes simplex esophagitis usually causes odynophagia, often with fever, sometimes with oral lesions, and would not be clustered in the midesophagus.

Practice Test 14
Questions

the pelvis, as well as superficial liver metastases, and ascites. She is considered to have what stage disease?

DIRECTIONS (Questions 1 through 50): Each of the numbered items or incomplete statements in this section is followed by answers or by completions of the statement. Select the ONE lettered answer or completion that is BEST in each case.

Items 1–4

A 63-year-old G1P0010 woman presents to your office with a 3-year history of abdominal pain, increasing abdominal distention, and weight loss. She denies any history of abnormal Pap smears and is in a long-term monogamous relationship. Her only pregnancy occurred at age 42 and resulted in a spontaneous abortion. She has a history of non–insulin-dependent diabetes and hypertension. On physical exam, she is found to be an obese white female in no acute distress. The abdomen appears symmetrically distended, and no masses are palpable, but seems to indicate intra-abdominal fluid. On pelvic exam, you are unable to palpate the uterus or adnexa due to distention and guarding.

1. The most helpful diagnostic test at this point would be

   (A) complete blood count (CBC) with differential
   (B) pelvic ultrasound
   (C) CA 125
   (D) barium enema
   (E) chest x-ray

2. She is brought to surgery for exploratory laparotomy. At that time, she is found to have tumor involving both ovaries and surface of the uterus, with peritoneal implants outside the pelvis, as well as superficial liver metastases, and ascites. She is considered to have what stage disease?

   (A) I
   (B) II
   (C) III
   (D) IV
   (E) V

3. The best treatment recommended at this time consists of

   (A) cytoreductive surgery
   (B) cytoreductive surgery plus radiation therapy
   (C) radiation therapy plus chemotherapy
   (D) cytoreductive surgery plus chemotherapy
   (E) cytoreductive surgery plus chemotherapy plus radiation therapy

4. With appropriate treatment, her 5-year survival rate is most likely to be

   (A) < 1%
   (B) 10%
   (C) 30%
   (D) 45%
   (E) > 99%

END OF SET

Items 5–7

An otherwise healthy 37-year-old woman is seen for intermittent, short episodes of chest pain that wake her up at night. Her physical exam is normal, and her resting electrocardiogram (ECG) is normal. She denies any drug use, and her family history is negative for heart disease. A fasting lipid profile was normal.

5. Appropriate diagnostic tests to request at this time include all of the following EXCEPT

   (A) exercise ECG
   (B) cardiac catheterization
   (C) 24-hour ambulatory monitor
   (D) stress echocardiogram

6. The results of all studies were normal. She is instructed to present to the emergency department (ED) in the event of pain to facilitate diagnosis. Thus, an episode of pain is witnessed in the ED and is associated with ST segment elevation on her ECG. Myocardial infarction (MI) is ruled out by enzymes, an echocardiogram is normal, and a toxicology screen is negative. What is the likely diagnosis?

   (A) coronary artery dissection
   (B) anomalous origin of a coronary artery
   (C) coronary artery spasm
   (D) occult cocaine use

7. Appropriate therapy for this patient might include

   (A) digoxin
   (B) clonidine
   (C) nifedipine
   (D) propranolol

END OF SET

8. A 67-year-old man with poor dentition presents with several weeks of fevers and night sweats, weight loss, and malaise. On exam he has a 3/6 mitral regurgitation murmur and his liver and spleen are enlarged. He reports anaphylaxis to an injection of penicillin 10 years ago. The blood cultures are positive for alpha-hemolytic streptococci *(Streptococcus*

viridans). What would be the most appropriate antibiotic to treat subacute endocarditis in this patient?

   (A) cefazolin
   (B) ceftriaxone
   (C) vancomycin
   (D) levofloxacin
   (E) erythromycin

9. A 42-year-old woman is seen in the ED with new-onset atrial fibrillation. She has had palpitations, mild shortness of breath, and fatigue for the past few months. She lost 30 pounds (14 kg) over 3 months. Physical examination shows height of 5′6″ (165 cm), weight of 240 pounds (109 kg), blood pressure of 140/64 mm Hg, and irregular pulse rate of 125/min. She has a stare, but no proptosis. Her thyroid gland is not palpable, but marked adiposity makes the examination difficult. There is a tremor of her hands and decreased muscle strength. Her laboratory studies show a serum thyroid-stimulating hormone (TSH) of < 0.01 μU/mL (N: 0.4–4.8), total thyroxine (T_4) of 1.2 μg/dL (N: 4.2–12), free thyroxine (free T_4) of 0.2 ng/dL (N: 0.7–1.6), and a total triiodothyronine (T_3) of 287 ng/dL (N: 90–200). Subsequent laboratory studies include a serum thyroglobulin of < 1 ng/mL (N: 1–30). The most likely cause of this woman's symptoms is

   (A) Graves' disease
   (B) subacute thyroiditis
   (C) factitious thyrotoxicosis
   (D) struma ovarii
   (E) T_3 toxicosis from a toxic nodule

10. A 26-year-old nonsmoking African-American woman from North Carolina presents with cough, arthralgias, and skin nodules. Chest radiograph reveals bilateral hilar adenopathy. What is the most likely diagnosis?

   (A) histoplasmosis
   (B) silicosis
   (C) sarcoidosis
   (D) adenocarcinoma
   (E) aspergillosis

11. A 65-year-old woman is found unresponsive at home by her family. Paramedics arrive and find her pulseless and without blood pressure. Her rectal temperature is 35.6° C (96.2° F). After 10 minutes, they are able to resuscitate her and transport her to the intensive care unit (ICU). A neurology consult is called 24 hours later. They find 6 mm, nonreactive pupils bilaterally and an absent corneal reflex. Neither "doll's-eye" maneuver nor injection of ice water into her auditory canal produces eye movements. An apnea test is negative. There is no decerebration but deep tendon reflexes are brisk and symmetric bilaterally with bilaterally positive Babinski reflex. The most likely diagnosis is

    (A) brain death
    (B) persistent vegetative state
    (C) acute left hemisphere stroke
    (D) postictal state
    (E) psychogenic coma

12. A 36-year-old man presents to the ED complaining of shortness of breath and dry cough for the past week. He is known to be human immunodeficiency virus (HIV) positive but has never been under medical care. His oxygen saturation is 92% on room air. Thrush is present in the oropharynx, and the lungs are essentially clear. His chest radiograph has extensive bilateral interstitial infiltrates. The white blood count (WBC) is $2.4/mm^3$ with 70% neutrophils and 8% lymphocytes. A lactate dehydrogenase (LDH) level is measured at 465 mg/dL. What is the likely etiology of his pneumonia?

    (A) *Streptococcus pneumoniae*
    (B) influenza
    (C) *Pneumocystis carinii*
    (D) *Pseudomonas aeruginosa*

13. All of the following statements regarding infection with *Pseudomonas aeruginosa* are true EXCEPT

    (A) it is a common cause of community-acquired pneumonia
    (B) it is frequently isolated in the sputum of patients with cystic fibrosis

    (C) bacteremia with *Pseudomonas* may occur in those receiving chemotherapy
    (D) *Pseudomonas aeruginosa* is associated with hot tub folliculitis
    (E) ecthyma gangrenosum lesions may be seen with *Pseudomonas aeruginosa* bacteremia

14. Which organism is most likely cultured from the ear canal in an uncomplicated case of otitis externa?

    (A) *Streptococcus pneumoniae*
    (B) *Staphylococcus epidermidis*
    (C) *Staphylococcus aureus*
    (D) *Pseudomonas aeruginosa*
    (E) *Haemophilus influenzae*

15. Which of the following patient history points are most illustrative of psychogenic erectile dysfunction?

    (A) absence of normal nocturnal erections
    (B) adequate erectile function with one partner and not another
    (C) inability to achieve an erection with long-term partner
    (D) inhibition of erectile function by medications such as antihypertensive medications

16. A 22-year-old woman is diagnosed with Graves' disease. Laboratory tests show a TSH of < 0.01 μU/mL (N: 0.4–4.8), free T_4 of 2.8 ng/dL (N: 0.7–1.6), and total T_3 of 256 ng/mL (N: 90–200). The patient elects therapy with radioactive iodine. Six weeks after treatment, her TSH is still undetectable, with a free T_4 of 0.6 ng/dL and a total T_3 of 95 ng/mL. What would you do?

    (A) Observe and recheck thyroid function tests in 6 weeks.
    (B) Observe and recheck thyroid function tests in 2 weeks.
    (C) Start levothyroxine.
    (D) Perform a 24-hour uptake and scan.
    (E) none of the above

17. A 70-year-old woman underwent lumpectomy, axillary node dissection, and breast radiotherapy for a 2.0-cm infiltrating breast cancer with no nodal involvement. It was estrogen receptor/progesterone receptor positive. She was placed on tamoxifen for 5 years to decrease the risk of recurrence. All of the following are side effects of tamoxifen EXCEPT

    (A) ocular toxicity

    (B) hot flashes

    (C) increased risk of endometrial cancer

    (D) increased risk for thromboembolic events

    (E) increased risk for hip fracture

18. The mean duration of pregnancy as calculated from the first day of the last menstrual period (LMP) is around

    (A) 280 days

    (B) 270 days

    (C) 290 days

    (D) 265 days

19. Which of the following is the preferred treatment for acute otitis media in a 3-year-old child?

    (A) oral antibiotics

    (B) topical otic drops

    (C) myringotomy with suctioning

    (D) myringotomy with tube placement

    (E) observation for resolution

20. A 58-year-old man presents with complaints of bothersome nocturia, intermittency, and a weak urinary stream. He has no history of urinary tract infections and exhibits normal renal function. Appropriate initial therapy includes all of the following EXCEPT

    (A) oral therapy with an alpha blocker such as terazosin or doxazosin

    (B) herbal agents such as saw palmetto

    (C) observation

    (D) transurethral prostatectomy

    (E) oral therapy with finasteride

21. What is the most effective surgical therapy for benign prostatic hypertrophy (BPH)-related voiding dysfunction?

    (A) transurethral prostatectomy (TURP)

    (B) transurethral microwave hyperthermia

    (C) transurethral laser prostatectomy

    (D) transurethral incision of the prostate

Items 22–23

A 78-year-old woman presents to the ED with double vision. The visual acuities are normal. The pupils react normally. Examination reveals a painless mass in the superotemporal quadrant within the orbit.

22. The LEAST likely diagnosis in this patient is

    (A) sarcoidosis

    (B) lymphoma

    (C) metastatic cancer

    (D) adenocystitis of the lacrimal gland

    (E) all of the above

23. Which of the following does not need to be performed?

    (A) chest x-ray

    (B) breast evaluation

    (C) magnetic resonance imaging (MRI)

    (D) tissue biopsy

    (E) gastroscopy

END OF SET

Items 24–25

A 6-year-old boy presents to the ED with a severe sore throat. He has been unable to eat or drink and has a fever of 38.8° C (102° F). On exam he is toxic appearing and has inspiratory stridor and paradoxic respirations.

24. What is the next most appropriate step?

    (A) immediate intubation in the ED

    (B) transport to ICU and intubate

    (C) intubation in an operating room

    (D) obtain blood gases

    (E) perform a thorough exam of the oropharynx

25. What is the characteristic radiographic appearance seen in the above disorder?

    (A) steeple sign
    (B) thumb sign
    (C) dumpling sign
    (D) tower sign
    (E) none of the above

                                    END OF SET

26. A young man has sustained blunt trauma in a motor vehicle collision. He appears anxious and diaphoretic. His BP is 80/60, with a pulse of 120. Neck veins are distended, and breath sounds are not heard on the left side. There is crepitus over the left anterior chest. His trachea is slightly deviated to the right. Heart tones are clear. Which of the following initial actions is most appropriate?

    (A) transfuse packed red blood cells (RBCs)
    (B) order a STAT portable chest x-ray
    (C) perform pericardiocentesis
    (D) needle decompression of the left hemithorax followed by chest tube placement
    (E) bedside ultrasound evaluation

27. All of the following statements regarding pericardial tamponade are correct EXCEPT

    (A) typical ECG findings include reduction of QRS voltage, flattening of T-waves, and electrical alternans
    (B) blunt injuries to the chest are the most common cause of traumatic pericardial tamponade
    (C) findings typically include jugular venous distention, narrow pulse pressure, and pulsus paradoxus
    (D) emergency management consists of rapid IV fluid loading followed by pericardiocentesis until definitive surgical intervention can be obtained
    (E) chest x-ray usually demonstrates an enlarged cardiac silhouette with clear lung fields

28. Dark-field microscopy is a useful examination for diagnosing which of the following sexually transmitted diseases?

    (A) herpes simplex
    (B) primary syphilis
    (C) chancroid
    (D) crab lice
    (E) chlamydia

29. Which infectious disease increases the chance of a cutaneous adverse reaction to trimethoprim–sulfamethoxazole?

    (A) acquired immune deficiency syndrome (AIDS)
    (B) sarcoidosis
    (C) cutaneous T-cell lymphoma
    (D) multiple myeloma
    (E) primary biliary cirrhosis

30. During a job physical, a 30-year-old African-American woman is found to be anemic. Further examination revealed mild splenomegaly and jaundice. Her hemoglobin was 11 g/dL, mean corpuscular volume (MCV) 96 fL, and a reticulocyte count was 4.7%. Additionally, she had an LDH of 316, a total bilirubin of 2.2 with 0.2 direct, and a nondetectable haptoglobin. The peripheral blood smear revealed target cells. What test would be useful to determine the diagnosis?

    (A) serum ferritin
    (B) hemoglobin electrophoresis
    (C) glucose-6-phosphate dehydrogenase (G6PD) deficiency assay
    (D) osmotic fragility test
    (E) 51 Cr red cell survival test

31. A 40-year-old man without previous health problems is seen in your office for a 6-month history of daily chest discomforts. These occur randomly during the day, unrelated to activity, eating, or position, and are substernal, "intense," and without radiation, nausea, dyspnea, or dizziness. He has tried antacids and over-the-counter H_2 blockers without relief. He is on no medications, does not smoke or drink, and has no risk factors for coronary artery disease (CAD). He is very physically active, and recently had a negative cardiac stress test. Which of the following is most likely to be diagnostic?

    (A) a proton-pump inhibitor, double-dose, before bed, for 3 weeks
    (B) endoscopy and esophageal biopsies
    (C) esophageal manometry
    (D) 24-hour pH probe
    (E) coronary arteriography

32. A 35-year-old G1P0 previously healthy woman undergoes a routine pelvic ultrasound exam during her third trimester of pregnancy. The examiner notes a 4-cm maximal diameter echogenic lesion in the right lobe of an otherwise unremarkable liver. The patient has no history of possible symptoms related to this lesion, has never been on birth-control pills, and has a history of normal liver function tests before this pregnancy, and several months postpartum, when she comes to your office. At delivery, her alkaline phosphatase (ALP) level is increased twofold over normal levels. Which of the following tests would you be LEAST likely to perform in order to make a diagnosis?

    (A) MRI
    (B) ultrasound-guided fine-needle biopsy
    (C) tagged RBC scan with single-photon emission computed tomography (SPECT)
    (D) bolus-enhanced CT scan
    (E) hepatic arteriography

33. Which of the following diagnostic tests is most specific for idiopathic achalasia?

    (A) grossly dilated body of esophagus on barium swallow
    (B) esophageal manometry with a hypertensive, nonrelaxing lower esophageal sphincter (LES) and aperistalsis of body
    (C) decreased air in stomach bubble on abdominal upright x-ray
    (D) endoscopy of esophagus with large amounts of old retained food

34. Which infectious agent has been most frequently implicated in the development of erythema multiforme?

    (A) *Trichophyton rubrum*
    (B) *Pseudomonas aeruginosa*
    (C) *Staphylococcus aureus*
    (D) herpes simplex
    (E) hepatitis A

35. Sildenafil (Viagra) is an acceptable treatment option for all of the following patients EXCEPT

    (A) a 65-year-old man with diabetes mellitus and hypertension
    (B) a 55-year-old man following a radical prostatectomy for prostate cancer
    (C) a 32-year-old man with erectile dysfunction with a new partner
    (D) a 68-year-old man with angina requiring nitrate-containing medications

36. In a child with nasal polyposis and pancreatic insufficiency, which is the most appropriate next diagnostic test?

    (A) CT scan of paranasal sinuses
    (B) sweat chloride test
    (C) ciliary biopsy
    (D) serum chloride level
    (E) radioimmunoassay

37. A 30-year-old man is admitted after a syncopal event. He had one similar prior event. His physical exam is normal, as are his labs. He has a family history of sudden death. His ECG is shown in Figure 14.1. Appropriate treatment includes

(A) cardiac catheterization

(B) exercise ECG

(C) implantation of an automatic defibrillator

(D) beta blocker therapy

Items 38–39

A 3-year-old child is seen with a history of acute pain and purulent otorrhea after 4 days of ear pain, hearing loss, and fever. Exam reveals purulent drainage in the ear canal and a tympanic membrane perforation, with poor landmarks visible on the drum.

38. The most appropriate diagnosis is

(A) cholesteatoma

(B) otitis externa

(C) traumatic tympanic membrane perforation

(D) perforated acute otitis media

(E) chronic suppurative otitis media

39. The most appropriate treatment is

(A) emergency mastoidectomy

(B) elective mastoidectomy

(C) tympanoplasty

(D) intravenous antibiotics

(E) observation

END OF SET

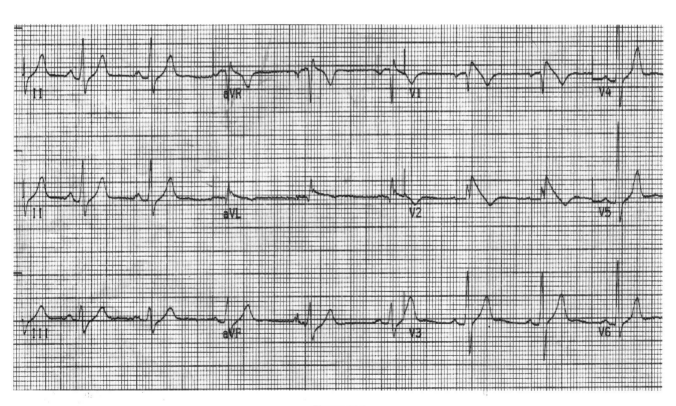

Figure 14.1

40. A 45-year-old man injured his right leg while playing basketball. He went up for a rebound, and when he came down, it felt as if someone stepped on his heel. He now has calf swelling and difficulty walking. On examination, he has moderate calf swelling, and manual compression of the calf does not produce plantar flexion of the foot. The most likely diagnosis is

(A) exercise-induced deep venous thrombosis (DVT)

(B) intramuscular hemorrhage

(C) ruptured Achilles tendon

(D) plantaris tendon rupture

41. A 75-year-old man presents with progressively decreased ability to ambulate. He states he cannot walk straight and that it has been getting worse for the past year. He has had a history of neck pain for years and has recently developed left arm pain. There is no history of vision, hearing, or speech changes. He states that after walking 20 feet his balance becomes worse and his legs feel weaker. On examination, repetitive finger-to-nose testing is normal. He has normal sensation and normal reflexes in his upper extremities. He has 50% loss of normal motion in his neck, but extremes of motion are painless. He has 1+ pulses in his feet and a normal sensory examination to light touch. Lower extremities are hyperreflexic. He ambulates in the hall, leaning against and holding onto the wall. Passive range of motion of all joints is normal. The most likely diagnosis is

(A) cerebellar space-occupying lesion

(B) cerebral vascular disease

(C) amyotrophic lateral sclerosis

(D) cervical myelopathy

(E) Parkinson's disease

42. A 64-year-old female nonsmoker is seen in your office for pulmonary infiltrates, cough, and dyspnea. Her symptoms started about 6 months ago and have been getting worse. She has otherwise been healthy except for systemic hypertension and recurrent urinary tract infections (UTIs). Medications include lisinopril 10 mg daily, metoprolol 50 mg twice daily, and nitrofurantoin daily for urinary tract prophylaxis. She has been on all medications for over a year. Physical exam reveals normal vital signs, SaO_2 of 89% on room air, normal S1 A2P2 and an S4, coarse bilateral Velcro crackles, and no clubbing or peripheral edema. Chest radiograph reveals predominantly basilar fibrotic infiltrates. What is the most likely cause of the infiltrates?

(A) restrictive cardiomyopathy

(B) drug toxicity

(C) idiopathic pulmonary fibrosis

(D) community-acquired pneumonia

(E) none of the above

43. A 2-year-old healthy male infant whose parents are nonsmokers presents to the ED with fever, cough, and nasal congestion. You diagnose the patient with croup. Which of the following is characteristically found on examination?

(A) diffuse macular rash

(B) inspiratory stridor

(C) vesicles in mouth

(D) barking "seal-like" cough

(E) all of the above

44. A dipstick urine analysis is performed in the office for a man with complaints of urinary frequency and dysuria. The test demonstrates 1+ RBCs, 2+ leukocytes, and is positive for nitrites. Appropriate intervention includes all of the following EXCEPT

(A) send a clean-catch urine sample for culture and sensitivity

(B) digital rectal examination

(C) empiric oral antibiotic therapy for a presumed UTI

(D) cystoscopy to evaluate the urethra

(E) delayed oral antibiotic therapy pending the results of the urine culture

45. A stuporous elderly man arrives via EMS with no other medical history available. He is moaning, opens his eyes when spoken to,

and is trying to pull out his IV. Initial exam shows no obvious trauma or active hemorrhage. Initial BP is 70/45 with a pulse of 100. The chest is clear. Which of the following represents the most appropriate initial action?

(A) Give a rapid 500 cc IV bolus of normal saline (NS) and then reassess the patient.

(B) Start a low-dose dopamine IV drip and titrate to bring the systolic BP above 90 mm Hg.

(C) Rapidly infuse 2 L of Ringer's lactate with 5% dextrose IV.

(D) Rapidly infuse one unit of packed RBCs type O negative.

(E) Order a 12-lead ECG.

46. A 48-year-old woman receiving chemotherapy for breast cancer with known metastases to the vertebrae develops worsening back pain with sudden onset of bilateral lower extremity weakness and inability to get out of bed. She has urinary incontinence and is noted to have hyperreflexia of both lower extremities. Which of the following represents the most appropriate immediate intervention for the patient?

(A) Order a noncontrast CT of the brain.

(B) Request an MRI of the spine.

(C) Administer IV dexamethasone.

(D) Order an x-ray of the thoracic and lumbar spine.

(E) Order a STAT CBC and erythrocyte sedimentation rate (ESR).

47. Nail pitting is a characteristic feature of

(A) psoriasis

(B) atopic dermatitis

(C) cutaneous T-cell lymphoma

(D) pityriasis rosea

(E) tinea versicolor

48. A 41-year-old man, previously healthy, is brought to the ED with a 6-hour history of hematemesis. His blood pressure is 130/80 supine and 125/72 upright, and his pulse is 84 and regular supine and 115 upright. The remainder of his physical exam is unremarkable. He takes ibuprofen for headaches, but does not smoke or drink. He is resuscitated with intravenous fluids. His hemoglobin prior to intravenous fluids is 13 g/dL. All of the following scenarios would require admission to the hospital EXCEPT

(A) at endoscopy, a gastric ulcer with an adherent clot is found

(B) at endoscopy, a duodenal ulcer with a flat black spot at its base is observed

(C) at endoscopy, a duodenal ulcer with a nonbleeding visible vessel is found

(D) at endoscopy, a duodenal ulcer with a bleeding visible vessel is observed, and the bleeding ceases with heater-probe therapy

(E) at endoscopy, a gastric ulcer with a clean base is identified, and the patient develops chest discomfort with ST elevations on ECG

49. Which mycobacteria infection is mostly likely to be seen in a patient who owns an aquarium?

(A) *M. ulcerans*

(B) *M. tuberculosis*

(C) *M. marinum*

(D) *M. avium*

(E) *M. intracellulare*

50. What is a common noncutaneous feature of Peutz–Jeghers syndrome (PJS)?

(A) coronary aneurysms

(B) small intestinal polyps

(C) glomerulonephritis

(D) cranial calcifications

(E) retinal pigmentation

Practice Test 14
Answers and Explanations

1. **(B)** This is a case of ovarian cancer. This is also a classic presentation whereby the patient presents with abdominal distention, ascites, and no other symptoms. The history of diabetes and hypertension are actually associated with endometrial rather than ovarian cancer. Nulliparity may be a risk factor for either ovarian or endometrial cancer. A history of abnormal Pap smears is related to cervical cancer, which is not the case here anyway. In light of the fact that she has ascites and abdominal distention, the pelvic viscera cannot be palpated, and therefore a pelvic ultrasound is the standard of care in order to better ascertain if there is any pelvic pathology. As part of the staging workup for ovarian cancer, one would obtain a CBC, barium enema, and chest x-ray, but they may or may not be abnormal. The CA 125 is certainly a tumor marker for epithelial ovarian carcinoma, but is usually used in following the course of disease and would not be as helpful as a pelvic ultrasound in this case scenario.

2. **(C)** This is the description for Stage III ovarian carcinoma (see Table 14.1). Most cases of ovarian cancer are not discovered until the patient is Stage III, as in this case scenario. Stage I is growth limited to the ovaries. Stage II is growth involving one or both ovaries with pelvic extension. Stage IV is growth involving one or both ovaries with distant metastases, malignant pleural effusion, or parenchymal liver metastases.

3. **(D)** The treatment of choice is cytoreductive surgery with postoperative adjuvant chemotherapy. The concept here is to debulk the tu-

mor mass to less than 1 cm in size. Partial omentectomy along with pelvic and periaortic node sampling is performed as well. There is only a limited role for radiation therapy in the management of ovarian cancer.

4. **(C)** The 5-year survival rate for Stage III ovarian cancer is about 30%, even with optimal treatment.

5. **(B)** Performing a study for ischemia evaluation is appropriate even though the symptoms are atypical in that they occur only at night. An exercise ECG is appropriate and can be done as a first step. It would also be appropriate to perform a stress echocardiogram, which provides functional anatomic information in addition to the electrocardiographic information. A 24-hour ambulatory monitor could reveal electrocardiographic abnormalities during symptoms. A limitation to ambulatory monitoring is that in patients with sporadic symptoms, a symptomatic episode might not occur during the recorded interval. Cardiac catheterization would be inappropriate at this time. This study gives anatomic but not functional information.

6. **(C)** Coronary dissection would result in MI. In general, anomalous origin of a coronary artery presents much earlier in life. Most will present in infancy with MI and heart failure. If a patient presents at a later age, symptoms are likely to be exertional, related to and caused by dynamic compression of the anomalous vessel. Cocaine use is unlikely in light of the patient's history and the negative toxicology screen. Most likely, the patient has

TABLE 14.1 FIGO Staging for Primary Carcinoma of the Ovary

Stage	Description
I	Growth limited to the ovaries
Ia	Growth limited to one ovary; no ascites containing malignant cells; no tumor on the external surface; capsule intact
Ib	Growth limited to both ovaries; no ascites containing malignant cells; no tumor on the external surface; capsule intact
Ic	Tumor either Stage Ia or Ib but with tumor on the surface of one or both ovaries; or with capsule ruptured, or with ascites present containing malignant cells, or with positive peritoneal washings
II	Growth involving one or both ovaries with pelvic extension
IIa	Extension and/or metastases to the uterus and/or tubes
IIb	Extension to other pelvic tissues
IIc	Tumor either Stage IIa or IIb but with tumor on the surface of one or both ovaries; or with capsule(s) ruptured, or with ascites present containing malignant cells, or with positive peritoneal washings
III	Tumor involving one or both ovaries with peritoneal implants outside the pelvic and/or positive retroperitoneal or inguinal nodes; superficial liver metastasis equals Stage III; tumor is limited to the true pelvis, but histologically proven malignant extension is to small bowel or omentum
IIIa	Tumor grossly limited to the true pelvis with negative nodes but with histologically confirmed microscopic seeding of abdominal peritoneal surfaces
IIIb	Tumor of one or both ovaries with histologically confirmed implants of abdominal peritoneal surface; none exceeding 2 cm in diameter; nodes negative
IIIc	Abdominal implants > 2 cm in diameter and/or positive retroperitoneal or inguinal nodes
IV	Growth involving one or both ovaries with distant metastasis; if pleural effusion is present, there must be positive cytologic test results to deem a case study IV; parenchymal liver metastasis equals Stage IV

coronary artery spasm. Pain tends to be cyclical, occurring at the same times of day. Spasm often occurs in arteries with atherosclerotic lesions but can occur in angiographically normal vessels.

7. **(C)** This patient is most likely suffering from transient episodes of coronary vasospasm. The spasm can be treated or prevented by coronary vasodilators like nitrates or calcium channel blockers. Nifedipine is a potent vasodilator. Propranolol, while effective for other forms of angina, does not relax coro-

nary artery smooth muscle. The other choices play no role in coronary vasospasm. PRN use of nitrates would also be useful.

8. **(C)** The drug of choice to treat alpha-hemolytic streptococci is penicillin, depending on minimal inhibitory concentration (MIC) results. In a patient who is penicillin allergic with true anaphylaxis, cephalosporins should be avoided. Vancomycin is used to treat serious infections due to *Streptococcus* species when a penicillin alternative is needed.

9. **(C)** Any thyrotoxic state is accompanied by an elevated serum thyroglobulin, which is co-released from the thyroid gland with T_4 and T_3; the only exception is ingestion of exogenous thyroid hormone preparations, which do not contain thyroglobulin. These thyroid hormone preparations can be used inappropriately by obese people in an attempt to lose weight; most commonly, patients will ingest levothyroxine (T_4) (Synthroid, Levoxyl), and occasionally, liothyronine (T_3) (Cytomel), as in this case in which high levels of T_3 (from Cytomel) suppressed TSH and subsequently the secretion of T_4 and thyroglobulin by the thyroid gland.

10. **(C)** Recognize a common presentation of sarcoidosis. Histoplasmosis would be unusual in this region of the United States. She has no exposure history for silicosis. In a young nonsmoker, lung cancer would be extremely rare.

11. **(A)** This patient has an absence of clinical brain stem activity and without evidence for hypothermia or central nervous system (CNS) depressants (such as barbiturate) meets the clinical criteria for brain death. Deep tendon reflexes are generated by the spinal cord and can persist in the setting of recent brain death. A vegetative state can be diagnosed only when 2 weeks have passed and is found in a patient who is awake but not aware of his or her surroundings. Brain stem reflexes are preserved in patients in the vegetative state who can survive with support for many years but who have a negligible chance for recovery. In most states and in

most hospitals, a confirmatory test for brain death is required (electroencephalogram [EEG], evoked potential, arteriogram).

12. **(C)** This is a typical presentation for *Pneumocystis carinii* pneumonia (PCP), with hypoxia, diffuse interstitial infiltrates, and elevated LDH. The radiographic appearance of the lungs is often much worse than what is appreciated on physical examination. Patients with HIV who have a CD4 count < 200/mm^3 should receive prophylaxis against *Pneumocystis*. Trimethoprim–sulfamethoxazole is the first-line agent for prophylaxis and treatment. Steroids are indicated for hypoxia with an arterial PO$_2$ < 70 mm Hg.

13. **(A)** *Pseudomonas aeruginosa* is a gram-negative organism that may be responsible for very serious infections, especially in those who are immunocompromised. Rarely does it cause pneumonia in an immunocompetent patient. Patients with cystic fibrosis are colonized with *Pseudomonas* at an early age and frequently develop pneumonia with resistant strains. Ecthyma gangrenosum is a cutaneous finding associated with *Pseudomonas* bacteremia. Folliculitis due to *Pseudomonas* acquired in hot tubs has been described.

14. **(D)** Even in immunocompetent adults, *Pseudomonas* is the organism typically cultured in otitis externa.

15. **(B)** Psychogenic erectile dysfunction often accompanies anatomic abnormalities such as vascular disease. However, if a man is able to achieve an adequate erection with one partner and not another, it is likely that the sexual dysfunction is related to psychogenic issues.

16. **(C)** Even when the patient becomes hypothyroid after radioactive iodine (low free T$_4$), the TSH can still be undetectable; it can take many months for the TSH to rise above normal. Levothyroxine should be started in patients whose serum levels of thyroid hormones are low or in the lower half of normal, even if the TSH is suppressed.

17. **(E)** Tamoxifen is a mixed estrogen agonist–antagonist. Thus, increased postmenopausal symptoms including hot flashes are common. A slight increased risk of endometrial cancers have been reported with the use of tamoxifen. A 1 to 2% chance of deep venous thrombosis (DVT) or pulmonary embolism (PE) is reported with its use. Some women appear to have an increased risk of cataracts and retinal changes. Since this acts as an estrogen agonist, bone density is usually improved in women on tamoxifen.

18. **(A)** 280 days is close to 40 weeks and has been shown to be the mean duration of normal pregnancy in several large studies of healthy pregnancies.

19. **(A)** Although even with observation alone the resolution rate is very high, oral antibiotics have been shown to decrease symptoms (fever and pain) and hasten the clearance of effusion from the middle ear.

20. **(D)** This patient is best treated with a trial of oral therapy, either with finasteride or alpha-blocking agents. A transurethral prostatectomy is likely to improve his symptoms but would be considered unnecessary at this time.

21. **(A)** TURP remains the gold standard for the treatment of BPH-related voiding dysfunction. However, the other options such as microwave hyperthermia represent new alternatives, which potentially offer fewer side effects than TURP.

22. **(D)** Adenocystitis of the lacrimal gland causes painful swelling within the orbit. Sarcoidosis, lymphoma, and metastatic cancer may all occur within the orbit and may be associated with diplopia.

23. **(E)** The workup of patients with an orbital mass includes an evaluation to rule out metastatic disease, systemic disease such as sarcoid or lymphoma, and local disease, often by tissue biopsy. Gastroscopy is not a primary procedure in the evaluation of orbital tumors.

24. **(C)** This patient has epiglottitis, which is a respiratory emergency. The incidence has decreased in recent years with use of the *Haemophilus* vaccination. This patient is tiring and needs his airway secured. However, the ideal situation would be to intubate him in a controlled environment by someone experienced in airway management with multiple backup plans available (e.g., an operating room). It is imperative not to stimulate the child by removing him from his parents, examining the throat, or obtaining lab work.

25. **(B)** Steeple sign is seen with croup. The thumb sign is seen on a soft tissue lateral neck radiograph and is associated with acute epiglottitis. The other signs do not exist.

26. **(D)** Treatable causes of shock in patients who sustain blunt trauma, which should be addressed during the primary survey, include hypovolemia due to hemorrhage, tension pneumothorax, hemothorax, and pericardial tamponade. The findings presented are suggestive of shock due to a tension pneumothorax. Unless this condition is rapidly recognized and treated, the patient will die. The indicated treatment is immediate decompression of the chest on the affected side, followed by chest tube placement. Waiting for confirmation by chest x-ray is inappropriate and quite dangerous.

27. **(B)** While traumatic pericardial tamponade may be due to blunt trauma, it is usually the result of a penetrating injury.

28. **(B)** Dark-field examination of the primary chancre is the most specific test for the diagnosis of syphilis. It offers immediate identification of the causative organism, *Treponema pallidum.*

29. **(A)** The incidence of drug reactions to trimethoprim–sulfamethoxazole is greater than tenfold higher in HIV-infected persons.

30. **(B)** This scenario represents hemolytic anemia. A serum ferritin would not be indicated due to hemolytic anemia. Red cell survival is not helpful, nor would osmotic fragility be useful because the smear shows target cells, not spherocytes. A hemoglobinopathy or thalassemia would be the most likely cause of the hemolytic anemia. Hb SC or Hb CC would be the most common findings on the hemoglobin electrophoresis in this clinical setting.

31. **(D)** The differential diagnosis in this case is atypical chest pain due to cardiovascular disease versus gastroesophageal reflux disease (GERD). The former is not likely, given the normal stress test and lack of risk factors. There is nothing to suggest an esophageal motility disorder, which very rarely is the cause of atypical chest pain; hence, esophageal manometry is unlikely to be diagnostic. Endoscopy with or without biopsy often is nondiagnostic in GERD patients presenting with atypical chest pain. A therapeutic trial of a proton-pump inhibitor, double-dose, for 1 to 4 weeks, can be diagnostic of GERD as the cause of atypical chest pains, once cardiovascular disease has been reasonably excluded, but would not be given before bed, when most persons are fasting. A 24-hour pH probe is likely to be diagnostic in this patient who has daily episodes of chest pain.

32. **(B)** This previously healthy woman with an asymptomatic single, solid lesion in the liver and normal liver function tests (LFTs) (during pregnancy, ALP from the placenta usually is elevated up to twofold and returns to normal several weeks to months postpartum) most likely has a hemangioma of the liver, the most common benign tumor of the liver. MRI, bolus-enhanced CT scan, and tagged red blood cell scan with SPECT all are likely to demonstrate findings highly consistent with hemangioma. A liver tumor (hepatoma), adenoma (birth-control pills are a risk), or metastatic lesion is unlikely. Arteriography, while more invasive, can be useful if noninvasive testing/scans are unclear. Biopsy would rarely be necessary, and there is some risk of bleeding even with thin needles. Ultrasound findings with hemangioma often are nonspecific, but the echogenicity would

not be typical of a cyst, for which ultrasound is a very sensitive diagnostic modality.

33. **(B)** All of these diagnostic test results are consistent with idiopathic achalasia, but a grossly dilated esophagus could be seen with obstruction (i.e., adenocarcinoma at gastroesophageal junction), decreased air in the gastric bubble with obstruction and/or decreased air swallowing, and endoscopic findings as indicated with severe esophageal dysmotility other than achalasia (e.g., connective tissue disease). Achalasia is defined manometrically by aperistalsis in the body of the esophagus and a hypertensive LES that fails to relax with swallowing. Like *all* motility abnormalities, structural lesions must be excluded (i.e., endoscopy to rule out lesion at gastroesophageal junction), and in the case of achalasia, secondary achalasia due to tumor infiltration about the gastroesophageal junction damaging inhibitory neurons to the LES, mimicking idiopathic achalasia.

34. **(D)** Herpes simplex infection is associated with recurrent bouts of erythema multiforme, and prophylactic antiviral therapy reduces the occurrence.

35. **(D)** Sildenafil is an acceptable first-line treatment option for most men with erectile dysfunction, including secondary to psychogenic cause. However, the drug is contraindicated in men with cardiac disease requiring treatment with nitrate-containing medications. Sildenafil can inhibit the metabolism of nitrates, resulting in elevated blood levels and hypotension.

36. **(B)** Nasal polyposis in a child should be considered due to cystic fibrosis until proven otherwise; the sweat chloride test is therefore the most appropriate next test.

37. **(C)** This patient has Brugada's syndrome, which is characterized by a right bundle branch block with ST segment elevation in V_1 to V_3. In these patients, syncope and sudden death are caused by fast polymorphic ventricular tachycardias or ventricular fibrilla-

tion, which occur without warning. Brugada's syndrome is hereditary, and the prognosis in symptomatic patients is very poor if left untreated. In these patients, the heart is structurally normal without coronary disease and there is no QT prolongation. These patients for the most part are ideal candidates for treatment with an implantable defibrillator, and it is recommended that symptomatic patients receive this device.

38. **(D)** This is a classic history for perforated acute otitis media, which is a natural sequela of otitis media.

39. **(E)** Of the choices, E is most correct. Perforation is the natural history of acute otitis media, and the infection is on its way toward resolution. If antibiotics are used, topical or oral are adequate. Mastoidectomy is not indicated since there is no evidence of mastoiditis or chronic infection, and tympanoplasty is rarely needed since the perforation usually heals without difficulty.

40. **(C)** A plantaris tendon rupture will produce a sharp snap-like calf pain with swelling. Manual compression of the calf will cause plantar flexion of the foot (Thompson's test). This test is best done with the patient prone. An exercise-induced DVT will also yield a negative Thompson's test. This patient gives a classic history for an Achilles tendon rupture. In the acute care setting, 25% of Achilles tendon ruptures are misdiagnosed.

41. **(D)** This patient has cervical myelopathy secondary to osteoarthritis. Severe degenerative changes producing large vertebral and posterior element osteophyte formation can produce a severe narrowing of the spinal canal, resulting in both a mechanical block to motor tracts in the cord and block to intraspinal blood flow. Ischemia to the involved area of the cord increases symptoms with ambulation. Spinal stenosis of this severity requires decompression. When severe, patients will often present with sustained lower extremity clonus.

42. **(B)** Recognize nitrofurantoin as a cause of drug-induced lung disease. It can present in two ways: acutely with fever, chest pain, dyspnea, cough, and pleural effusion or in the chronic form as described in the question. Treatment is withdrawal of the drug.

43. **(D)** A barking cough is characteristic of croup. It notoriously goes away on the way to the ED or doctors office.

44. **(D)** A clean-catch urine sample can identify the bacterial organism in this setting of a presumed UTI and specify appropriate oral antibiotic therapy. A digital rectal examination will rule out acute prostatitis. Empiric antibiotic therapy may be initiated pending the urine culture but may be safely delayed in the absence of signs of systemic infection. However, a cystoscopy is not yet indicated for this patient.

45. **(A)** The first treatment for hypotensive patients seen in the ED who have clear lungs on auscultation is rapid IV infusion of NS or Ringer's lactate to a total of 20 cc/kg for children or 2 L for adults. Particular caution is required, however, when treating elderly patients or those with a known history of congestive heart failure (CHF) who may be at increased risk of fluid overload. Other patients at risk include those with hypothermia and drug intoxication as well as pregnant patients. For these patients, we should infuse fluid in 250- to 500-cc aliquots and carefully reexamine the patient for signs of fluid overload (neck veins, auscultation of lungs, vital signs) following each infusion before giving more fluid.

46. **(C)** Spinal cord compression is a medical emergency. IV dexamethasone should be administered as soon as possible, and then an MRI of the spine should be ordered. Plain films of the spine are of little value in this situation.

47. **(A)** Nail pitting is the most common nail finding in psoriasis. It consists of discrete, punched-out depressions in the nail surface.

48. **(B)** Persons with substantial, acute upper gastrointestinal tract bleeding (e.g., orthostatic changes in pulse or blood pressure) after medical stabilization should undergo endoscopy, which helps determine the severity of the problem and offers therapy as well. Ongoing bleeding, visible vessels (even without bleeding), and adherent clots all require admission to the hospital postendoscopy, as the risk of further hemorrhage is considerable. Ulcers with clean bases or flat, pigmented spots in their bases do not portend a significant risk of rebleeding and allow discharge from the ED of patients who otherwise are healthy and have rapid access to medical care in case they do rebleed. Patients with comorbidities (i.e., significant cardiac, vascular, pulmonary, renal, or liver disease; anticoagulated patients) and patients with complications (chest pain and acute ECG changes) or other endoscopic findings (very large and deep ulcers, particularly in the posterior duodenal bulb and upper body of the lesser curvature) merit admission to the hospital.

49. **(C)** *M. marinum* is ubiquitous in aquatic environments, including fresh and salt water. The organism is inoculated into the skin through small cuts or abrasions.

50. **(B)** Aside from pigmented mucosal lesions, patients with PJS also have multiple polyps in the small intestine.

Practice Test 15
Questions

DIRECTIONS (Questions 1 through 50): Each of the numbered items or incomplete statements in this section is followed by answers or by completions of the statement. Select the ONE lettered answer or completion that is BEST in each case.

1. A 35-year-old woman presents to your office with gradually increasing dyspnea over 8 months' duration to the point she is now requiring oxygen to maintain saturations. She has had an exhaustive workup including spirometry, chest radiograph, computed tomography (CT) scans, antinuclear antibody (ANA), and echocardiogram, which have been reported as normal. Physical exam reveals normal vital signs, clear lung fields, normal S_1 and A2 with a prominent P2; there are no gallop sounds and no clubbing. An arterial blood gas (ABG) reveals an A-a gradient of 60 mm Hg on 2 L of oxygen. What is the diagnosis?

   (A) pulmonary fibrosis
   (B) congestive heart failure (CHF)
   (C) primary pulmonary hypertension
   (D) asthma
   (E) none of the above

2. A 52-year-old postmenopausal woman presents with an acute myocardial infarction (MI). She had episodes of pain occurring with greater frequency and severity for the 2 days prior to coming to the emergency department (ED). The most recent episode occurred at rest and lasted 45 minutes. It was relieved by nitroglycerin in the ED. She has no prior history of any electrocardiographic (ECG) abnormalities, and her current tracing is shown in Figure 15.1. On physical exam, rales are present two thirds of the way up and she has a prominent S_3. Her cardiac enzymes are normal. Her short-term risk level of death or nonfatal MI is

   (A) high
   (B) intermediate
   (C) low

3. A 52-year-old man complains of erectile dysfunction. You change his antihypertensive medications but the patient returns without any evidence of improvement following the change in medications. He has also tried sildenafil samples from a friend without success. He is not under stress and a serum testosterone is normal. The next best step is

   (A) increase dose of sildenafil to 100 mg
   (B) refer for psychological therapy
   (C) perform intracavernous injection of vasoactive agent with duplex ultrasound
   (D) prescribe systemic testosterone gel or patch
   (E) refer for penile prosthesis placement

4. A 55-year-old auto mechanic presents to your office with gradually worsening dyspnea and cough. Lung examination is normal. His chest radiograph is seen in Figure 15.2. The most likely diagnosis is

   (A) silicosis
   (B) bagassosis
   (C) asbestosis
   (D) coal worker's pneumoconiosis
   (E) none of the above

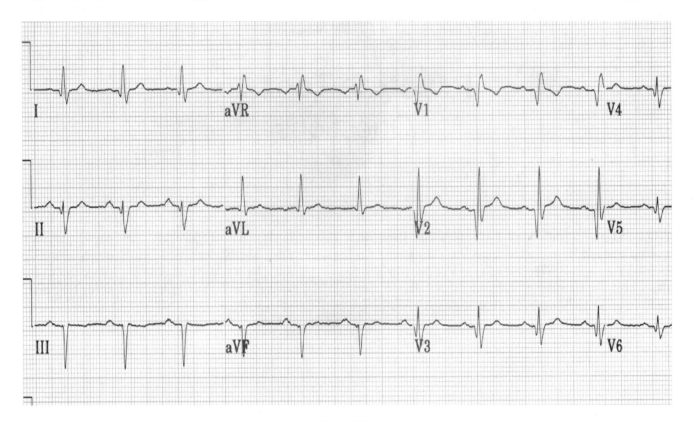

Figure 15.1

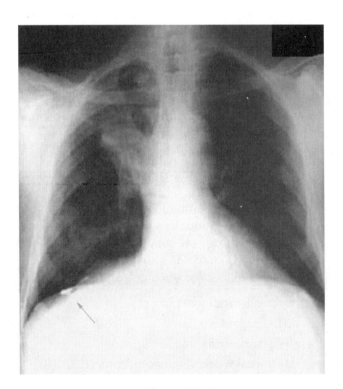

Figure 15.2

5. A 41-year-old woman with a history of acquired immune deficiency syndrome (AIDS) ($CD4 = 36/mm^3$) has just been started on didanosine (DDI), stavudine (D4T), and nelfinavir. She comes to the HIV clinic complaining of nausea/vomiting and severe left upper quadrant (LUQ) pain. Her amylase and lipase are both elevated. All of the following are potential causes of her pancreatitis EXCEPT

(A) DDI
(B) D4T
(C) nelfinavir
(D) *Cryptosporidium*
(E) cytomegalovirus

6. A 24-year-old man presents to the ED complaining of chest pain after smoking crack cocaine. He is moderately agitated, with temperature 38.5° C (101.3° F), pulse 120, and BP 220/120. His lungs are clear and his heart sounds are normal with no murmur present. ECG shows sinus tachycardia and changes

suggestive of early repolarization. Nursing staff has placed him on oxygen, established an IV line, and connected the patient to a cardiac monitor. Each of the following medications would now be appropriate EXCEPT

(A) aspirin

(B) nitroglycerin

(C) metoprolol

(D) lorazepam

(E) phentolamine

Items 7–8

A 26-year-old heterosexual man presents with an expanding rash on his lower extremity. The man is HIV positive and you make the diagnosis of Kaposi's sarcoma.

7. The most likely location of visceral involvement is

(A) bones

(B) brain

(C) gastrointestinal (GI) tract

(D) lungs

(E) kidneys

8. Which of the following is most likely to be present in a patient with acanthosis nigricans?

(A) hyperthyroidism

(B) diabetes mellitus

(C) hepatitis

(D) cutaneous T-cell lymphoma

(E) human immunodeficiency virus (HIV) infection

END OF SET

9. A 22-year-old woman is being evaluated for a history of several months of large-volume watery diarrhea. There is no history of weight loss, abdominal pain, or fever. Stool cultures for bacteria, parasites, and *Clostridium difficile* are negative. There is no gross or

occult blood in the stool and no fecal leukocytes. A stool specimen reveals: measured osmolality 230 mOsm/kg water, stool sodium 30 mEq/L, stool potassium 80 mEq/L. The best explanation for this person's diarrhea is

(A) secretory diarrhea

(B) osmotic diarrhea

(C) factitious diarrhea

(D) inflammatory diarrhea

(E) potassium-secreting large villous adenoma of rectum

10. A 24-year-old woman 3 months postpartum presents with severe anxiety. She stopped nursing 1 month ago. She now weighs 10 pounds less than before her pregnancy. She is having difficulty sleeping and is aware of palpitations. She tells you that at age 13, she was diagnosed with Graves' disease. She was treated with methimazole for 2 years and was euthyroid thereafter. On physical examination, her pulse rate is 120/min, stare and lid lag are evident, and her thyroid gland is slightly enlarged. Laboratory studies show a free thyroxine (T_4) of 3.2 ng/dL (N: 0.7–1.6), with a thyroid-stimulating hormone (TSH) of < 0.01 μU/mL (N: 0.4–4.8). What is the most appropriate next step?

(A) begin methimazole (Tapazole)

(B) treat with propranolol and reassure

(C) radioactive iodine treatment

(D) 24-hour radioactive iodine uptake and scan

(E) thyroglobulin level

11. A 56-year-old woman presents with malignant ascites. Which of the following is a potential curable cancer?

(A) breast

(B) ovarian

(C) gastric

(D) colon

12. A 53-year-old man presents with a several-month history of left hip pain. There is no history of trauma. Most of his pain is at night. Examination of his hip is unremarkable. He complains of mild groin pain with ambulation in the office. X-rays of his hip are shown in Figure 15.3A and B. Further diagnostic workup should include

(A) chest CT scan
(B) long-bone skeletal survey x-rays
(C) bone scan
(D) serum protein electrophoresis
(E) all of the above

Items 13–15

A 45-year-old woman is admitted with hypotension, chest pain, and a rapid pulse. A 12-lead ECG is performed (see Figure 15.4).

13. What is the rhythm disturbance?

(A) atrial fibrillation with rapid ventricular response and aberration
(B) ventricular tachycardia
(C) atrioventricular (AV) node reentrant tachycardia
(D) sinus tachycardia

14. The patient becomes progressively short of breath, clammy, and hypotensive. Correct treatment is

(A) lidocaine
(B) intravenous (IV) diltiazem
(C) IV amiodarone
(D) IV ibutilide
(E) direct current cardioversion

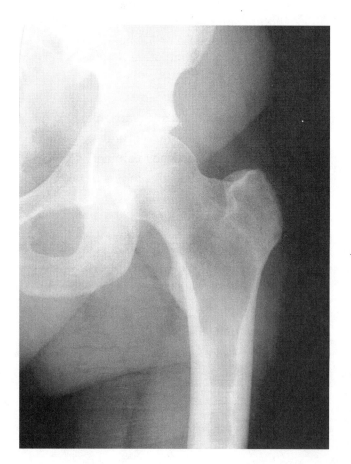
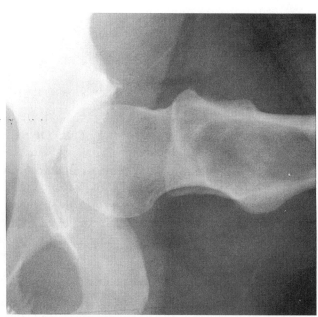

Figure 15.3 A and B

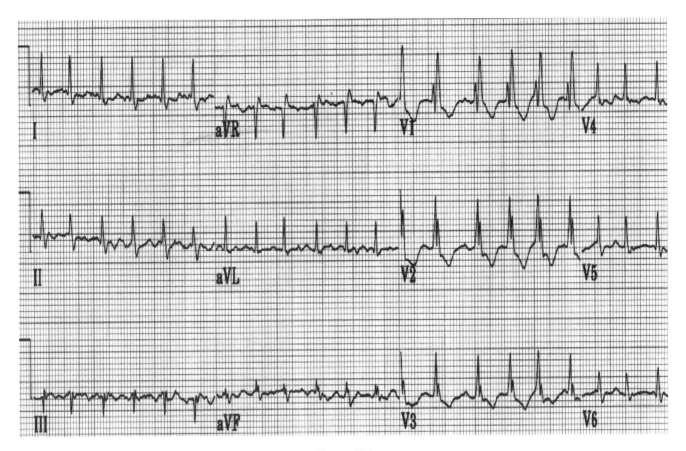

Figure 15.4

15. After stabilization, an echocardiogram is performed (see Figure 15.5). What is the patient's condition?

(A) aortic stenosis

(B) obstructive hypertrophic cardiomyopathy

(C) mitral stenosis

(D) cannot be determined from the echocardiogram

END OF SET

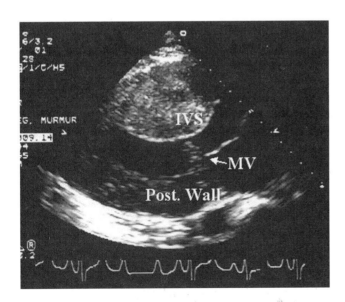

Figure 15.5

16. A 21-year-old patient presents with a 3-day history of worsening throat pain, painful swallowing, muffled voice, and fever. Exam reveals bilateral white exudate on the tonsils, with edema of the right soft palate and the uvula deviated toward the left. What is the most appropriate course of action?

    (A) intraoral drainage
    (B) external approach to drainage
    (C) IV antibiotics
    (D) lateral neck soft tissue x-ray
    (E) placement of an oral airway

17. Allogeneic bone marrow transplant is the only potential curative therapy in a 40-year-old man with

    (A) acute lymphocytic leukemia (ALL) in first remission
    (B) chronic lymphocytic leukemia (CLL) at diagnosis
    (C) acute myeloid leukemia (AML) in first remission
    (D) chronic myelogenous leukemia (CML) in chronic phase

18. A 64-year-old woman with Type 2 diabetes mellitus had increasingly severe angina pectoris not relieved by nitrates. Coronary catheterization shows significant three-vessel disease. Coronary bypass surgery is scheduled soon. On physical examination, her weight is 132 pounds (60 kg), and her thyroid gland is enlarged. The serum total T_4 is 3 μg/dL (N: 4.2–12) and the serum TSH is 60 μU/mL (N: 0.4–4.8). For further management, you would

    (A) give levothyroxine 100 μg/day (1.6 μg/kg)
    (B) give levothyroxine 25 μg/day and increase the dose gradually until the patient is euthyroid before doing bypass surgery
    (C) give levothyroxine 12.5 μg/day and increase the dose gradually until the patient is euthyroid before doing bypass surgery

    (D) proceed with coronary bypass surgery and treat the hypothyroidism postoperatively
    (E) give triiodothyronine (T_3) 25 μg twice a day for 3 days, then perform surgery

19. A 55-year-old man presents with a mass in his palm and "drawing" of his little and ring fingers. The mass started out as a small nodule about 10 years ago. There is no history of a puncture wound or other trauma. He has some pain in his hand with heavy use (see Figure 15.6). Your advice to this patient is

    (A) metastatic workup
    (B) needle biopsy of the mass
    (C) reassurance and the suggestion that he have a surgical release if he desires
    (D) amputation of the little and ring finger rays, including the metacarpals

20. Voiding symptoms related to benign prostatic hyperplasia (BPH) include all of the following EXCEPT

    (A) nocturia
    (B) intermittent stream
    (C) urgency with urge incontinence
    (D) pelvic pain
    (E) urinary frequency

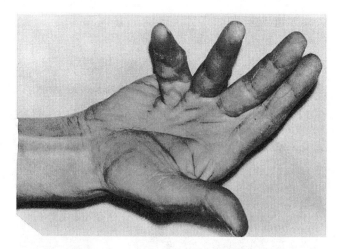

Figure 15.6
(Reproduced, with permission, from Calandruccio JH: Dupytrens contracture. In Canale ST (ed.). *Campbell's Operative Orthopedics*, 9th ed. St. Louis, MO: Mosby, 1998.)

Items 21–22

A 3-year-old child is seen with a marked esotropia. There appears to be no useful vision in the esotropic eye. The external extraocular movements are full.

21. The differential diagnoses of esotropia include all of the following EXCEPT

   (A) rhabdomyosarcoma
   (B) Coats' disease
   (C) retinoblastoma
   (D) amblyopia
   (E) retinal detachment

22. Which test must be done immediately before any other test?

   (A) magnetic resonance imaging (MRI)
   (B) CT scan
   (C) refraction
   (D) dilated ocular exam
   (E) ultrasonography

END OF SET

23. An intravenous drug abuser presents with a fever, heart murmur, and multiple tender erythematous papules on the palmar aspect of his digits. What is the most likely diagnosis?

   (A) Roth spots
   (B) Lisch nodules
   (C) Gottron's papules
   (D) Osler's nodes
   (E) Janeway lesions

24. A 29-year-old man with a long history of alcohol consumption and several episodes of alcoholic hepatitis undergoes endoscopy to see if he has varices, and indeed, esophageal varices are found in the distal esophagus. All of the following pathophysiologically increase the risk of his varices bleeding EXCEPT

   (A) directly measured portal venous pressure of 16 mm Hg
   (B) large varices

   (C) history of frequent acid reflux symptoms
   (D) red wale markings
   (E) binge drinking

25. All of the following increase the risk of formation of cholesterol gallstones within the gallbladder EXCEPT

   (A) decreased gallbladder ejection fraction
   (B) elevated biliary calcium concentration
   (C) elevated biliary cholesterol concentration
   (D) diminished biliary phospholipid concentration
   (E) diminished biliary bile salt concentration

Items 26–29

A 24-year-old woman comes to your office with a complaint of painful bowel movements for the past several days. She notes some mucus and bright red blood when she wipes. There is a history of an anal fissure twice in the past, and intermittent loose bowel movements with lower abdominal cramping, which has been worse in the last 6 weeks.

26. All of the following would be consistent with an uncomplicated, simple anal fissure EXCEPT

   (A) bright red blood on the toilet paper
   (B) mucus on the toilet paper
   (C) history of previous anal fissure
   (D) painful bowel movements
   (E) anal fissure on physical exam, lateral side of anus (3 o'clock)

27. The patient undergoes a flexible sigmoid-oscopy, which reveals an anal fissure, as well as aphthous ulcers in the midsigmoid colon. Biopsies in this region demonstrate focal acute inflammation and focal architectural changes, including branched glands. Stool culture for bacteria and stool exam for ova and parasites are negative. A small bowel barium x-ray is unremarkable. A complete blood count (CBC), sedimentation rate, and urinalysis are normal. Given the clinical history, findings at sigmoidoscopy, pathology results, and laboratory findings, which of the following would best be used to initially manage this patient?

(A) prednisone, 30 mg, PO q A.M.
(B) prednisone, 30 mg, PO q A.M., plus aza-thioprine, 2 mg/kg, PO q A.M.
(C) Pentasa, 1 g, PO qid
(D) Asacol, 800 mg, PO tid
(E) Anti–tumor necrosis factor (TNF)-alpha antibody (infliximab) infusion

28. Two weeks after starting therapy on ol-salazine, her diarrhea and cramps resolve, but she develops a severe, constant, bandlike pain across the top of her abdomen, with nausea. Which of the following most likely is responsible for this new problem?

(A) olsalazine-medicated chloride secretion from the small bowel
(B) Crohn's fistula with abscess
(C) mesalamine-induced pancreatitis
(D) Crohn's disease of the antrum and duo-denum
(E) duodenal ulcer

29. This patient's clinical course waxed and waned over the years. At age 27, she sud-denly discovered she was pregnant. All of the following could be used to treat her Crohn's disease, if necessary, during her pregnancy EXCEPT

(A) olsalazine
(B) Asacol
(C) azathioprine
(D) prednisone

(E) methotrexate
(F) Pentasa

END OF SET

30. What is the pathologic process seen in ery-thema nodosum?

(A) vasculitis
(B) thrombosis
(C) panniculitis
(D) hyperkeratosis

31. All of the following are part of initial lab work obtained on a healthy pregnant woman EXCEPT

(A) blood type and Rh
(B) rubella antibody
(C) hepatitis B surface antigen
(D) liver function tests
(E) rapid plasma reagin (RPR)

Items 32–34

A 26-year-old nulligravida presents to your office with primary infertility and a history of regular 28-day cycles with 4 days of menstrual flow. She and her partner have been together for 4 years and hav-ing unprotected intercourse at midcycle. Other-wise, her past medical history is significant for two episodes of chlamydia infection.

32. The test with the highest diagnostic yield at this time would be

(A) hysterosalpingogram (HSG)
(B) basal body temperature (BBT) charting
(C) endometrial biopsy
(D) progesterone level
(E) postcoital test

33. The best time to perform the above test would be at what point in her menstrual cy-cle (see Figure 15.7)?

(A) day 2
(B) day 8
(C) day 14
(D) day 22
(E) day 27

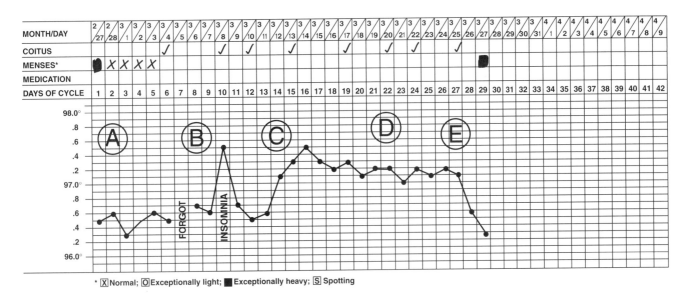

MONTH/DAY	2/27	2/28	3/1	3/2	3/3	3/4	3/5	3/6	3/7	3/8	3/9	3/10	3/11	3/12	3/13	3/14	3/15	3/16	3/17	3/18	3/19	3/20	3/21	3/22	3/23	3/24	3/25	3/26	3/27	3/28	3/29	3/30	3/31	4/1	4/2	4/3	4/4	4/5	4/6	4/7	4/8	4/9
COITUS				✓			✓		✓			✓				✓			✓			✓			✓																	
MENSES*	■	X	X	X	X																							■														
MEDICATION																																										
DAYS OF CYCLE	1	2	3	4	5	6	7	8	9	10	11	12	13	14	15	16	17	18	19	20	21	22	23	24	25	26	27	28	29	30	31	32	33	34	35	36	37	38	39	40	41	42

* ⊠ Normal; Ⓞ Exceptionally light; ■ Exceptionally heavy; Ⓢ Spotting

Figure 15.7

34. All of the following factors would be consistent with presumptive ovulation EXCEPT

    (A) regular 28-day cycles
    (B) biphasic BBT chart
    (C) endometrial biopsy with secretory endometrium
    (D) HSG showing bilateral occlusion
    (E) positive serum human chorionic gonadotropin (hCG)

END OF SET

35. A 36-year-old woman presents with a cough, rhinorrhea, and myalgia for 48 hours. Both her husband and child have similar symptoms. She states she has been afebrile and without shaking chills. The patient, however, had stage II nodular sclerosing Hodgkin's disease 2 years ago with bilateral neck and mediastinal adenopathy and received mantle field radiation as well as radiation of the para-aortic fields and splenic bed after undergoing splenectomy during a staging laparotomy. On exam, she is well appearing without palpable nodes. A chest x-ray is obtained and is found to be abnormal in the mediastinum. What is the most appropriate therapy?

    (A) antibiotics
    (B) chemotherapy
    (C) biopsy of the mediastinum
    (D) steroids
    (E) none of the above

36. An 8-year-old boy who has recurrent copious sputum production and digital clubbing presents for a second opinion regarding his asthma. What test do you recommend to make the diagnosis?

    (A) methacholine challenge
    (B) sputum eosinophils
    (C) pulmonary function tests
    (D) sweat chloride test
    (E) none of the above

37. A 57-year-old man has a history of MI. He is seen in your office for the first time, stating that his blood pressure was found to be elevated at a work physical and again in the nurses' office weekly for 4 weeks. On physical exam, his blood pressure was 180/90. There were no signs or symptoms of ischemia or heart failure but his ECG confirmed an old lateral wall infarction. His only medications are aspirin and atorvastatin calcium, 20 mg daily. Appropriate treatment for his hypertension would include

   (A) nifedipine
   (B) metoprolol
   (C) isosorbide dinitrate
   (D) magnesium

38. A 53-year-old patient has been started on medications for tuberculosis. A week later he presents to the health department complaining of severe bilateral lower extremity neuropathic pain. Which medication is responsible for his neuropathy?

   (A) rifampin
   (B) ethambutol
   (C) isoniazid (INH)
   (D) pyrazinamide

39. A 35-year-old man presents with a 4-day history of pain and swelling of the long finger after being "finned" by a catfish in a local lake. His finger is swollen, and he holds it flexed. There is tenderness over the flexor tendon sheath, and he complains bitterly when passive extension of the finger is attempted. The appropriate treatment is

   (A) ED IV antibiotics, a prescription for oral antibiotics, and instructions to see you for follow-up in 2 days
   (B) admission to the hospital, elevation of the hand, and IV antibiotics
   (C) ED drainage and outpatient IV antibiotics
   (D) admission to the hospital, emergency operative irrigation of the sheath (either open or closed through), and IV antibiotics

40. An 85-year-old man presents with urinary hesitancy and frequency over a 1-year period. He has no bony pain or joint discomfort. An exam is performed, revealing an enlarged prostate and a prostate-specific antigen (PSA) of 56 ng/mL, with an elevated alkaline phosphatase and normal blood counts. Transurethral resection relieves the patient's obstructive symptoms, and biopsies from this reveal Gleason's grade 3/10 prostate cancer. An abdominal/pelvic CT is obtained for staging, with no evidence of local adenopathy. A bone scan reveals two "hot spots" in the iliac bone suggestive of blastic lesions on x-ray. What is the optimal management strategy in this patient?

   (A) orchiectomy
   (B) radiation to the pelvis
   (C) luteinizing hormone-releasing hormone (LHRH) agonist plus flutamide
   (D) diethylstilbestrol (DES)
   (E) serial observation with treatment delayed until symptoms develop

41. Medical indications for prostate surgery for BPH include all of the following EXCEPT

   (A) recurrent urinary tract infections (UTIs)
   (B) urinary retention
   (C) elevated serum creatinine
   (D) urge-related incontinence
   (E) bladder calculi

42. A 28-year-old woman presents with a 2-day history of flulike symptoms, including weakness, myalgias, nonproductive cough, and low-grade fever. She takes no medications except birth-control pills. Prior history is remarkable for idiopathic thrombocytopenic purpura at age 15 for which she underwent splenectomy. Exam shows the patient to have a rattling cough but no respiratory distress with a temperature of 38.5° C (101.3° F), pulse 100, respirations 20, BP 118/60, and pulse oximetry normal on room air. Exam of head, eyes, ears, nose, and throat (HEENT) shows serous nasal drainage. Lungs are clear to auscultation. The most appropriate management for the patient at this time is

(A) provided a chest x-ray shows no infiltrates, management should include increased oral fluids, acetaminophen, and follow-up with her primary care physician if unimproved in 48 hours

(B) a short course of oral steroids and an inhaled beta agonist should be prescribed

(C) if the chest x-ray is clear, request a ventilation-perfusion of the lungs

(D) empiric antibiotic therapy should be started

(E) if the chest x-ray is negative, a Waters view of the sinuses should be ordered

43. What type drug is most likely to have caused the fat pad on this patient's upper back (see Figure 15.8)?

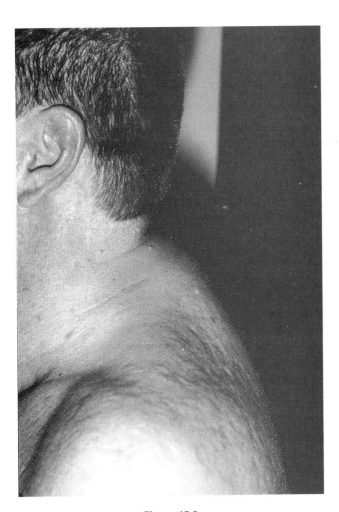

Figure 15.8

(A) protease inhibitor
(B) calcium channel blocker
(C) antiandrogen
(D) beta blocker
(E) retinoid

44. Lichen planus is most commonly seen in association with

(A) hepatitis A
(B) hepatitis B
(C) hepatitis C
(D) Epstein–Barr virus
(E) cytomegalovirus

45. A 48-year-old man undergoes a routine checkup. He has never been ill, does not smoke or drink, and there is no family history available, as he was adopted. A routine CBC and smear reveals a microcytic, hypochromic anemia, most consistent with iron deficiency. His serum ferritin is low, three separate stools for occult blood are negative, and a flexible sigmoidoscopy to 70 cm is normal. Which of the following is the best course of action?

(A) iron supplementation until stores are repleted or hemoglobin is normalized
(B) recheck hemoglobin 3 months later
(C) small bowel biopsy to rule out celiac disease
(D) endoscopy
(E) colonoscopy
(F) barium enema

46. A 65-year-old man with a history of ulcers many years ago is seen in the ED after an episode of large-volume, painless hematemesis. He is on antihypertensive medications and occasional ibuprofen. He once had elective surgery for an abdominal aortic aneurysm. After volume resuscitation, his physical exam is unremarkable, and an extended upper endoscopy is performed, with this finding in the proximal third portion of the duodenum (see Figure 15.9). The best course of action is

(A) epinephrine injection and thermal coagulation

(B) six to eight biopsies of this lesion, including the edges *and* the center

(C) surgical consultation

(D) CT scan of the abdomen

(E) abdominal visceral angiography

(F) colonoscopy

47. A 52-year-old woman with recurrent episodes of painless melena requiring intermittent blood transfusions is seen for a second opinion. Previous evaluation has included normal colonoscopy, small-bowel enteroclysis, abdominal CT scan, and upper GI series. The following was noted in the antrum on upper endoscopy (see Figure 15.10). Twice-daily H_2-blocker therapy has not been

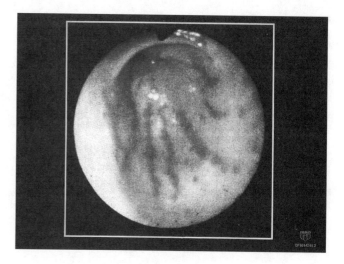

Figure 15.10

helpful. Which of the following is the best course of action?

(A) repeat colonoscopy

(B) argon plasma coagulation therapy at upper endoscopy

(C) intraoperative small-bowel panendoscopy

(D) visceral angiography

(E) high-dose proton-pump inhibitor therapy

48. A 42-year-old man presents with an acute GI bleed, manifested by hematemesis and melena. He has a 2-month history of fever, night sweats, 15-pound weight loss, anorexia, and epigastric aching pains. Prior to this, he was well. After volume resuscitation, the following is noted at upper endoscopy on a retroflexed view of the gastric fundus (see Figure 15.11). What is the most likely diagnosis?

(A) benign gastric ulcer

(B) gastric leiomyoma

(C) gastric lymphoma

(D) gastric adenocarcinoma

(E) Dieulafoy's lesion

49. A 35-year-old woman develops severe periumbilical pain over the last 2 days. Previously, she has been well and is on no medica-

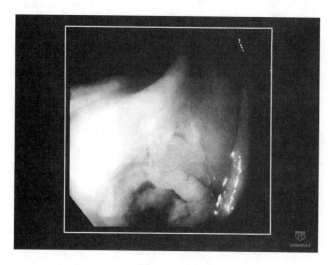

Figure 15.9

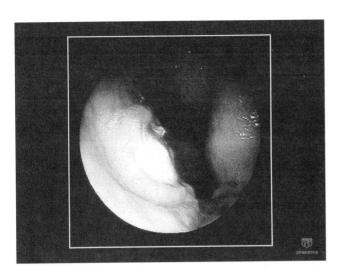

Figure 15.11

tions. Her family history is unremarkable. In the ED, her blood pressure is 160/195, pulse rate 108 and regular, and her physical exam is remarkable for severe abdominal pain with minimal tenderness on exam. An abdominal x-ray and CT scan of the abdomen are both unremarkable. Her CBC is normal, sedimentation rate 92, and serum creatinine 2.5 mg/dL. Emergency abdominal visceral arteriography is performed. Which of the following diagnoses is most likely to be confirmed by the arteriogram?

(A) mesenteric arterial thrombosis

(B) intussusception

(C) mesenteric venous thrombosis

(D) mesenteric vasculitis

(E) mesenteric arterial embolism

50. A 42-year-old HIV-infected physician who has been doing very well on three-drug anti-HIV therapy recently develops new esophageal dysphagia, intermittently, for bulky solids only. She denies fever, chills, oral ulcers, odynophagia, abdominal pain, diarrhea, bleeding, or weight loss. Her medications are zidovudine, lamivudine, indinavir, a multivitamin, and occasional acetaminophen and ibuprofen. She does not smoke or drink. A CBC and serum chemistries are normal. Which of the following is the most likely cause of her new dysphagia?

(A) Kaposi's sarcoma of the esophagus

(B) non-Hodgkin's lymphoma of the esophagus

(C) *Candida* esophagitis

(D) cytomegalovirus (CMV) esophagitis

(E) gastroesophageal reflux disease (GERD)

Practice Test 15
Answers and Explanations

1. **(C)** With the exhaustive workup and no cause identified, pulmonary hypertension is the most likely suspect. The elevated A-a gradient is indicative of a pulmonary parenchymal or vascular process. It is difficult to get an accurate measurement of right-sided pressures on echocardiogram except by experienced operators and that is why the echocardiogram was reportedly "normal." The next step would be right heart catheterization to document severity of pulmonary hypertension.

2. **(A)** Patients with prolonged episodes occurring with an accelerated pattern who present with heart failure are at very high risk. The following table is a categorization of patients presenting with unstable angina.

	High Risk	Intermediate Risk	Low Risk
Feature	≥ 1 of the following present	≥ 1 of the following present	May have any of the following
History	> 20 minutes while at rest and ongoing	Prior MI, peripheral or cerebrovascular disease, prior coronary artery bypass graft (CABG), prior use of aspirin	
Character of pain	> 20 minutes while at rest and ongoing	>20 minutes at rest now resolved. Moderate or high chance patient has coronary artery disease (CAD)	New-onset class III or IV angina in past 2 weeks. Moderate or high likelihood of CAD

	High Risk	Intermediate Risk	Low Risk
Clinical findings	Pulmonary edema, new mitral regurgitation murmur, S_3, hypotension, bradycardia, tachycardia, > 75 years old	> 70 years old	
ECG findings	Transient ST changes > 0.05 mV, new bundle branch block, sustained ventricular tachycardia	T-wave inversions > 0.05 mV. Pathologic Q waves	Normal or unchanged ECG during chest pain

Table adapted from Braunwald et al: *ACC/AHA Guidelines for Unstable Angina.*

3. **(C)** Although another trial of sildenafil may be successful, it is now likely that this patient has either a venous leak syndrome or vascular disease, which is not responsive to oral therapy. Intracavernous injection of a vasoactive agent such as prostaglandin E1 in conjunction with a duplex ultrasound can aid in the identification of the etiology of his erectile dysfunction.

4. **(C)** Asbestos exposure in mechanics is usually related to working with brakes. The radiographic pattern reveals irregular peripheral interstitial infiltrates mostly in the bases with pleural plaques and is virtually diagnostic of the disease but can also be seen in mesothelioma and tuberculosis.

5. **(C)** Pancreatitis in a patient with AIDS has a lengthy differential diagnosis. In addition to the common etiologies (i.e., gallstones and al-

cohol), drugs and infections must be considered. Some of the medications used to treat HIV may cause pancreatitis such as DDI and zalcitabine. Many of the opportunistic infections such as cytomegalovirus (CMV) infection, *Cryptosporidium,* and *Mycobacterium avium* complex can also involve the pancreas. Nelfinavir is usually well tolerated with few side effects and has not been reported to cause pancreatitis.

6. **(C)** While the majority of patients who present to the ED with chest pain associated with the use of cocaine do not have acute MI, it is an ideal agent for causing cardiac ischemia and MI and has this potential even in young, otherwise healthy individuals. We must, therefore, take the complaint of chest pain seriously in individuals who have used cocaine. Aspirin and nitroglycerin are first-line agents for these patients. Benzodiazepines like lorazepam can reduce the agitation often seen in these patients. Highly agitated patients who have been abusing cocaine may have high fever, tachycardia, and major BP elevation due to massive adrenergic discharge. Both alpha and beta receptors are maximally stimulated. Administration of a beta blocker like metoprolol runs the risk of unopposed alpha stimulation and may make the patient's condition worse. Phentolamine is now considered the agent of choice for such cases.

7. **(C)** The most frequent sites of internal involvement in AIDS-associated Kaposi's sarcoma are the GI tract and lymph nodes.

8. **(B)** Acanthosis nigricans occurs in insulin-resistant states such as diabetes mellitus.

9. **(C)** Measured stool osmolality is always 290 mOsm/kg water, as stool by definition is iso-osmotic. If a stool specimen is left out for a period of time postevacuation and then measured, the osmolality can *increase* (bacterial metabolism outside the body creates more osmoles). Hypo-osmolar stool is found when water is added, postevacuation, to simulate diarrhea. The lack of fever, pain, bleed-

ing, and fecal leukocytes makes inflammatory diarrhea unlikely. Potassium-secreting adenomas should increase the stool potassium (N: 90 mEq/L), osmotic diarrheas create a gap (290-(stool sodium plus potassium, times 2)) of > 50 mOsm/kg water. The stool sodium and potassium in this case are both slightly decreased because of the (factitious) addition of water. With secretory diarrhea, the osmotic gap is < 50.

10. **(D)** In this case, the differential diagnosis is between postpartum thyroiditis and Graves' disease. Postpartum thyroiditis occurs in 5 to 10% of women after delivery. It begins with an initial phase of hyperthyroidism within 4 months postpartum, followed by hypothyroidism between 3 and 7 months postpartum. Subsequently, there is a spontaneous recovery of thyroid function in most patients; few remain permanently hypothyroid. Graves' disease, like any other autoimmune disease, can flare up in the postpartum period, usually between 3 and 6 months postpartum. The only way to make a final and definite diagnosis is to get a 24-hour uptake and scan, the uptake being high in Graves' and low in postpartum thyroiditis. Making a diagnosis is important because treatment is different: For Graves', options are antithyroid agents or radioactive iodine; for postpartum thyroiditis, treatment is symptomatic with beta blockers, because the hyperthyroid phase is self-limited.

11. **(B)** In general, ovarian cancer is usually diagnosed at more advanced stages since women are unaware unless they have symptoms of abdominal discomfort or distention. Combination chemotherapy with platinum-based and paclitaxel-based chemotherapy and aggressive debulking surgery can result in long-term survival in Stage III ovarian cancer. The presence of malignant ascites and breast, colon, or gastric spread represents Stage IV disease, and chemotherapy in this setting to date has been merely palliative.

12. **(E)** This large lytic lesion has the appearance of multiple myeloma. Lesions from meta-

static carcinoma usually have a moth-eaten appearance. Although often cold on bone scan, this test is still necessary in workup. Lesions half the diameter of a long bone or larger should be considered for prophylactic stabilization before fracture. If a serum protein electrophoresis is indicative of myeloma, a serum calcium level and a bone marrow aspirate should also be performed.

13. **(A)** Although the complexes are wide, the rhythm is grossly irregular, consistent with atrial fibrillation. The aberration may be rate related, or the patient may have a conduction defect. In general, ventricular tachycardia is regular, as is AV node reentry. Sinus tachycardia should have visible P waves.

14. **(E)** Regardless the nature of the arrhythmia, with hemodynamic compromise, cardioversion should be performed. Although the arrhythmia is atrial fibrillation, IV diltiazem could lead to profound hypotension and ibutilide is too slow. Lidocaine, a Class Ib antiarrhythmic, does not affect atrial fibrillation.

15. **(B)** The marked thickness of the left ventricular walls and the systolic anterior motion of the mitral valve are consistent with the diagnosis. In aortic stenosis, there can be compensatory left ventricular hypertrophy but rarely to the extent seen in hypertrophic cardiomyopathy and the aortic valve would be visibly abnormal. There would not be marked hypertrophy with mitral stenosis and the mitral valve would be visibly abnormal.

16. **(A)** The physical findings are classic for tonsillitis with a peritonsillar abscess. Appropriate treatment is intraoral drainage of the abscess.

17. **(D)** To date, 60% of those with CML who have undergone allogeneic bone marrow transplant have been cured. Allogeneic transplant has not been shown to be superior in ALL and CLL. Allogeneic transplant is favored in AML in first remission. Those patients having favorable cytogenetics, which include t8,21, t15,17, and inv16, are generally treated with chemotherapy alone, whereas those with less favorable cytogenetic patterns are offered allogeneic transplant.

18. **(D)** Several retrospective studies have shown that hypothyroidism does not greatly increase the risk of surgery. In this patient with unstable coronary artery disease, therapy with thyroid hormone could increase myocardial metabolic demands and precipitate myocardial infarction. Therefore, the best approach would be to proceed with bypass surgery and then cautiously treat the hypothyroidism postoperatively. Nevertheless, in the absence of severe coronary artery disease (CAD), it is preferable to restore a euthyroid state before elective surgery. Urgent surgery need not be postponed because of hypothyroidism.

19. **(C)** Dupuytren's contracture is due to a proliferative fibroplasia of the subcutaneous palmar tissue, occurring in the form of nodules and cords. Initially, the mass is small, firm, and fixed to the overlying palmar skin with dimpling. With progression, fixed flexion contractures occur. Contractile myofibroblasts producing increased type 3 collagen are the predominant cell type. Dupuytren's disease occurs 10 times more frequently in males than females and begins in middle age. It is most common in those of Celtic and Scandinavian origin. Treatment is a partial fasciotomy. Recurrence is possible.

20. **(D)** Bladder outlet obstruction from an enlarged prostate can result in any alteration in the normal voiding pattern including those listed above. However, BPH is an unlikely cause of pelvic or prostatic pain.

21. **(A)** Rhabdomyosarcoma is a malignant tumor of the orbit usually seen in children. When present, there is limitation of the extraocular movements and fullness to the orbit. Conditions such as Coats' disease, retinoblastoma, and retinal detachment can cause esotropia and exotropia due to lack of central fixation. In amblyopia, the ocular findings may be normal, or there may be a

difference in the refractive error between the two eyes.

22. **(D)** While all of the examinations listed may be necessary in the workup of a child with loss of central vision, a dilated ocular examination is the first step in the evaluation of these patients. Intraocular pathology, such as retinoblastoma, retinal detachment, and Coats' disease, will be diagnosed by doing a dilated ocular examination. An amblyopic eye will be essentially normal on dilated examination, although unilateral myopia can sometimes be identified.

23. **(D)** Osler's nodes are tender lesions that occur on distal digital tufts in the setting of subacute bacterial endocarditis (SBE). Histologically, they demonstrate a vasculitis without microabscess formation. (Janeway lesions also occur in the setting of SBE, but usually are nontender and involve the palms and soles.)

24. **(C)** By LaPlace's Law, the greater the diameter of the varix (size), the inverse of the thickness of the wall (signs of mural thinning/abnormalities), and the greater the pressure of the fluid within the tube (and hence intramural pressure as a result of episodes of alcoholic hepatitis with even greater portal venous pressure), the more likely it will explode. Acid reflux is not a risk factor for variceal bleeding, as varices explode but do not erode.

25. **(B)** Elevated biliary calcium is a risk for pigment stone formation but not cholesterol stone formation. Gallbladder stasis, elevated biliary cholesterol, and diminished biliary bile salts and phospholipid increase the risk of cholesterol gallstone formation.

26. **(E)** Most uncomplicated, simple anal fissures are at 6 or 12 o'clock. Fissures in other locations are more suggestive of other pathogeneses, such as Crohn's disease. Simple anal fissures commonly present with pain on passage of bowel movements, often with some mucus or bright red blood on the toilet paper,

and they may recur, especially in persons with an abnormal bowel habit (e.g., hard stools and straining, loose stools).

27. **(D)** This patient has clinical, sigmoidoscopic, pathologic findings consistent with mild Crohn's disease of the colon. The small bowel is normal radiographically. Asacol would be the best therapeutic choice. She is not sick enough to require prednisone, immunomodulatory therapy (azathioprine), or anti–TNF-alpha antibody therapy. Since the small bowel is not involved, Pentasa, which, in contrast to Asacol, is active against small bowel as well as colonic inflammation in Crohn's disease, is not required.

28. **(C)** All mesalamine compounds have the potential for the complication of acute pancreatitis, which usually presents with constant, severe upper abdominal pain, often with nausea and/or vomiting. Azathioprine and 6-mercaptopurine, used in Crohn's disease, also can cause acute pancreatitis. A duodenal ulcer would be unlikely in this young patient (low prevalence of *Helicobacter pylori*). Patients with inflammatory bowel disease (IBD) usually are cautioned to avoid nonsteroidal anti-inflammatory drugs (NSAIDs), which rarely exacerbate IBD. The clinical scenario, as described in this patient, is not typical of ulcer pain or Crohn's fistula with abscess. Crohn's disease of the upper GI tract is rare, usually with concomitant terminal ileal disease, and would be likely to present more like ulcer disease with intermittent upper abdominal pain, with or without anorexia, pain after eating, nausea, or vomiting. Olsalazine is the one mesalamine derivative that can *cause* diarrhea, which this patient no longer has. This would not cause upper abdominal pain, as this patient experienced.

29. **(E)** Most medications used to treat Crohn's disease, including mesalamine derivatives, prednisone, and azathioprine (or 6-mercaptopurine), are believed to be safe during pregnancy. Methotrexate is absolutely contraindicated. Ciprofloxacin also should not be used during pregnancy, and metronidazole

should not be used during the first trimester. There is little available information on the use of anti–TNF-alpha antibody infusion therapy during pregnancy.

30. **(C)** Erythema nodosum is a hypersensitivity reaction that arises in response to a variety of stimuli. Its primary pathologic feature is that of a panniculitis.

31. **(D)** Type and Rh determination is crucial in the prevention of Rh sensitization. Rubella antibody allows identification and immunization of nonimmune women postpartum. Identification of hepatitis B carrier status allows optimal management of infants immediately postpartum to prevent perinatal hepatitis B infection. Detection and treatment of syphilis helps prevent congenital syphilis in the fetus as well as future complications of syphilis in the mother.

32. **(A)** This patient is at risk for tubal disease in light of her history of sexually transmitted infections with chlamydia. The rest of her gynecologic history is essentially unremarkable, and definitely consistent with regular ovulatory cycles. The only test for tubal patency listed among the choices given is the HSG. BBT charting is used to document the physiologic rise in temperature associated with postovulatory progesterone production. This results in a "biphasic" temperature graph as seen in Figure 15.7. In women who do not ovulate, the resulting BBT is "monophasic" (i. e., without the physiologic rise in temperature). An endometrial biopsy is done in the late luteal phase and is used as a bioassay for progesterone effect on the endometrium, thus resulting in secretory endometrium. In women who are anovulatory, the endometrial biopsy will show proliferative endometrium, an effect of estrogen. A serum progesterone level may be measured approximately 7 days postovulation in order to analyze the "adequacy" of the luteal phase. Finally, the postcoital test looks at the interaction between the sperm and the cervical mucus just prior to ovulation. There is no reason to suspect any abnormality in cervical mu-

cous production (e.g., DES, cervical conization, etc.).

33. **(B)** Day 8 would be the best time to perform an HSG in light of regular 28-day cycles with 4 days of bleeding. An HSG should not be performed during menses (day 2) because of the theoretical risk of iatrogenic endometriosis secondary to retrograde seeding. Additionally, an HSG should not be performed at ovulation or thereafter because of the risk of interrupting a potential pregnancy.

34. **(D)** An HSG does not evaluate for the presence or absence of ovulation. It is only able to evaluate the shape of the uterine cavity and tubal status. All of the other choices are associated with ovulatory cycles (e.g., *regular* cycles), biphasic BBTs, secretory endometrium, and, of course, a positive pregnancy test.

35. **(E)** As with most patients who receive radiation therapy, those patients who have received radiation to the mediastinum for Hodgkin's lymphoma indefinitely have abnormal x-rays due to residual abnormality in the tumor mass and scarring secondary to the radiation. The use of CT scan, MRI, and gallium 67 scans and now positron-emission tomography (PET) scans have been extensively evaluated for predictive accuracy in this setting. Gallium and PET appear most predictive. The most important action would be to compare prior x-rays with the above film. If there is evidence of disease progression, then restaging should be pursued. If recurrence happens, it is generally within the first 2 to 3 years after therapy.

36. **(D)** Copious sputum production and digital clubbing are not typical of asthma. They are more typical of bronchiectasis, and in a child this age, cystic fibrosis would be high on the differential. Pulmonary function testing would show an obstructive pattern in both asthma and cystic fibrosis.

37. **(B)** In patients with coronary disease and hypertension, there has been noted to be a slight increase in the occurrence of MI. While

it is difficult to determine this from the natural history of the disease, use of nifedipine as a first-line agent for hypertension in a patient with known CAD is not recommended. Isosorbide dinitrate is rarely added as an adjunct treatment for patients with CAD, angina, and hypertension but would not be an appropriate first-line drug. Magnesium offers no benefit. Metoprolol would be ideal since it has been shown to decrease post-MI mortality and is an effective antihypertensive.

38. **(C)** Peripheral neuropathy secondary to INH is known to occur and vitamin B_6 (pyridoxine) should be given to patients receiving INH to prevent the neuropathy. Those with concurrent malnutrition are at increased risk, especially chronic alcoholics.

39. **(D)** The four "cardinal" signs of suppurative tenosynovitis are: tenderness over the involved sheath, rigid positioning of the finger in flexion, swelling of the finger, and pain on attempted passive hyperextension of the finger. Infection results from spread from the adjacent pulp or from puncture wounds of the flexor creases. When early tenosynovitis is suspected, immediate treatment with IV antibiotics and splinting can abort the spread of infection if the patient's symptoms have been present for < 48 hours. If drainage and irrigation are necessary, the prognosis for return of normal function is poor.

40. **(E)** This is an asymptomatic man except for urinary obstructive symptoms that were relieved by transurethral resection. He has no pain in the pelvic area despite these "hot spots." Since randomized trials show no survival advantage for delayed rather than immediate endocrine therapy, observation with delayed treatment until symptoms develop is acceptable. Bilateral orchiectomy or LHRH agonist with androgen blockade might be considered at the time of progression. DES is not indicated in the elderly. Again, radiation is not indicated with lack of symptoms.

41. **(D)** Although bothersome, urge incontinence is not an absolute indication for surgical intervention for BPH. A bladder outlet procedure on the prostate is indicated for acute urinary retention, recurrent infections, azotemia, and the presence of bladder calculi.

42. **(D)** Splenectomized patients are at high risk for sepsis due to encapsulated organisms, especially *Streptococcus pneumoniae*. This includes most adult sickle cell patients who are functionally asplenic due to previous splenic infarction. Febrile illness must be taken seriously in this patient population, and antibiotic coverage for *S. pneumoniae* should be routinely provided. Once again, the value of a thorough history and physical exam cannot be overemphasized. Physicians often mismanage these patients with disastrous results because they failed to obtain the prior history of splenectomy or did not do an abdominal exam to identify the surgical scar.

43. **(A)** The subcutaneous mass on the patient's upper back is consistent with HIV lipodystrophy due to protease inhibitor therapy.

44. **(C)** Several epidemiologic studies have shown a higher prevalence of hepatitis C virus infection in patients with lichen planus than in normal control subjects.

45. **(E)** A male patient of this age group with iron deficiency anemia has colon cancer until proven otherwise. Flexible sigmoidoscopy, stools for occult blood, and barium enemas alone or in combination can be used as screening tests, but are not the best tests when bleeding and/or iron deficiency anemia is present. If this patient's colonoscopy were done and negative, consideration would then need to be given to an upper GI source or celiac disease with malabsorption of iron.

46. **(C)** In a patient with a major bleed and a history of surgery for an abdominal aortic aneurysm, fistula from the graft to bowel is

the diagnosis of greatest risk (exsanguination) to the patient. Indeed, the extended upper endoscopy shows an unusual area of ulceration in the third portion of the duodenum, the most typical site of aortoenteric fistula formation. CT scans and visceral arteriography can miss the diagnosis and, in the absence of another obvious source for this patient's hematemesis, are not indicated and could be fatal if surgery is delayed. Colonoscopy in this setting (hematemesis) is not indicated. Biopsies or thermal coagulation of this lesion are not indicated and could precipitate exsanguination. The third part of the duodenum is an unusual site for a benign or malignant ulcer.

47. **(B)** The presentation is most consistent with upper GI or small bowel bleeding. The endoscopic image demonstrates multiple, linear erythematous streaks in the antrum, diagnostic of watermelon stomach or gastric antral vascular ectasia (GAVE). Endoscopic thermal coagulation usually stops the intermittent small- and/or large-volume bleeding. Thus, options A, C, and D are not necessary. Acid-lowering therapies do not help bleeding from GAVE.

48. **(C)** The endoscopic image is that of a mass lesion, protruding from the wall of the fundus, with extensive central ulceration, as well as a small visible vessel. Both options B and D could look like this, but the history, with night sweats and fever, best fits lymphoma. A benign gastric ulcer would not protrude from the wall of the stomach (the ulcer would be deep to the mucosa) within a mass lesion. A Dieulafoy's lesion would be a visible vessel without mass, ulceration, weight loss, pain, fever, or sweats. A gastric leiomyoma could protrude from the wall of the stomach, but ulceration would be more focal, at the tip, if present. The history alone strongly suggests a malignant lymphoma.

49. **(D)** The patient's history of acute abdominal pain out of proportion to the physical findings suggests mesenteric ischemia. The normal CT scan makes mesenteric venous thrombosis, which can be seen in younger persons with a personal or family history of coagulopathy, unlikely. Her age and lack of medical history make mesenteric arterial thrombosis or embolism unlikely. Intussusception should have been evident on CT scan and abdominal x-ray (obstructive features). Mesenteric vasculitis, such as polyarteritis nodosa, is most likely, given the elevated blood pressure, serum creatinine, and sedimentation rate, and would be diagnosed by finding multiple, segmental microaneurysms on visceral angiography.

50. **(E)** This patient with HIV infection is doing very well on triple anti-HIV therapy, and presumably is not immunosuppressed. This, and her lack of other symptoms, makes options A, B, and D highly unlikely, and C very unlikely. Pill esophagitis would also be possible, but she does not have odynophagia. Successfully treated HIV-infected patients with GI symptoms are likely to have the same, common GI problems nonimmunosuppressed HIV-negative persons develop, with the added risk of medication-related problems (e.g., diarrhea).

NOTES

NOTES

NOTES

NOTES

NOTES

NOTES

NOTES

NOTES

NOTES

NOTES